Current Techniques in Arthroscopy

Current Techniques in Arthroscopy

Third Edition

Edited by

J. Serge Parisien, MD, FACS

Chief
Arthroscopic Surgery Service
Hospital for Joint Diseases Orthopaedic Institute;
Clinical Professor
Department of Orthopaedic Surgery
New York University Medical School
New York, New York, USA

With 34 contributors

1998

Thieme

New York • Stuttgart

Developed by Current Medicine, Inc., Philadelphia

Current Medicine

400 Market Street
Suite 700
Philadelphia, PA 19106

MANAGING EDITOR: . . . . Lori J. Bainbridge

DEVELOPMENTAL EDITOR:. . . . . Danielle Shaw

EDITORIAL ASSISTANT: . . . . Jennifer Schafhauser

ART DIRECTOR: . . . . Paul Fennessy

DESIGN AND LAYOUT:. . . . . Patrick Whelan

ILLUSTRATION DIRECTOR:. . . . . Ann Saydlowski

ILLUSTRATORS: Wiesia Langenfeld, Larry Ward, and Debra Wertz

PRODUCTION MANAGER: . . . . Lori Holland

PRODUCTION ASSOCIATE: . . . . Sally Nicholson

INDEXER:. . . . . David Amundson

Printed in the United States by Quebecor

10 9 8 7 6 5 4 3 2 1

ISBN:0-86577-738-1
ISSN:1068-4107

Preface

Since the publication of the first two editions of *Current Techniques in Arthroscopy*, we have witnessed the refinement of some established arthroscopic procedures and the advent of a number of innovative techniques in this field. This third edition is intended to provide the reader with cutting-edge information in this rapidly developing field, and is designed to be a companion of the first two editions of this series.

To this end, the chapters on arthroscopic techniques on the wrist, elbow, and ankle have been revisited with emphasis placed on recent developments. New chapters have been added on such topics as outpatient surgery for the anterior cruciate ligament deficient knee, revision of the failed anterior cruciate ligament reconstruction, the use of allograft in ligament surgery, the management of avascular meniscal tears, and the reconstruction of the anterior cruciate ligament in the skeletally immature patient. Furthermore, we have discussed the role of arthroscopy in the management of pyarthrosis and the dysfunctional total knee replacement. Chapters on shoulder surgery include innovative and promising techniques for repair of the torn rotator cuff, an update on suture anchors, and the pitfalls and possible complications of arthroscopic shoulder procedures. New topics also include the value of arthroscopy in the treatment of some disorders of the hip and subtalar joints, of the plantar fascia, and of the intervertebral disc. Thanks to the outstanding work of a distinguished panel of contributors, we believe that the goals of this publication have been reached.

I wish to express my sincere gratitude to my guests for their enriching contributions. I am also indebted to Dr. Ronald Moscovich and Dr. Donald Rose from the Hospital for Joint Diseases staff for their invaluable editorial assistance. Above all, I am very grateful to the editors at Current Medicine and their staff for bringing this new endeavor to a successful and timely completion.

J. Serge Parisien, MD, FACS

Contributors

JAMES A. ARNOLD, MD
Associate Clinical Professor
Department of Orthopaedics
University of Arkansas for Medical
  Sciences
Little Rock, Arkansas, USA;
Chief
Arnold Orthopedic Associates, PA
Fayetteville, Arkansas, USA

MARíA LAURA CLARO, MD
La Plata Institute of Arthroscopy
La Plata, Argentina

JAMES D. DALTON, JR., MD
Shoulder and Sports Fellow
Department of Orthopaedic Surgery
University of Pittsburgh School of
  Medicine
Pittsburgh, Pennsylvania, USA

DANIEL JULIO DE ANTONI, MD
Teaching Fellow
Department of Medical Sciences
National University of La Plata;
Medical Director
La Plata Institute of Arthroscopy
La Plata, Argentina

GREGORY C. FANELLI, MD
Chief
Orthopaedic Sports Medicine and
  Arthroscopic Surgery Services
Geisinger Medical Center
Danville, Pennsylvania, USA

DANIEL D. FELDMANN, MD
Orthopaedic Surgery Resident
Geisinger Medical Center
Danville, Pennsylvania, USA

LARRY D. FIELD, MD
Co-director
Upper Extremity Service
Mississippi Sports Medicine
Jackson, Mississippi, USA

MARK FIELD, MD
Fellow in Sports Medicine
Mississippi Sports Medicine
Jackson, Mississippi, USA

BASIM A. FLEEGA, MD
Chief
Shoulder Service;
Director
Godesberger Orthopedic Hospital
Bonn, Germany

MARK H. GETELMAN, MD
Southern California Orthopedic Institute
Van Nuys, California, USA

ALEXANDER I. GLOGAU, MD
Attending Physician
Fellowship Director
Arthroscopy and Sports Medicine Fellowship
Associated Orthopaedics and Sports Medicine
Plano, Texas, USA

GREGORY J. HANKER, MD
Assistant Clinical Professor
Department of Plastic and Reconstructive Surgery
University of Southern California School of
  Medicine
Los Angeles, California, USA;
Attending Physician
Southern California Orthopedic Institute
Van Nuys, California, USA

KELLY B. HANKER
Research Medical Assistant
Harvard-Westlake School
North Hollywood, California, USA

CHRISTOPHER D. HARNER, MD
Associate Professor
Department of Orthopaedic Surgery
University of Pittsburgh School of Medicine
Pittsburgh, Pennsylvania, USA

PETER C. KWONG, MD
Associated Orthopaedics and Sports Medicine
Plano, Texas, USA

PETER D. LAIMINS, MD
Southern California Permanente Medical Group
Panorama City, California, USA

ROGER V. LARSON, MD
Associate Professor
Department of Orthopaedic Surgery
University of Washington School of Medicine
Seattle, Washington, USA

JOEL LOBO, MD
University of Toronto Faculty of Medicine
Toronto Western Hospital
Toronto, Ontario, Canada

JESS H. LONNER, MD
Assistant Professor
Department of Orthopaedic Surgery
University of Pennsylvania School of Medicine;
Attending Orthopaedic Surgeon
Penn Musculoskeletal Institute
Hospital of the University of Pennsylvania
Philadelphia, Pennsylvania, USA

HOWARD J. LUKS, MD
Instructor
Director of Sports Medicine
Department of Orthopaedic Surgery
New York Medical College
Valhalla, New York, USA

GREGORY G. MARKARIAN, MD
Orthopedic Associates of Naperville
Naperville, Illinois, USA

MICHAEL H. METCALF, MD
Resident
Department of Orthopaedic Surgery
University of Washington School of Medicine
Seattle, Washington, USA

DARRELL J. OGILVIE-HARRIS, MB, CHB, MSc, FRCS
Associate Professor
Department of Orthopaedic Surgery
University of Toronto Faculty of Medicine;
Director
Sports Medicine Specialists
Toronto Western Hospital
Toronto, Ontario, Canada

J. SERGE PARISIEN, MD, FACS
Chief
Arthroscopic Surgery Service
Hospital for Joint Diseases Orthopaedic Institute;
Clinical Professor
Department of Orthopaedic Surgery
New York University Medical School
New York, New York, USA

ANDREW H.N. ROBINSON, FRCS
Senior Registrar
Department of Orthopaedics
Addenbrooke's Hospital
Cambridge, England, United Kingdom

JOHN S. ROGERSON, MD
Assistant Clinical Professor
Department of Orthopaedics;
Physicians Plus Medical Group
Madison, Wisconsin, USA

FELIX H. SAVOIE III, MD
Co-director
Upper Extremity Service
Mississippi Sports Medicine
Jackson, Mississippi, USA

KEVIN P. SHEA, MD
Associate Professor
Department of Orthopedics
University of Connecticut School of Medicine
Farmington, Connecticut, USA

STEPHEN J. SNYDER, MD
Southern California Orthopedic Institute
Van Nuys, California, USA

JAMES P. TASTO, MD
Associate Clinical Professor
University of California, San Diego, School of Medicine
San Diego Sports Medicine and Orthopaedic Center
San Diego, California, USA

JOHN W. URIBE, MD
Chief
Department of Sports Medicine;
Associate Professor
Department of Orthopedic Surgery
University of Miami School of Medicine
Miami, Florida, USA

RICHARD N. VILLAR, MS, FRCS
Consultant
Department of Orthopaedic Surgery
Cambridge University;
Cambridge Hip and Knee Unit
Cambridge Lea Hospital
Cambridge, England, United Kingdom

EUGENE M. WOLF, MD
Associate Clinical Professor
Department of Orthopedic Surgery
University of California, San Francisco, School of Medicine;
California Pacific Medical Center
San Francisco, California, USA

ZHONGNAN ZHANG, MD, PHD
Arnold Orthopedic Associates, PA
Fayetteville, Arkansas, USA

Contents

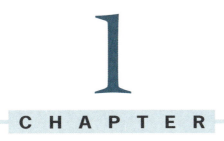

CHAPTER 1

Endoscopic Plantar Fascial Release: A New Treatment For An Old Nemesis

DARRELL J. OGILVIE-HARRIS AND JOEL LOBO

Plantar fasciitis is an enthesopathy of the insertion of the plantar fascia at the medial calcaneal tubercle. It occurs commonly in healthy people who are involved with activities involving jumping and in those of advancing age, and can be associated with many seronegative spondyloarthropathies. Pain resulting from plantar fasciitis is typically located over the medial calcaneal tubercle and occurs in the morning or at the start of an activity involving weight bearing. Radiographs often reveal a bony spur at the insertion of the plantar fascia onto the medial calcaneal tubercle. However, the spur represents a reactive formation of bone in this inflammatory process and is not the cause of foot pain *per se*. This pain responds to conservative therapy approximately 90% of the time. Footwear with adequate heel cup support, stretching exercises, and rest are the mainstays of conservative therapy. In many cases of failed conservative therapy, local corticosteroid injection often relieves the intractable pain of plantar fasciitis. For those patients who do not respond to these methods of conservative therapy after 6 to 12 months, surgery may be an option. Plantar fasciotomy for the treatment of plantar fasciitis refractory to an adequate trial of conservative therapy is the last resort for such patients.

Recently, a technique has been described whereby the plantar fasciotomy can be done endoscopically. The endoscopic procedure requires less time and allows patients to return to their daily lifestyles earlier than with an open procedure and often with better functional results. This paper first provides a background to the etiology, diagnosis, and management of plantar fasciitis and then discusses the merits and indications for endoscopic plantar fasciotomy for intractable plantar fasciitis

STRUCTURE OF THE FOOT

The sole of the foot is divided into six layers. These are, from superficial to deep, skin and superficial fascia, plantar fascia, and the four muscular layers of the sole.

Skin covering the sole of the foot is fixed to the underlying tissue by dense fibers. It is thicker about the heel, lateral margin, and metatarsals. Subcutaneous tissue about the heel consists of a spiral network of fibrous fat-filled septa. A subcutaneous bursa is also present subcalcaneally. In the anterior foot, vertical fibers form a similar fat-filled network and connect the dermis to the plantar fascia. The end result is a complex network of fibers and fat that serves to anchor the skin to the plantar fascia and to provide shock absorption [1].

Lateral cutaneous sensation over the heel is provided by two calcaneal branches of the sural nerve. Sensation to the medial heel and posterior third of the sole are supplied by the posterior medial and anterior medial calcaneal nerves, respectively (Fig. 1-1). These are branches of the medial calcaneal nerve (a branch of the posterior tibial nerve) that lie superficial to the plantar fascia [1]. It is these nerves that are at risk during a plantar fasciotomy.

The posterior tibial nerve continues into the second muscular layer before bifurcating into the medial and lateral plantar nerves. Whereas the medial plantar nerve provides cutaneous sensation to the medial two thirds of the anterior sole, the lateral plantar nerve innervates the anterolateral sole.

The plantar aponeurosis is a fibrous structure divided in three parts: lateral, medial, and central. The lateral part of the plantar aponeurosis is thicker posteriorly and thinner anteriorly, covering the abductor digiti minimi muscle. It runs from the lateral margin of the medial calcaneal tubercule and bifurcates into a lateral component, which inserts on the base of the fifth metatarsal, and a medial deep component, which inserts into the fourth toe. The medial component is thinner posteriorly and thicker anteriorly. It covers the abductor hallucis muscle and is continuous with the dorsal aponeurosis of the foot. The central band of the plantar aponeurosis is the most important. It is thick posteriorly where it originates from the posteromedial calcaneal tubercle. The central band fans out anteriorly into five slips that insert subcutaneously with superficial fibers at the ball of the foot and deep fibers that cover the flexor tendons of the foot. In addition to this fibrous network, two intermuscular septa extend from the medial and lateral margins of the central component. These allow the sole of the foot to be compartmentalized into lateral, medial, and central compartments.

Deep to the plantar fascia lies the first layer of plantar muscles. The most medial of these is the abductor hallucis, followed centrally by the large flexor digitorum brevis. Finally, the abductor digiti minimi muscle is found laterally in the first layer of plantar muscles [1]. Three more layers of plantar muscles are present, but they are not discussed in this chapter.

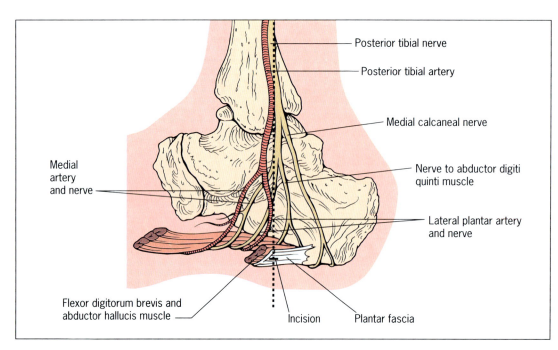

Medial artery and nerve

Flexor digitorum brevis and abductor hallucis muscle

Posterior tibial nerve

Posterior tibial artery

Medial calcaneal nerve

Nerve to abductor digiti quinti muscle

Lateral plantar artery and nerve

Incision

Plantar fascia

Figure 1-1.
Anatomy of the medial border of the foot. Neurovascular structures are not at risk when the portal is correctly placed. The *dotted line* runs along the posterior border of the medial malleolus.

FUNCTION OF THE FOOT

The foot serves two main functions: it supports body weight during stance and walking and serves as a lever with which the body propels itself during walking. Teleologically, both these functions could be accommodated with a simple lever, which could be composed of a single-jointed ankle and solid foot. The disadvantage of this system, however, would be an inability of the foot to accommodate itself to uneven ground. It is for this reason that the multijointed foot makes teleologic sense [2].

The division of the foot into multiple segments suggests that it can only bear weight if it is built in the form of an arch. Stability of the foot can be accounted for by its three arches and supporting structures. These are the medial longitudinal, lateral longitudinal, and transverse arches. The medial longitudinal arch, perhaps the most important stabilizer, consists of the calcaneus, talus, navicular, cuneiforms, and the first three metatarsals. The lateral longitudinal arch runs through the calcaneus, cuboid, and metatarsals four and five. The transverse arch runs through the bases of the metatarsals, cuboid, and cuneiforms. The plantar ligaments hold these components together and reinforce the stability of the arches. Finally, the plantar fascia prevents sagging of the arch during loading by connecting its ends inferiorly.

Understanding the biomechanics of walking is vital to comprehension of the function of the plantar fascia. During heel strike, the foot pronates. This complex movement involves internal rotation of the tibia on a fixed foot, eversion at the subtalar joint, dorsiflexion of the ankle, and abduction of the forefoot [3••]. The foot is most flexible in this position and thus adapts to uneven ground. The swing phase of walking proceeds through midstance and toe-off. It is during toe-off that the subtalar joint locks and the foot supinates. The tibia externally rotates on the fixed foot, the foot inverts at the subtalar joint, and the ankle is plantar flexed with an adducted forefoot. In addition, the toes are extended at the metatarsophalangeal joints. This position stretches the plantar fascia and thus stabilizes the medial longitudinal arch.

Toe-off is a passive action that involves the windlass mechanism [4••]. A windlass is a nautical device similar to a winch. Working in the same way, hyper-extension of the toes "hoists" the plantar fascia over a metatarsal pulley. It can, therefore, stabilize the medial longitudinal arch by taking up the slack between its metatarsal and calcaneal ends.

Thus, the foot's main functions of weight bearing and forward propulsion over uneven terrain are accommodated by its multijointed design and stabilized by the plantar fascia.

TREATMENT OF PLANTAR FASCIITIS

The treatment of chronic heel pain caused by plantar fasciitis should first involve conservative measures. The first line of treatment is always prevention. In the case of plantar fasciitis, education of those at greatest risk for developing the condition is essential. Heel cord and plantar fascia stretching before activity minimizes the microtrauma associated with running. Good quality athletic shoes that are comfortable, fit well, and have good heel supports are essential [5].

The simplest treatment is rest. The patient should rest his or her feet as necessitated by the degree of pain felt. In addition to rest, icing the foot for 15 minutes several times a day reduces inflammation associated with plantar fasciitis [6]. Some experts have advocated the application of heat to the sole of the foot to relieve pain [6]. As mentioned, proper footwear is essential to minimize the pain of plantar fasciitis. Shoes should have adequate support and cushioning for the heel, which may be possible by using orthotics and heel pads. Orthotic support devices should have a heel cup to support and stabilize the heel and subtalar joint on impact at heel strike. In addition to heel cups, arch supports are also useful to stabilize the medial longitudinal arch during toe-off and stance. The easiest solution is to change footwear (or change back to footwear worn previously). Brand-name running shoes are usually the best choice; a knowledgeable salesperson is invaluably helpful in finding the patient comfortable and well-fitting shoes.

A change in activity is also usually helpful. While the foot heals, activities such as swimming and cycling may be substituted for running and jumping. Physiotherapy may be a useful adjunct to pre-activity stretching, including stretching of the Achilles tendon and gastrocnemius-soleus muscles. Toe exercises may help to strengthen intrinsic muscles of the foot for support, which lessens stress on the plantar fascia and promotes healing through "rest."

Nonsteroidal anti-inflammatory medications may be helpful in the acute phase of plantar fasciitis [7], as well as long-term adjuvant treatment. Cortisone injections are the last line of conservative management; they are diagnostic as well as therapeutic and will relieve inflammation associated with plantar fasciitis, but not alleviate pain from other possible causes in the differential diagnosis. Controversy exists surrounding the area of injection of the corticosteroids. Some experts advocate injection of anesthetic plus steroid into the origin of the plantar fascia. Others have injected steroids directly into the fat pad itself. Some concern remains, however, about fat necrosis resulting from steroid injection. In the heel pad, this could be disastrous, since the fat-filled fibrous network of the heel pad would be destroyed, and with it, the cushioning effect of this structure. No more than two injections of steroid are given for fear of plantar fascial rupture [3••].

Conservative treatment should be given a 6-month course before moving onto surgical treatment. Bordelon [8] has found that 95% of patients who are treated conservatively respond to treatment within 6 to 10 months.

Surgical management of plantar fasciitis is a last resort and should only be considered after exhausting conservative treatment measures. The procedure involves division of the plantar fascia distal to the medial calcaneal tubercle. In the open procedure, the incision is made medially and in a plantar direction, the plantar nerves are avoided, and the fascia are divided completely.

Some surgeons advocate removal of any associated bone spur. Removal of the bone spur, however, may prolong healing time and increase postoperative pain. Such removal was done when bone spur was thought to be associated with pain caused by plantar fasciitis. It is now known that this is untrue. Therefore, removal of the spur, unless it impinges on nerves, is not recommended. During an open plantar fasciotomy, the patient is placed in a fixed ankle cast and is non–weight bearing for 2 to 3 weeks. Stretching and exercises are resumed at this point, and sports are resumed 4 to 6 weeks postoperatively. Whereas fasciotomy for pain refractory to conservative management of plantar fasciitis is felt to be successful about half the time, the other half of patients continue to have the same amount of pain as before, or more.

ENDOSCOPIC PLANTAR FASCIOTOMY

A technique that is gaining more popularity than open plantar fasciotomy is endoscopic plantar fasciotomy [9••]. In its early stages, this technique involved insertion of a cannula through a 1-cm incision on the medial side of the heel through to the lateral side. The incision site was determined by examining radiographs and by entering the heel 1 cm anterior to the medial calcaneal tubercle or heel spur. Using an endoscope on one end of the portal and a knife on the other, the plantar fascia was divided completely under endoscopic view. This outpatient procedure requires about 15 minutes, and patients are able to bear full weight within 3 to 4 days. Follow-up studies show that 80% of the pain is alleviated by 6.3 weeks with the endoscopic technique versus 10.3 weeks with the open technique [10]. Patients who have been in pain for longer periods also seem to do better with the endoscopic technique than with open surgical release. Complications are related mostly to the technical aspects of the surgery, injury to nerves on the medial side of the heel, pes planus following complete fascial release, and refractory postoperative pain.

In a recent study by the authors, it was found that radiography is often unnecessary to delineate the portals. It was demonstrated that a line extended from the posterior border of the medial malleolus is a reproducible bony landmark. This line is extended to the sole of the foot (Fig. 1-2). With the foot in neutral dorsiflexion, the medial portal is developed on this line approximately 1 cm deep to the skin on the sole of the foot. This safely avoids the important neurovascular structures in the sole of the foot. As with the technique

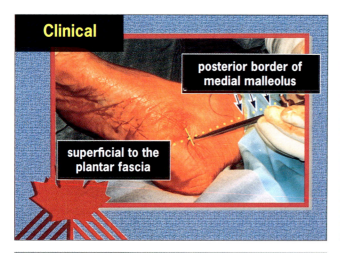

Figure 1-2. Line extending from the posterior border of the medial malleolus to the sole. This line establishes the landmark for the medial portal. The foot is placed in neutral dorsiflexion. The medial portal is placed on this line 1 cm deep to the skin, superficial to the plantar fascia.

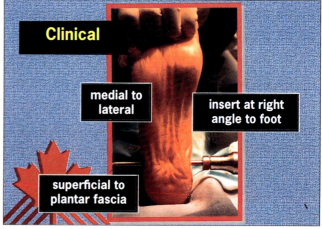

Figure 1-3. The medial portal is made on a line extending from the posterior border of the medial malleolus about 1 cm deep to the skin. The foot must be in neutral dorsiflexion. The slotted cannula is introduced from medial to lateral at right angles to the long axis of the foot.

of Barrett and Day [11], the authors use an incision on the medial side of the heel and insert a cannula through to the lateral side. The cannula must pass at right angles to the long axis of the foot (Fig. 1-3).

The authors use the endoscopic carpal tunnel equipment manufactured by Smith & Nephew Donjoy (Boston, MA). A small spatula is introduced into the endoscopic portal and used to palpate the plantar fascia, which will be proximal to the incision. The open slotted cannula is then passed from medial to lateral as described previously. The slot in the cannula faces proximally, as it is superficial to the fascia. The videoscope is then introduced from the lateral side (Fig. 1-4).

A small triangular bladed knife is then passed from the medial portal. The plantar fascia is palpated, visualized, and divided (Fig. 1-5). The knife blade is used to sharply divide the fascia until the underlying muscle can be seen. The muscle must be seen so the

surgeon will know that division is complete (Fig. 1-6). The cut edges of the fascia are palpated with a probe to ensure that division is total, and further efforts are made if necessary.

Postoperatively, patients are allowed immediate weight bearing. However, they are not allowed to partake in activities involving impact for at least 6 weeks. They should carry out a rehabilitation program with exercises appropriate for plantar fasciitis. The authors also routinely prescribe soft orthotics, since there is some loss of height of the plantar arch associated with the procedure.

Controversy remains surrounding total versus partial release of the plantar fascia. Barrett and Day [11] currently release the medial two thirds of the plantar fascia. Stability of the arch is believed to be lost with complete release. Until now, however, no biomechanical evidence exists. A recent study [12] was done by

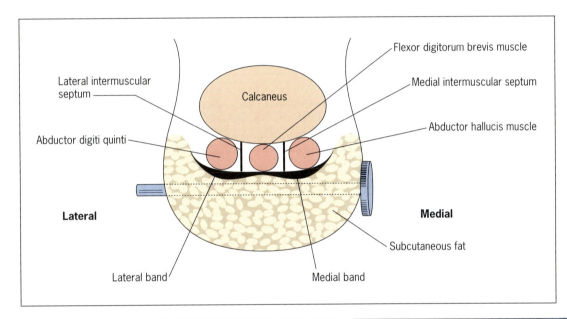

Figure 1-4. The position of the slotted cannula overlying the plantar fascia. The fascia is to be divided from superficial to deep.

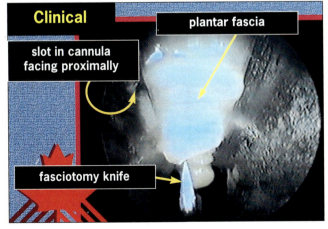

Figure 1-5. Endoscopic view of the plantar fascia. This is a "heads-up" view so the top of the picture is proximal. The fascia is clearly visualized prior to division.

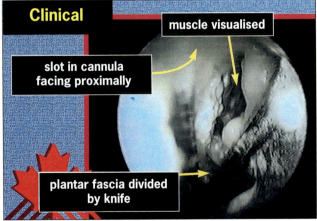

Figure 1-6. The divided fascia. The muscle fibers are visible beneath it. The fascial area must be palpated after division to ensure that all fibers have been divided.

the authors of this chapter to determine the biomechanical characteristics of the plantar fascia before and after partial and total plantar fasciotomy. Six cadaveric feet were sequentially mounted in a custom-made holder and tested on a biomechanical apparatus to derive the stiffness of the plantar fascia from force-displacement curves. Three separate measurements were made: stiffness of the intact plantar fascia, stiffness following selective plantar fasciotomy of either the central or lateral band, and stiffness after total plantar fasciotomy. The study found that a significant difference existed between the stiffness of the intact plantar fascia and that following selective partial plantar fasciotomy. However, no significant difference was found between the decrease in stiffness whether the central band or the lateral band was cut. Furthermore, no significant difference was present in stiffness between partial and total plantar fasciotomy [12]. This led to the conclusion that both partial and total plantar fasciotomy decreased stability of the medial plantar arch. From this finding, it was apparent that both the central and lateral bands of the plantar fascia were equally important to biomechanical stability of this arch. Division of either band decreased stiffness of the medial plantar arch, but no statistically significant difference was found between selective central or lateral partial plantar fasciotomy. From these conclusions, it may be argued that if no significant difference exists between partial and total plantar fasciotomy, the latter should be performed to provide adequate pain relief in the treatment of plantar fasciitis.

The authors' study looked at a consecutive series of 40 feet in which there were symptoms for at least 6 months. All had had an endoscopic plantar fascia release as outpatients. Patients were observed for an average of 18 months (6 months to 4 years). Results were assessed by the junior author using the criteria of pain, stiffness, and functional recovery for work and sports. Overall, 88% had no pain and 88% had full recovery of all daily activities. Only 76% returned to sporting activities with no restrictions. No complications ensued, although a single patient had residual tenderness around the medial portal. One patient failed to benefit at all from the procedure.

CONCLUSION

Plantar fasciotomy has been proven beneficial in the treatment of foot pain resulting from plantar fasciitis refractory to conservative therapy alone. Studies have shown that endoscopic plantar fasciotomy is associated with a lower morbidity, better functional outcome, and faster recovery time than with an open procedure. The endoscopic procedure is still in its early stages; many aspects of the surgery will require refinement once further biomechanical and functional studies are completed. Despite its novelty, endoscopic plantar fasciotomy may prove to be the treatment of choice for plantar fasciitis in patients who have failed conservative therapy and are willing to undergo a short surgical procedure to relieve their intractable foot pain.

REFERENCES AND RECOMMENDED READING

Recently published papers of particular interest have been highlighted as:
•• Of outstanding interest

1. Sarrafian SK: *Anatomy of the Foot and Ankle: Descriptive, Topographic, Functional.* Philadelphia: JB Lippincott; 1993:127–137.

2. Snell RS: *Clinical Anatomy for Medical Students,* edn 4. Toronto: Little, Brown; 1992:681–686.

3.•• Karr SD: Subcalcaneal heel pain. *Orth Clin North Am* 1994, 25:161–175.
Excellent overview of pathology, diagnosis, and treatment.

4.•• Seto JL, Brewster CE: Treatment approaches following foot and ankle injury. *Clin Sports Med* 1994, 13:695–718.
Excellent review of management techniques.

5. Leach RE, Seavey MS, Salter DK: Results of surgery in athletes with plantar fasciitis. *Foot Ankle* 1986, 7:156–161.

6. Clarfield M, Bull C: *Plantar Fasciitis.* Anaprox Sports Injuries Series. Toronto: Syntex Incorporated; 1994.

7. Schepsis AA, Leach RE, Gorzyca J: Plantar fasciitis: etiology, surgical results, and review of the literature. *Clin Orthop* 1991, 266:196.

8. Bordelon RL: *Heel Pain: Surgery of the Foot and Ankle.* Edited by Mann RA. St. Louis: Mosby; 1993:837–847.

9.•• Barrett SL: Endoscopic plantar fasciotomy. *Clin Podiatr Med Surg* 1994, 11:469–481.
Surgical technique and results are discussed.

10. Kinley S, Frascone S, Calderone E, *et al.*: Endoscopic plantar fasciotomy versus traditional heel spur surgery: a prospective study. *J Foot Ankle Surg* 1993, 32:595–603.

11. Barrett SL, Day SV: Endoscopic plantar fasciotomy: two portal endoscopic surgical techniques—clinical results of 65 procedures. *J Foot Ankle Surg* 1993, 32:248–256.

12. Ogilvie-Harris DJ, Lobo JJ, Woodside T: Work in progress. Paper presented at Arthroscopy Association of North America. San Diego, CA; April, 1997.

2
CHAPTER

Management of Avascular Meniscal Tears

ZHONGNAN ZHANG AND JAMES A. ARNOLD

In 1936, King [1] published his classic experiment on meniscal healing in dogs. He found that peripheral meniscal tears could be spontaneously healed, yet injuries in other areas did not heal. It was concluded that to be biologically healed, meniscal lesions must communicate with the peripheral blood supply. Using the ink-injection technique, Arnoczky and Warren [2] demonstrated that approximately 20% to 25% of the meniscus at the peripheral position has blood supply and the other 75% to 80% of it is avascular (Fig. 2-1). The healing potential of meniscal tears relies on the degree of the vascularization [1–3,4•]. Partial meniscectomy of avascular meniscal tears is a popular orthopedic procedure. However, surgeons and researchers agree that the injured meniscus should be preserved whenever possible because of its vital function to the knee joint

[5–13]. In the past, pedicle flaps have been grafted from the synovium and placed into meniscal tears [14–18]. This grafting helped in meniscal healing but would be a difficult procedure under arthroscopy. In addition, peripheral meniscal synovium has been abraded to promote the healing of meniscal injury. However, this technique was not effective for tears in the avascular zone [19]. It might be possible to heal avascular meniscal tears by injection of fibrin clot into the lesion [20–22]. However, it is unknown whether healing strength is sufficient enough, since there is no blood supply involved in the healing process when fibrin clotting is used.

An animal study [4•]of trephination plus suturing to treat longitudinal injuries was conducted in the avascular area of the meniscus in 20 goats. All 20 samples of the trephination plus suturing group showed obvious macroscopic signs of healing. At 25 weeks, the mean maximum tensile strength of five samples in this group was 40.4 kg/cm². Also at 25 weeks, some collagen fibers in the healing tissue in the trephination plus suturing group were aligned along the predominantly circumferential distribution of meniscal collagen fibers. In contrast, only three samples (one in each period) of the suturing only group were partly healed, but they were too fragile to be tested for tensile strength. The rest of this group had no gross healing noted at all. The difference in healing time between the two groups was statistically significant. Thus, the study indicated that trephination plus suturing can significantly promote the healing of meniscal tears in the avascular area.

On the basis of animal studies [3,4•], an arthroscopic surgical system and procedure of trephination plus suturing were designed for clinical practice. A total of 36 patients with meniscal tears underwent arthroscopic trephination plus suturing, and 28 patients had suturing only. The minimum follow-up period was 3 years. Two symptomatic re-tears occurred in the trephination plus suturing group, and seven occurred in the suturing only group. The symptomatic re-tear rate of the trephination plus suturing group was significantly smaller than that of the suturing only group (P < 0.01). Therefore, these studies indicate that the patients treated with trephination have fewer symptoms and a lower clinical failure rate [23••]. The authors now routinely perform arthroscopic trephination plus suturing for patients with medial longitudinal meniscal tears.

INDICATIONS FOR TREPHINATION AND SUTURING

Trephination and suturing together are indicated in longitudinal avascular (white zone) tears of the medial meniscus, longitudinal avascular-vascular (white-red zone) tears of the medial meniscus, and chronic peripheral (red zone) meniscal tears. Complex, horizontal, radial, and macroscopic degenerative tears are not indications and should be treated by arthroscopic partial meniscectomy.

OPERATIVE TECHNIQUE

The trephination system consists of a trephine, a power handle, and a guide. The trephine is characterized by its toothlike tip and diameter of 2.2 mm (Fig. 2-2). The remainder of the trephine is similar to a motorized arthroscopic shaver. Any manufacturer's arthroscopic motorized driver may be used as the power device (Fig. 2-3). The guide consists of a sheath with a handle and a blunt trocar (Fig. 2-4).

The arthroscope is inserted through anterolateral portal, and the medial meniscus is probed with a nerve hook through the anteromedial portal. After a longitudinal tear is found in the avascular area of the medial meniscus (Fig. 2-5), the sheath with a blunt trocar is introduced into the knee joint through the anterior medial approach (Fig. 2-6). The trocar is withdrawn after the blunt tip reaches

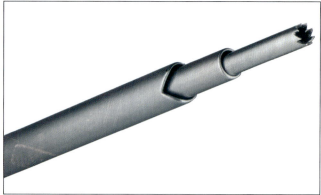

Figure 2-2. The sawtooth tip of the trephine.

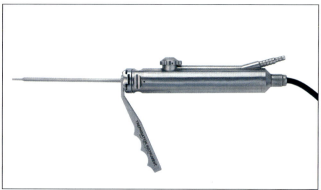

Figure 2-3. Power handle (*right*) with trephine and guide (*left*).

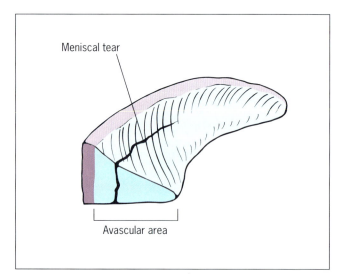

Figure 2-1. Meniscal tear at the avascular area (white zone).

the tear either superior or inferior to the meniscus. The trephine, connected to the power handle (*see* Fig. 2-3), is introduced through the sheath to the outer wall of the tear (Fig. 2-7). A core of meniscal tissue is cut by motorized rotation of the trephine and removed by suction through the power handle (Fig. 2-8). A tunnel diameter of 2.2 mm is created from the tear of the white zone to the periphery of the meniscus. The length of the trephine outside the sheath is 15 mm (*see* Fig. 2-2). One tunnel is drilled for every 4 to 5 mm of tear. Two tunnels, for example, may be needed for a tear 8 to 10 mm long. The portal for the arthroscope is changed from lateral to medial, and a suturing instrument is inserted through the medial portal. Two means of fixation of the meniscal tear can be used: 1) horizontal sutures are placed inside-out by either a double or single needle guide (*see* Fig. 2-8) through a vertical posterior-medial incision, and the 2-0 nonabsorbable sutures are tied outside to the capsule (Fig. 2-9), or 2) bioabsorbable arrows are

inserted across the tear, and the repaired tear is probed with a nerve hook to test for security of fixation.

REHABILITATION

In patients with meniscus repairs alone without reconstruction, full extension is achieved before weight bearing is allowed. Immediate range of motion is recommended, and weight bearing is resumed as tolerated when extension is achieved. Patients with isolated meniscal injuries are allowed to return to sports as soon as 4 to 6 weeks following repair; however, patients with unstable peripheral longitudinal tears without anterior cruciate ligament (ACL) reconstruction are instructed to not resume competitive or high-demand recreational activities. This patient population is rare because most patients choose to have the ACL reconstruction with clinical instability. After ACL reconstruction, a similar accelerated rehabilitation program is allowed. Limited time

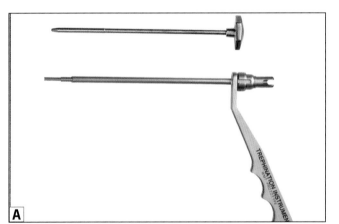 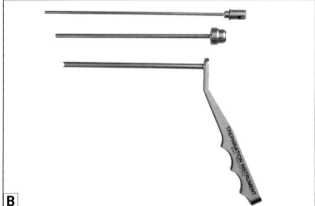

Figure 2-4. A, Trephination guide with trochar (*top*) and trephine (*bottom*). **B,** Trephine (*top*), sheath of trephine (*middle*), and trephination guide (*bottom*).

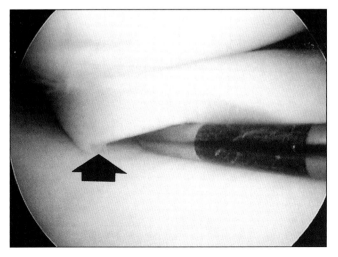

Figure 2-5. Meniscal tear (*arrow*) at the white zone probed with a nerve hook.

on crutches is recommended to restore full range of motion more quickly.

DISCUSSION

Zhang et al. [3] and Gershuni et al. [24] have separately proven that preparation of vascular tunnels by trephination may promote the healing of avascular tears. A normal healing process requires blood supply and stability of the injured segments. Trephination may bring blood supply to the injury [3,4•], and it is doubtful whether an unstable or large meniscal tear could be healed by trephination only [3]. The authors add suturing to the trephination because combined blood supply and stabilization are necessary for the healing process.

In a preliminary animal experiment [3], the senior author failed to develop a channel with a biopsy needle because the channel tended to close after needle withdrawal. Henning et al. [20] experienced the same problem clinically. The trephine designed by the senior author has a sawtooth tip that enables the surgeon to harvest a meniscal core by rotating the trephine to penetrate the meniscus (see Fig. 2-1). The channel created does not collapse and does allow much better vascularity to the avascular meniscus. A trephine designed for surgery can be adapted to an ordinary power handle and used

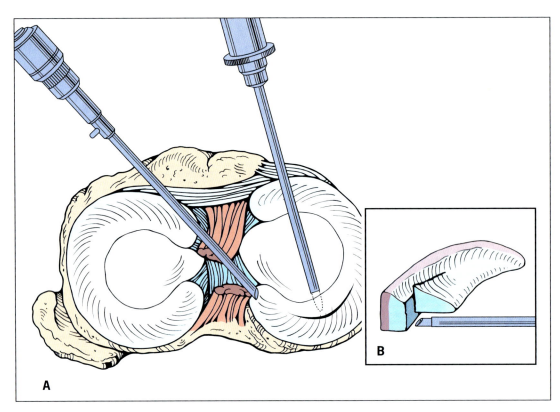

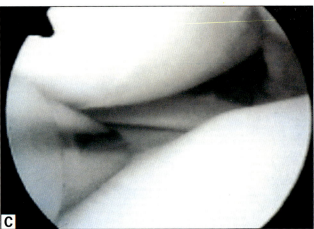

Figure 2-6. The trephination guide is inserted into the knee joint through the standard anterior-medial portal (**A**), and the guide with blunt trochar is inserted through the space inferior to the meniscus (**B**). **C**, Arthroscopic view of the insertion of the trephination guide.

in trephination and suturing surgery (*see* Fig. 2-2). The rotation of the trephine is motorized, making the inside-out cut fast and easy. The core of meniscal tissue cut by the trephine is evacuated by suction through the trephine tip and power handle so that blockage of the tunnel by the meniscal core is no longer a problem.

The trocar guide for trephination may easily introduce the trephine to the tear and prevent the articular cartilage from abrasion by the sharp tooth of the trephine (*see* Fig. 2-5). The tip of trephine outside the trocar is 15 mm, which is the maximal depth of the trephination. The tip of the sheath can be used as a mark of measurement to control the depth of the cut to protect the posterior neurovasculature of the knee (*see* Fig. 2-2). The authors do not trephine tears of the lateral meniscus because the posterolateral popliteal tendon limits the use of the peripheral vascular area for vascularization of the tears [25]. The technique introduced in this chapter is for tears of the posterior and middle sections of the medial meniscus. Of course, most longitudinal meniscal tears occur posteriorly. There is a concern about potential damage to the outer rim of the meniscus by trephination, but the animal and clinical studies do not support this hypothesis [3,4•,15,23••].

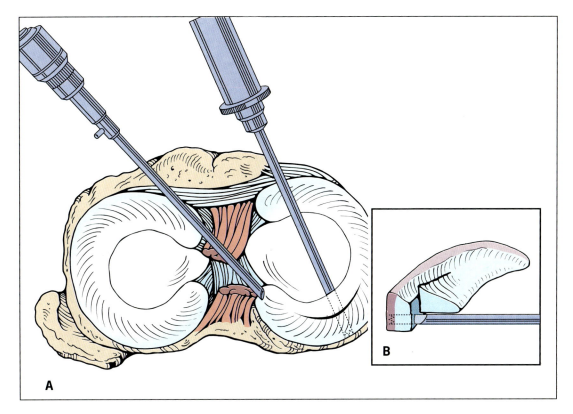

A

B

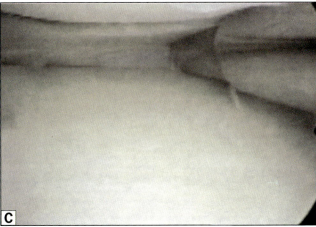

C

Figure 2-7. The trephine is inserted through the guide to the tear (**A**), and a tunnel to the periphery of the meniscus is created by the trephine (**B**). **C,** Arthroscopic view of the trephination.

Rehabilitation after meniscal repair and trephination has evolved as confidence in theses repairs has been obtained. In the past, weight bearing was restricted for 4 to 6 weeks, with the knee blocked from extension. Sports were not allowed for 3 to 6 months. However, in recent years, rehabilitation after ACL reconstruction, as well as meniscal repair without reconstruction, have evolved significantly. Although no satisfactory studies have been performed showing that repair of menisci function as well as normal menisci, our results with more aggressive rehabilitation appear to be encouraging and come from anecdotal experience.

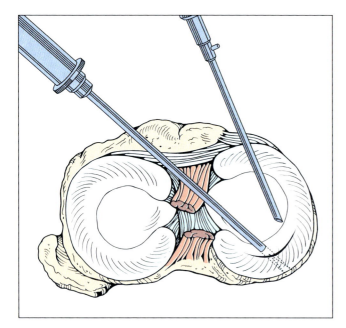

Figure 2-8. Needles are inserted into the joint through either the anterior-medial or anterior-lateral portal to repair the meniscal tear.

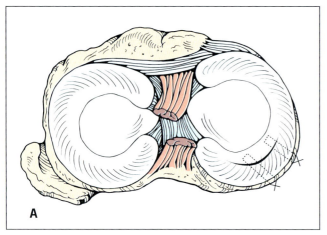
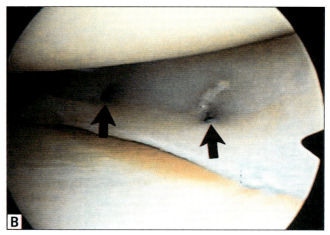

Figure 2-9. A, The sutures tied to the capsule. **B,** Meniscal tear fixed with sutures (*arrows*).

REFERENCES AND RECOMMENDED READING

Recently published papers of particular interest have been highlighted as:

• Of interest

•• Of outstanding interest

1. King D: The healing of semilunar cartilages. *J Bone Joint Surg* 1936,18:333–342.

2. Arnoczky SP, Warren RF: The microvasculature of the meniscus and its response to injury: an experimental study in the dog. *Am J Sports Med* 1983, 11:131–141.

3. Zhang ZN, Tu KY, Xu YK, *et al.*: Treatment of longitudinal injuries in avascular area of meniscus in dogs by trephination. *Arthroscopy* 1988, 4:151–159.

4.• Zhang ZN, Arnold AJ, Williams T., *et al.*: Repairs by trephination and suturing of longitudinal injuries in the avascular area of the meniscus in goats. *Am J Sports Med* 1995, 23:35–41.

Preclinical study showing trephination and suturing for meniscal repair.

5. Baratz ME, Fu FH, Mengato R: Meniscal tears: the effect of meniscectomy and of repair on intraarticular contact areas and stress in the human knee. A preliminary report. *Am J Sports Med* 1986, 14:270–275.

6. Baratz ME, Rehak DC, Fu FH: Peripheral tears of the meniscus: the effect of open versus arthroscopic repair on intraarticular contact stresses in the human knee. *Am J Sports Med* 1988, 16:1–6.

7. DeHaven KE: Rational for meniscus repair of excision. *Clin Sports Med* 1985, 4:267–273.

8. Fairbank TJ: Knee joint changes after meniscectomy. *J Bone Joint Surg* 1948, 30(suppl B):664–670.

9. Hede A, Svalastoga E, Reimann I: Articular cartilage changes following meniscal lesions: repair and meniscectomy studied in the rabbit knee. *Acta Orthop Scand* 1991, 62:319–322.

10. Larson RL: The knee—the physiological joint. *J Bone Joint Surg* 1983, 65(suppl A):143–144.

11. Seedhom BB: Transmission of the load in the joint with special reference to the role of the menisci. *N Engl J Med* 1979, 8:220.

12. Sommerlath K, Gillquist J: Knee function after meniscus repair and total meniscectomy: a seven-year follow-up study. *Arthroscopy* 1987, 3:166–169.

13. Strand T, Engesaxter LB, Molster AO: Meniscus repair in knee ligament injuries. *Acta Orthop Scand* 1985, 56:130–132.

14. Cisa J, Basora J, Madarnas P, *et al.*: Meniscal repair by synovial flap transfer: healing of the avascular zone in rabbits. *Acta Orthop Scand* 1995, 66:38–40.

15. Gao JZ: Experimental study on healing of old tear in the avascular portion of menisci in dogs. *Chung Hua Wai Ko Tsa Chih* 1990, 28:726–729, 782.

16. Ghanially FN, Wedge JH, LaLonde A: Experimental methods of repairing injured menisci. *J Bone Joint Surg* 1986, 68(suppl B):106–110.

17. Klompmaker J, Jansen HW, Veth RP: Pouous polymer implant for repair of meniscal lesions: a preliminary study in dogs. *Biomaterials* 1991, 12:810–816.

18. Sekiya H: Free synovium grafting for the repair of the avascular portion of canine knee joint meniscus. *Nippon Seikeigeka Gakkai Zasshi* 1992, 66:50–60.

19. Nakhostine M, Gershuni DH, Anderson R: Effects of abrasion therapy on tears in the avascular region of sheep menisci. *Arthroscopy* 1990, 6:280–287.

20. Henning CE, Lynch MA, Yearout KM: Arthroscopic meniscal repair using an exogenous fibrin clot. *Clin Orthop* 1990, 252:64–72.

21. Ishimura M, Tamai S, Fujisawa Y: Arthroscopic meniscal repair with fibrin glue. *Arthroscopy* 1991, 7:177–181.

22. Nakhostine M, Gershuni DH, Danzig LA: Effects of an in-substance conduit with injection of a blood clot on tears in the avascular region of the meniscus. *Acta Orthop Belg* 1991, 57:242–246.

23.•• Zhang ZN, Arnold JA: Trephination and suturing of avascular meniscal tears: A clinical study of the trephination procedure. *Arthroscopy* 1996, 12:726–731.

Clinical study showing the trephination procedure for meniscal repair.

24. Gershuni DH, Skyhar MJ, Danzig LA: Experimental models to promote healing of tears in the avascular segment of canine knee menisci. *J Bone Joint Surg* 1989, 71(suppl A):1363–1370.

25. Horibe S, Shino K, Maeda A, *et al.*: Results of isolated meniscal repair evaluated by second-look arthroscopy. *Arthroscopy* 1996, 12:150–155.

3

Outpatient Anterior Cruciate Ligament Reconstruction

ALEXANDER I. GLOGAU AND PETER C. KWONG

Arthroscopy of the knee is one of the most common orthopedic procedures currently performed. There are thousands done yearly. Many involve reconstruction of the anterior cruciate ligament (ACL). Historically, this procedure has evolved from a major open joint case requiring an inpatient hospital stay lasting from 5 to 7 days to the arthroscopically assisted approach using one or two incisions with a bone–patellar tendon–bone (BPTB) or hamstring autograft requiring only an overnight stay. The procedure is also done on an outpatient basis.

In this era of managed care and highly competitive contracting, many surgical procedures that used to be performed on an inpatient basis are now being performed on an outpatient basis. All surgical specialists have been forced into an economic mode that constrains operative time, equipment, use of inpa-

tient facilities, and physician and facility fees. The trend has certainly been for the majority of orthopedic surgeons to avoid inpatient hospital stays and to develop ACL reconstruction into an outpatient surgical procedure that is safe, comfortable, convenient, and economically attractive to the ACL-deficient patient and to third-party payers.

The Associated Arthroscopy Institute (AAI) in Plano, TX has taken this one step further. To increase the economic efficiency and reduce direct patient cost while increasing convenience for both the patient and physician, ACL reconstructions are now performed in an office-based ambulatory surgical center (ASC). AAI's primary goal for office ACL reconstruction is to provide the same quality of care as in the hospital setting or hospital-based ASC. AAI's operative theater is of the same standard as a hospital's operative suite, and AAI provides equivalent anesthesia standards and preoperative and postoperative monitoring that are of equally high quality. The advantages of performing office-based ACL surgery are the tremendous economic savings as well as the possibility of providing a much more comfortable and less intimidating environment for the patient. This chapter outlines AAI's protocol for office-based outpatient ACL reconstruction.

PATIENT SELECTION

Of course, not every patient with a ruptured ACL needs reconstruction. This decision should be based on the patient's age, activity status, grade of instability, and level of motivation, along with concomitant injuries to the knee. As the procedure has become less invasive, less morbid, and more sophisticated, indications for this procedure are expanding to both younger patients with open physeal plates to more active individuals in their fourth and fifth decades who want to continue playing competitive sports with significant rotational stress. After the need for an ACL reconstruction has been established, a decision must also be made to determine if the patient is an appropriate candidate for an outpatient ACL procedure. Of course, the subset of patients with ACL-deficient knees requiring surgery is relatively young (under 45 years of age), in good to excellent physical condition, and highly motivated, which makes the decision for an outpatient procedure that much easier. Of the factors involved in this process, the most important to ensure a successful outcome is patient education. The patient must be informed about what to expect preoperatively, during the procedure, and postoperatively. The first postoperative night must be carefully explained, including use of prescription drugs, a continuous passive motion (CPM) unit if used, and a cryotherapy unit, which may be very beneficial.

The ideal candidate for an outpatient ACL reconstruction must be a mature individual, with a normal to high level of pain tolerance, without any significant psychologic overlay, and with a satisfactory support group at home. Patients with anxiety disorders or depression should probably be excluded for outpatient ACL reconstruction. Logistic problems such as the patient living in a second story apartment or driving a manual transmission automobile must be discussed. The type of work a patient does and how long he or she will not be able to work should be mentioned along with the intense physical therapy regimen required for a successful outcome. These well-discussed points will make the outpatient surgical experience much more pleasant for the patient.

PREOPERATIVE EVALUATION AT THE CLINIC

At AAI, a complete orthopedic evaluation is performed before the patient arrives for formal preoperative testing. A full series of radiographs will already have been performed on the ACL-deficient patient. Magnetic resonance imaging (MRI) is not routinely performed unless a question exists about other intra-articular injuries or the grade of the ACL injury. Preoperative evaluation includes a complete history and physical examination, determination of the patient's anesthetic-class level based on past medical history, underlying medical problems, social history, and current medications. A completely separate visit is important for several reasons. First, this is when much of the patient education process is performed. Second, repetitive questioning of the patient during a complete history and physical examination provides a measure of safety in determining any possible medical problems that may elevate a patient from Class I or II anesthetic risk to Class III, which may be inappropriate for the in-office ambulatory surgical setting. Table 3-1 provides an explanation of physical status levels according to the American Society of Anesthesiologists (ASA) [1].

For Class I anesthetic-risk patients, no preoperative urinalysis or blood work is performed. A chest radiograph is only necessary if the patient has a history of current or recent smoking. This radiographic film is read by an outside radiologist to rule out any significant pulmonary problems. An electrocardiogram (ECG) is only ordered if the patient has a history of cardiac disease or is older than 45 years of age. Diabetes with or without a history of hypertension immediately elevates a patient to a higher risk level, at which point a more complete workup is performed. For any Class II or higher individuals undergoing ACL reconstruction, consideration for outpatient surgery in the acute care hospital setting may be in order to ensure appropriate consultant physician availability.

It is necessary to routinely obtain results of pregnancy tests for women of child-bearing age. Patients are also specifically asked about the use of the newer dietary agents, fenfluramine, phentermine hydrochloride, and dexfenfluramine, which may cause a patient to enter into a hypotensive crisis while under general anesthesia. This complication has been explained as a decreased response of the adrenal gland and resultant depression of catecholamine release. A minimum 2-week hiatus between cessation of this type of medication and the general anesthesia must elapse for this procedure to be considered safe by the ASA. For the surgeon's protection, consent is obtained from the patient for preoperative human immunodeficiency virus (HIV) testing. At AAI, some of the surgeons forgo this test and its attendant high cost, consider all patients as potential transmitters of the virus, and always take appropriate precautions to avoid contamination.

Finally, patients are again instructed in detail about their behavior the night before surgery, which includes the last time they may eat or drink, and about the careful shaving of their knee. The patient is informed of the time to arrive for surgery, what to expect on arrival, and a projected schedule for the day. This is of the utmost importance for personal service for the patients, especially in the office ASC setting. The completed clinical documentation at AAI includes a thorough history and filled-out physical form, preoperative orders, standardized consent form, and copies of the most recent office notes.

INSURANCE PRECERTIFICATION

From the moment a physician at AAI has filled out a surgical scheduling slip for an upcoming ACL reconstruction, it is referred to AAI's office staff for insurance precertification. AAI is still in the process of convincing some insurance carriers of the benefits of the office-based outpatient surgical procedure. Insurance precertification may take several days. For the benefit of the patient and to reduce costly and time-consuming phone calls, a global precertification process has been started at AAI. With one phone call, AAI staff tries to determine the benefits for a patient on a particular plan regarding physician fees, surgical fees, facility and hardware fees, postoperative and functional braces, anesthesia fees, and the amount of physical therapy allowed. These are some of the most confusing aspects of the entire experience for patient and staff alike. If this information is all available before surgery, patients are better informed and definitely happier at not receiving unexpected bills.

PATIENT PREOPERATIVE PREPARATION

At AAI, the patient arrives approximately 1 hour before his or her scheduled surgical time, compared

Table 3-1	Ambulatory Surgery Patient Selection Criteria

I. American Society of Anesthesiologists physical status classifications

A. Physical status I

   1. Healthy patient, no systemic disease

B. Physical status II

   1. Mild systemic disease without functional limitations

   2. Examples: chronic bronchitis, moderate obesity, diet-controlled diabetes mellitus, previous myocardial infarction, mild hypertension

C. Physical status III

   1. Severe systemic disease associated with definite functional limitations

   2. Examples: coronary artery disease with angina, insulin-dependent diabetes mellitus, morbid obesity, moderate to severe pulmonary insufficiency

D. Physical Status IV—**not candidate for ambulatory surgery**

   1. Severe systemic disease that is a constant threat to life

   2. Examples: organic heart disease with marked cardiac insufficiency, persisting angina, intractable arrhythmia; advanced pulmonary, renal, hepatic, or endocrine insufficiency

E. Physical status V—**not candidate for ambulatory surgery**

   1. Moribund patient who is not expected to survive without the operation

   2. Examples: ruptured abdominal aneurysm with profound shock

F. Physical status VI—**not candidate for ambulatory surgery**

   1. A declared brain-dead patient whose organs are being removed for donor purposes

G. Physical status E (emergency)

   1. Used to denote presumed poorer physical status of any patient in one of these categories who is operated on on an emergency basis

II. Physician and patient preference

III. Positive motivation

IV. General good health

V. Well-controlled systemic disease

VI. Adequate or appropriate support systems

VII. Requirements of patient's insurance

VIII. Extent of surgical procedure

XI. Premature infant or older infant born prematurely who need postoperative apnea monitoring—**not candidates for ambulatory surgery**

Adapted from Litwack [1].

with 2 to 3 hours before surgery in the hospital outpatient setting. In the locker room, the patient changes into a surgical gown and then is led to the gurney in the preoperative holding area. An intravenous tube is placed, from which the patient receives 1 g of cefazolin sodium. Patients with a history of a reaction to penicillin still receive cephalosporin; no adverse reactions have occurred for any of AAI's arthroscopy patients. Patients strongly allergic to cephalosporins receive intravenous ciprofloxacin, which is not nearly as cost-effective an agent. All ACL patients receive preoperative local anesthesia despite the use of light general anesthesia. The use of local anesthesia significantly reduces the amount of anesthetic needed for the outpatient ACL reconstruction and therefore limits postoperative nausea and vomiting. This also indirectly reduces anesthesia expense. At AAI, 50 to 60 mL of a 50% mixture of 2% lidocaine and 0.25% bupivacaine with epinephrine (Fig. 3-1) are used. As many authors agree, including McGuire *et al.* [2], Kao *et al.* [3••], and Friedman [4], control of postoperative pain is very important for the ACL procedure performed in the outpatient setting. The patients, when fully prepared, actually walk independently from the preoperative area directly to the operating suite.

ANESTHETIC CONSIDERATIONS

For any surgical procedure requiring general anesthesia performed at AAI, a board-certified anesthesiologist is engaged. Some local plastic surgeons and podiatrists use certified nurse anesthetists, and even though use of this type of ancillary health-care professional is more cost-effective, it may put the surgeon at too great a risk in the office-based ASC. General anesthesia is achieved by either endotracheal intubation or use of a laryngeal mask airway (LMA). The LMA is certainly more comfortable for the patient but does not give full control of the airway to the anesthesiologist and may be associated with increased incidence of aspiration. Full monitoring is achieved with pulse oximetry, automatic intermittent blood pressure readings, and continuous ECG and CO_2 readings.

Use of intravenous propofol and the inhalation agent desflurane, both with extremely fast elimination times, has revolutionized the rapid control of patient responsiveness for the anesthesiologist. AAI therefore routinely uses general anesthesia for outpatient ACL surgery. Many other anesthetic techniques may be used for outpatient ACL reconstructions. Meade *et al.* [5] advocate use of a preoperative femoral nerve block. At the Southern California Orthopedic Institute, Friedman [4] reports that 50% of the ACL outpatients elect to have an epidural anesthetic; occasionally, the catheter is allowed to remain in place to supply additional postoperative analgesia.

Ketorolac tromethamine is an excellent adjunct for the control of postoperative pain. McGuire *et al.* [2] reported in 1993 that for outpatient ACL patients, ketorolac was as or more efficacious than the opioids meperidine or morphine without the adverse side affects or the higher cost. At AAI, surgeons routinely give 60 mg intramuscularly 30 minutes before the end of the procedure. However, care must be taken with the use of ketorolac. Reports have been made of vascular effects from this drug, which may cause bleeding in patients with a previous history of ulcer disease or other bleeding disorders.

SURGICAL PROCEDURE

After general anesthesia has been achieved, examination under anesthesia is performed. A tourniquet is

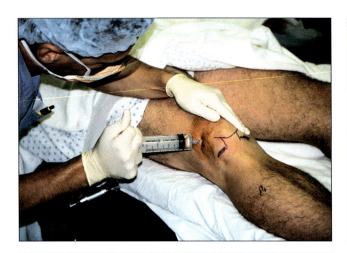

Figure 3-1. Preoperative local anesthesia with sterile intra-articular injection of bupivacaine and lidocaine mixture with epinephrine.

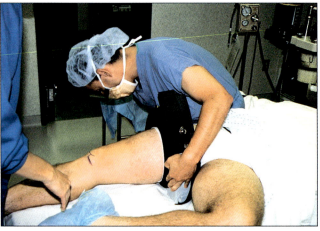

Figure 3-2. Positioning and placement of leg holder with tourniquet, which is not immediately inflated.

applied to the affected lower extremity (Fig. 3-2), but not immediately inflated. The upper thigh is then placed into a carefully padded leg holder, and the opposite limb is padded and protected. The knee, leg, and foot are prepared using Duraprep (3M Health Care, St. Paul, MN) (Fig. 3-3), an easily applied, long-lasting antibacterial and antiviral agent. A sterile arthroscopy pack has been designed for AAI, which includes full sterile drapes, gowns, tubing, basin, sponges, towels, needles, #11 blade, and dressings required for the entire procedure. This has been very carefully thought out to minimize wastage of any single-use items during the procedure.

Tourniquet time is minimized by performing the diagnostic arthroscopy, arthroscopic meniscal resection or repair, ACL remnant excision, and notchplasty without tourniquet. This attempts to limit tourniquet time to 1 hour or less. Prolonged tourniquet times have been shown to increase immediate postoperative pain and paresthesias significantly. In fact, many of these outpatient ACL operations have been done without a tourniquet. This does tend to add at least 15 minutes to the procedure because of poorer visualization and therefore may not be cost effective or beneficial to the patient. For most patients, 3 to 4 cc of epinephrine 1:1000 is added to each 5-liter bag of irrigating fluid to help control capillary bleeding into the joint. During much of the endoscopic portion of the ACL procedure, the knee remains *dry*. For in-office ASC meniscal repairs, the meniscal arrows made by Bionix (Toledo, OH) are very helpful. They can usually be quickly placed through preexisting portals and do not require posteromedial or lateral incision for suture passage or tying.

The diagnostic arthroscopy is performed through two standard inferior patellar portals. Inflow is through the arthroscope sheath. During the past few years the nitrogen-driven Davol (Cranston, RI) arthroscopy pump has been very effective. It is simple to use and keeps up satisfactory flow with a multitude of different shavers and burrs, including the Dyonics (Smith & Nephew Endoscopy, Inc, Andover, MA), Linvatec (Largo, FL), and Arthrex (Naples, FL) systems. A full evaluation of the patella, gutters, medial and lateral compartments, and ACL and posterior cruciate ligament (PCL) is made with the 30° arthroscope. If indicated, a 70° arthroscope is inserted through the notch to evaluate the posterior compartment, menisci, and PCL. Any pathology, excluding that of the ACL, is addressed at this time.

The ACL is carefully examined and probed. If it is attenuated or torn, it is removed using an arthroscopic shaver. Notchplasty is also performed using a combination of curettes, full-radius resector, and an arthro-

scopic burr, either round or flame shaped. Care is taken to clean the posterolateral corner of the notch to reveal the over-the-top position and not be fooled by the resident's ridge. The inferolateral portion of the notch must also be adequately expanded to avoid graft impingement in this region. Some authors, including Clancy [6], have recently advocated a trend toward minimizing this portion of the procedure. With the endoscopic approach, there must be adequate visualization for passage of the femoral interference screw. The stump of the ACL may remain for use of the tibial drill guide but should be removed before completion of the procedure to avoid the formation of a cyclops lesion.

Arthroscopic instrumentation is now removed, and graft harvesting is begun. Quite often at this time, the leg is exsanguinated and the tourniquet is inflated. However, in many instances, bleeding is not substantial and the entire procedure is performed without inflation of the tourniquet. At AAI, the majority of the grafts are BPTB constructs, but medial hamstrings are also used when they are indicated. Patellar tendon allografts obtained through Cryolife yield consistently excellent results when they are available. (They are sometimes unavailable because of increasing usage and diminishing supply.) Use of an allograft in selected patients does increase overall cost by $1500, but significantly decreases operative time and postoperative patient morbidity. It is an ideal procedure for the office-based outpatient surgical setting.

If a BPTB construct is to be used, a midline incision approximately 6 to 9 cm long is made. This is fashioned from the inferior pole of the patella to the medial side of the tibial tubercle. Careful dissection is

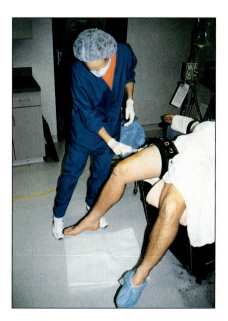

Figure 3-3. Preoperative preparation using Duraprep (3M Health Care, St. Paul, MN)

taken down through the peritenon of the patellar tendon. The width of the tendon is measured, and the central third is marked. Using the Linvatec captured oscillating saw guide system (Fig. 3-4), the patellar and tibial tubercle plugs are cut, and then a fresh #10 blade is used to incise the tendon between the two plugs. The harvested graft is carefully brought to the back table to be prepared for passage and measurement. The shorter of the two plugs is chosen for the femoral tunnel. The Linvatec system has predrilled holes in the bone plugs. Two heavy gauge Ticron (Sherwood-Davis & Geck, St. Louis, MO) sutures are placed through the tibial bone plug to be used for traction and tensioning later. A partially threaded guidewire from the Synthes (Paoli, PA) 6.5-mm cannulated screw system is then drilled into the tendon end of the femoral bone plug to be used in a popsicle-stick fashion to pass the graft through the joint and into the femoral tunnel. This is another small step to decrease postoperative levels of pain by avoiding the use of a transosseous tunnel and creation of a thigh wound. The graft construct is shaped to pass through the appropriate size tunnel and also pre-tensioned using the Arthrex tensioning device (Fig. 3-5).

At this point, the knee is revisited arthroscopically to prepare the tibial and femoral bone tunnels. Using the Linvatec or Arthrex POP (posterior cruciate ligament–oriented placement guide) anterior tibial guide set at 55° to 60°, depending on the overall graft length, a tibial tunnel is created (Fig. 3-6). The Arthrex cannulated coring reamer works quite well, providing an excellent source of bone for grafting the donor sites at the end of the procedure and putting much less bony debris into the joint during the drilling process. Landmarks used for the

placement of the tibial tunnel are the ACL footprint, anterior horn of the lateral meniscus, medial tibial spine, and the PCL. The entry point into the joint should be about 5 to 7 mm anterior to the PCL. The POP guide is quite helpful in selecting this point of entry. The tibial tunnel is then cleaned with a shaver and a rasp to smooth all edges and remove all loose bony fragments.

The femoral tunnel is created with the knee in 90° of flexion. A 7-mm offset over-the-top guide is inserted through the tibial tunnel and into the posterior notch at the anatomic origin of the ACL. The 7-mm offset allows for a 2-mm posterior wall at the level of the joint. Rarely, breakout through the posterior wall occurs. Simply converting this single-incision ACL reconstruction into a two-incision type usually changes the obliquity of the femoral tunnel enough to allow for adequate interference fixation. The femoral tunnel is drilled to a depth 5 mm greater than the measured femoral bone plug to allow for adequate seating of the plug as closely as possible to the isometric position. The 11 o'clock and 1 o'clock positions are used for placement of the tunnels in the left and right knees, respectively. The Arthrex cannulated reamer also has measurement markings at its proximal end that can be read while reaming in order to make adjustments in the depth of the femoral tunnel to avoid any graft-tunnel length mismatch.

Metal interference screws have not been used at AAI. The bioabsorbable screws made from polylactic acid have been found to work as well or better than the permanent interference screws. These screws have a pullout strength, stiffness, and insertion torque comparable with that of titanium screws. They also have a slow reabsorption pattern lasting

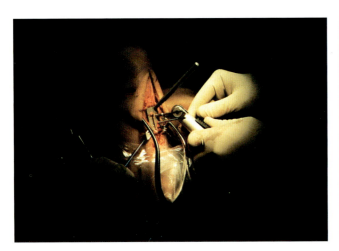

Figure 3-4. Captured guide system for creation of bone plugs.

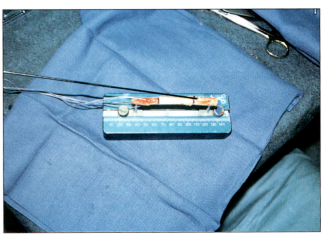

Figure 3-5. Prepared bone–patellar tendon–bone autograft with distal traction sutures and a partially threaded popsicle stick in the femoral bone plug.

longer than 2 years [7••], and they have worked well in the allograft cases, providing excellent interference purchase. These screws do require a better starting point for endoscopic passage. Both Linvatec and Arthrex have available notchmakers for ease of femoral screw placement. These screws have a characteristic squeak upon tightening that confirms an excellent interference fit.

The prepared BPTB graft is passed in popsicle-stick fashion through the tibial tunnel, transarticularly, and into the femoral tunnel. The passing guidewire is removed. With the knee in a hyperflexed position to maintain parallelism of the wire and bone plug, a Nitinol flexible guidewire (Bard Radiology Div.,Covington, GA) is placed through the patellar tendon defect into the previously formed notch in the femoral tunnel. A biodegradable screw with protective sheath is then passed along the guidewire and driven into the femoral tunnel by hand tightening (Fig. 3-7). Slight tension is placed on the nonabsorbable sutures on the tibial end to avoid the catching of redundant fibers in the threads of the interference screw. The screwdriver and guidewire are removed. The graft is visualized arthroscopically, and the knee is taken through a full range of motion with tension on the graft. Any potential areas of impingement are addressed at this time with a shaver, rasp, or burr if needed. Care must be taken to not injure the newly placed graft. Full extension and flexion must be easily reached during this check for impingement.

With the knee in 15° to 30° of flexion, a second guidewire is passed through the tibial tunnel and visualized arthroscopically anterior to the graft. Placement of the screw in this manner ensures that the plug is along the posterior half of the tibial tunnel and

helps avoid any potential anterior impingement problems. The tibial biodegradable interference screw is then passed with a posterior draw on the tibia and appropriate tension on the graft. The graft is then examined arthroscopically, and the knee is checked for stability. The patellar tendon defect is closed with multiple #1 Vicryl (Ethicon, Somerville, NJ) sutures, and the subcutaneous tissue, and skin are closed in the usual fashion. Portals and wound are injected with 30 mL of additional bupivacaine for longer-term postoperative pain relief. Portals are allowed to remain open for drainage. A sterile pressure dressing is applied. A hinged postoperative brace is applied, which allows full range of motion.

POSTOPERATIVE MANAGEMENT

Under the light general anesthesia used at AAI, patients are extubated before transfer into the recovery room. After an in-office ACL procedure, the patient is monitored for a period of at least 1 to 2 hours. When stabilized, patients are transferred into a postoperative recliner. Pain management is through a combination of intravenous and intramuscular meperidine hydrochloride. Postoperative nausea is controlled with intravenous ondansetron hydrochloride, which is an excellent agent with minimal side effects and quick antiemetic relief for the patient; however, it is quite expensive. For breakthrough pain, ketorolac tromethamine is effective when given intravenously after surgery. In the postoperative recovery room, patients are carefully monitored, and mental status is checked along with the neurovascular status of the lower extremity on a regular basis. Patients are discharged after they have obtained an Aldrete [8] score of

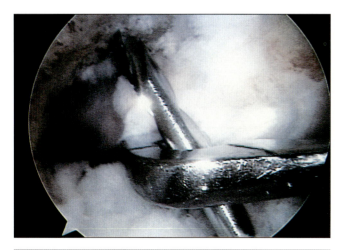

Figure 3-6. Intra-articular photograph of anterior tibial guide being used adjacent to posterior cruciate ligament.

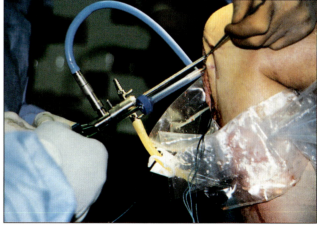

Figure 3-7. Entry of the sheath into the joint.

eight or better in the recovery room, based on activity, respiration, circulation, consciousness, and color (Table 3-2.)

Patients are sent home with prescriptions for hydrocodone, ketorolac tromethamine, and 4 days of oral antibiotics (Keflex 500, one tablet four times a day). The patients are instructed to use the hydrocodone and ketorolac tromethamine in an alternating fashion, which seems to be quite effective. The patients do not receive medications requiring triplicate prescriptions. It is essential to educate the patient about the increasing discomfort that will occur after the intraoperative block has worn off. It is also necessary to advise patients to keep ahead of the pain and avoid reaching the point at which nothing seems to provide relief. None of AAI's ACL patients have been readmitted because of uncontrollable pain.

Immediately after surgery, patients, using crutches, are allowed to put as much weight as they can tolerate on the affected limb. They are encouraged to discontinue the use of crutches as soon as the pain allows. All patients fill out a complete evaluation of the ASC and the entire procedure during their first postoperative visit, which occurs within 3 to 5 days.

A home CPM unit, with detailed instructions for its use, is usually delivered the night before surgery. If pain permits, the patient should start at 0° to 60° on the night of surgery. Patients are encouraged to increase this daily by 3° to 5°. This includes going to a hyperextended position of -3° to -5° to help achieve

Table 3-2	Associated Arthroscopy Institute* Postoperative Discharge Requirements:Score of 8 or Above				

Postanesthesia Recovery Score	In	15	30	45	Out
Activity					
Able to move voluntarily or on command					
4 extremities = 2 pts					
2 extremities = 1 pt					
0 extremities = 0 pts					
Respiration					
Able to breathe deeply and cough freely = 2 pts					
+ Dyspnea shallow or limited breathing = 1 pt					
Apneic = 0 pts					
Circulation					
BP = 20 mm Hg of preanesthesia = 2 pts					
BP = 20–50 mm Hg of preanesthesia = 1 pt					
Preoperative BP - BP = 50 mm Hg of preanesthesia = 0 pts					
Consciousness					
Fully awake = 2 pts					
Rousable on calling = 1 pt					
Not responding = 0 pts					
Color					
Normal = 2 pts					
Pale, dusky, blotchy, jaundiced, other = 1 pt					
Cyanotic = 0 pts					
Total Score					

* Plano, TX.
BP—blood pressure.
Adapted from Aldrete and Kroulik [8].

full extension quickly. After 2 postoperative weeks, most patients have already achieved full range of motion, and the unit is no longer needed. Patients benefit from this device, as it aids them in achieving full range of motion in a shorter time and helps with pain control while they are using it, especially at night.

Cryotherapy is not routinely used at AAI, primarily because of insurance prohibitions. In the small group of patients in whom cryotherapy has been used, the response has been very positive. A recent presentation by Barber *et al.* [9] at the AANA meeting in San Diego reported significant improvement in postoperative pain levels when this adjunctive therapy was used.

The hinged postoperative brace is recommended for 3 to 4 weeks. Rehabilitation is begun on the first postoperative day following an aggressive protocol. Many patients are ready to run during the second postoperative month.

ASSOCIATED ARTHROSCOPY INSTITUTE DATA

The group of 13 patients who have had ACL reconstructions at AAI was composed of 12 men and one woman. Patients ranged from 17 to 38 years old, with the average age of 31.6 years. All patients received general anesthesia. Tourniquet times ranged from 75 minutes to 145 minutes, with an average time of 104 minutes. The patients received, on average, two injections of meperidine and hydroxyzine hydrochloride or meperidine and promethazine hydrochloride. Operating time ranged from 85 minutes to 180 minutes, with an average

time of 148 minutes. Time in the recovery room ranged from 70 minutes to 270 minutes, with an average recovery room time of 125 minutes. The total time in AAI ranged from 250 minutes to 445 minutes, with an average total time of 336 minutes (5.6 hours). All patients receive a postoperative phone call. There were no major complications. There have been no transfers to a hospital immediately postoperatively or any admissions within the first 24 to 48 hours for pain control, infection, or deep venous thrombosis. Patient reviews of the procedure describe the significant pain involved in the first 24 to 48 hours, but overall, they said that the procedure was satisfactory and that they would go through it again on an outpatient basis.

ECONOMIC CONSIDERATIONS

Recent literature (Table 3-3) supports two different ways of increasing the economic efficiency of an ACL reconstruction. The first involves surgical technique, that is, endoscopic single-incision versus the popular two-incision approach. The second consideration is performing ACL reconstructions on an outpatient versus inpatient basis.

In 1988, Jackson and Jennings [10] were the first surgeons to describe a two-incision, arthroscopically assisted ACL reconstruction technique, which was further modified by Karzel and Friedman [11], who published their results in 1990. In the same year, Rosenberg *et al.* [12] described an endoscopic single-incision technique, and now most ACL procedures performed in this country are done arthroscopically,

| Table 3-3 | Cost Comparisons |

Study	Inpatient Hospital, dollars	Outpatient Hospital, dollars	ASC, dollars	In-office ASC	Maximum Savings, %
Nogalski *et al.* [14]	15,000	13,520	—	—	9.86
Malek *et al.* [15] (one incision)	9132	7600	—	—	16.77
Malek *et al.* [15] (two incisions)	12,711	—	—	—	—
Friedman [4]	8900	7700	4640	—	47.87
Zoellner and Richter [17]	6900	4300	—	—	37.68
Kao *et al.* [3••]	9200	3905	—	—	57.55
Novak *et al.* [21]	12,000	8800	3800	—	68.33
AAI	—	8100	5300	4700	41.98
Average	10,549	7704	4580	4700	56.58

AAI—Associated Arthroscopy Institute (Plano, TX); ASC—ambulatory surgical center.

assisted either through the two-incision or one-incision approach. The percentage of two-incision versus one-incision ACL procedures and the percentage of inpatient or outpatient ACL procedures is not easily ascertained. From an economic standpoint, the most advantageous method of performing an ACL reconstruction is an outpatient procedure through a single incision with minimal utilization of single-use items.

In 1994, Sgaglione and Schwartz [13••] compared 45 procedures using a two-incision technique, with 45 procedures done endoscopically. The endoscopic procedures averaged 2.1 fewer hospital days, which had a significant financial impact. They concluded that the lateral thigh incision did increase postoperative pain and, therefore, indirectly increased cost.

The financial implications of single-incision endoscopic procedures are impressive. Nogalski et al. [14] in 1995 reviewed their two-incision versus one-incision technique and found significantly shorter hospital stays and lower charges. The two-incision technique averages 2.8 hospital days versus 1.6 hospital days for the one-incision method. The difference in charges was greater than $2000, with over $15,000 in charges for the two-incision versus $13,520 for the one-incision technique.

In 1996, Malek et al. [15] again confirmed that the two-incision technique was much more expensive than the one-incision technique, with hospital charges of $12,711 and $9132, respectively. These were inpatient procedures. When compared with their outpatient single-incision endoscopic technique, this dropped down to a $7600 procedure. Losee et al. [16] and others performed outpatient ACL surgery on 314 patients. They did not use intramuscular or intravenous narcotic postoperative analgesia. There were no unusual complications, and there was an estimated savings of $5900 per patient.

In 1995, Friedman [4] presented his results on ACL reconstruction costs. He contrasted the cost of performing ACL reconstructions with a 23-hour hospital stay, hospital outpatient procedure, and ASC-based procedure. These charges were $8900, $7700, and $4640, respectively. This yields a 30% savings for hospital outpatient procedures and a 48% savings for ASC procedures. He thought that the key to outpatient success was preoperative education and postoperative instructions that were quite detailed. He also uses CPM for only 1 week, along with cryotherapy. He uses the pain medications hydrocodone and ketorolac tromethamine, and he also uses methocarbamol as a muscle relaxant.

Even with considerations of a one-incision versus a two-incision approach aside, outpatient versus inpatient settings demonstrate large variances in costs. Multiple presentations to AANA have dealt specifically with outpatient cost savings. Zoellner and Richter [17] compared inpatient versus outpatient BPTB reconstructions with respect to nausea, vertigo, itching, pain, and postoperative analgesic use. Overall price differences included inpatient costs of $6900 versus outpatient costs of $4300, a savings of 37%. They performed a total of 700 procedures, 180 inpatient and 520 outpatient. There were four outpatient readmissions (one for nausea, two for pain, and one for acute hypertension). However, there was no significant difference in the incidence of nausea or postoperative analgesic use in outpatient versus inpatient patients. In fact, complications were greater for inpatients, with a higher incidence of vertigo and itching. They concluded that the outpatient procedure was highly successful and efficacious.

In 1996, Scranton et al. [18] presented the outcomes of more than 100 endoscopic quadruple-hamstring ACL procedures, which were low in cost and highly successful as outpatient procedures. They concluded that this was due to a combination of good postoperative pain control and the use of a hamstring graft, which significantly decreased pain because it required a smaller incision and less dissection. They used home CPM, cryotherapy, and an inexpensive hinged-type brace.

In 1995, Kao [3••] followed up with 37 patients with BPTB ACL reconstructions. The outpatient average charge was $3905 versus an inpatient charge of $9200. This is a 58% savings through outpatient services. The visual analog pain differences that were measured showed no significant changes between patients who underwent inpatient and outpatient procedures. They did believe, however, that for successful outpatient procedures, patient appropriateness must be determined prior to surgery through a detailed patient interview. In 1996, Williams et al. [19] compared outpatient pain levels in endoscopic ACL procedures versus arthroscopy for non-ACL procedures. Of course, there were significant pain differences. However, all 28 patients involved tolerated their outpatient ACL procedure. They were satisfied with the process and said they would do it again. There were no admissions, readmissions, or emergency department visits for these patients.

In the same year, Meade et al. [5] presented outcomes for the use of a femoral nerve block for outpatient ACL reconstructions in 206 patients. The femoral nerve block lasts an average of 36 hours, which gives excellent postoperative analgesia for the first 1 to 1.5 postoperative days. Only two of 206 patients required readmission for 23-hour observation for pain problems. There was a reported $6000 saving per patient. Meade predicted that outpatient ACL surgery using the femoral nerve block technique would become the standard of care in the near future. Felger and Pritchard [20] followed up with 48 patients who had had ACL reconstructions. A total of 94% of the patients were pleased with their outcome. There was a cost savings of $3000 per patient.

Novak *et al.* [21] presented the results of 74 endoscopic BPTB ACL reconstructions. Of these, 45 were done on an outpatient basis and 29 on an inpatient basis. The ASC cost was $3800, the outpatient hospital cost was $8800, and the hospital inpatient cost for a 1-day elective stay was $12,000. The day surgery unit resulted in savings over hospital outpatient and inpatient services of 56% and 67%, respectively. Novak *et al* thought that their successful outpatient procedures could be attributed to a strong commitment to preoperative patient education; the use of epidural anesthesia; the use of propofol for general anesthesia, combined with the use of intramuscular ketorolac tromethamine injections; the use of injectable local anesthetics postoperatively, with limited or no use of a tourniquet; and postoperative cryotherapy.

CONCLUSION

As already discussed, many authors are coming to the same conclusion. In an ASA physical status I patient, it is no longer necessary to perform an ACL reconstruction on an inpatient basis. This is consistent with the way patients are treated at AAI. More than 16 ACL reconstructions have been performed at AAI in 1997. With hospital outpatient cost currently at $8100, hospital day surgery unit's at $5300, and AAI's at $4700, this yields a 34% and 41% savings, respectively. Table 3-3 provides a summary of these charges, as well as an average for inpatient hospital ACL reconstruction cost of $10,549, an outpatient hospital setting cost of $7704, an ASC cost of $4580, and AAI's in-office ASC cost of $4700. The overall savings figure comparing these averages is 56.6%. These studies show the importance, from a practical standpoint, of not only outpatient versus inpatient settings but also of a single-incision versus a two-incision technique for outpatient ACL reconstructions. The next major step in physician independence and control should be the development of in-office ASCs. A state-of-the-art, in-office ASC, such as that at AAI, can provide excellent, safe, convenient, comfortable, and cost-effective care for outpatient ACL patients.

REFERENCES AND RECOMMENDED READING

Recently published papers of particular interest have been highlighted as:
•• Of outstanding interest

1. Litwack K: *Core Curriculum for Post Anesthesia Nursing Practice.* Philadelphia: WB Saunders; 1995:624–625.

2. McGuire DA, Sanders K, Hendricks SD: Comparison of ketorolac and opioid analgesics in postoperative ACL reconstruction outpatient pain control. *Arthroscopy* 1993, 9:653–661.

3.•• Kao JT, Giangarra SE, Singer G, Martin S: A comparison of outpatient and inpatient anterior cruciate ligament reconstruction surgery. *Arthroscopy,* 1995, 11:151–156.
Well-done study providing convincing evidence about the advantages of outpatient anterior cruciate ligament surgery.

4. Friedman M: Outpatient ACL reconstruction. Presented at the AANA Fall Course. Palm Desert, CA; December 7–10, 1995.

5. Meade TD, Lee RS, Ferry K, *et al.:* Preoperative femoral nerve block for outpatient ACL reconstruction. Abstract presented at the AANA Annual Meeting. Washington, DC; April 11–14, 1996.

6. Clancy WG: Anatomic endoscopic ACL reconstruction with autogenous patellar tendon graft. *Orthopedics* 1997; 20:397–400.

7.•• Weiler A, Hoffman R, Windhagen H, *et al.:* Biomechanical evaluation of different biodegradable interference screws. Abstract presented at the AANA Annual Meeting. San Diego, CA; April 23–26, 1997:38–40.
Excellent, rigorous report on the pullout strength and failure of different bioabsorbable sutures.

8. Aldrete J, Kroulik D: A post anesthetic recovery score. *Anesth Analg* 1970, 49:924–933.

9. Barber FA, McGuire D, Click S: Continuous flow cold therapy for outpatient ACL reconstruction. Paper presented at AANA Annual Meeting. San Diego, CA; April 23–26, 1997:33–34.

10. Jackson DW, Jennings LD: Arthroscopically-assisted reconstruction of the anterior cruciate ligament using a patellar tendon bone autograft. *Clin Sports Med* 1988, 7:785–800.

11. Karzel RP, Friedman MJ: Arthroscopic diagnosis and treatment of cruciate and collateral ligament injuries. *Arthroscopy of the Knee.* Philadelphia: WB Saunders; 1990:131–154.

12. Rosenberg TD, Paulos LE, Parker RD, *et al.:* Arthroscopic surgery of the knee. In *Operative Orthopaedics.* Edited by Chapman MW. Philadelphia: JB Lippincott; 1988:1585–1604.

13.•• Sgaglione NA, Schwartz RE: Arthroscopically assisted reconstruction of the anterior cruciate ligament: initial clinical experience and minimal 2-year follow-up comparing endoscopic transtibial and two incision techniques. *Arthroscopy* 1997, 13:156–165.
Good controlled study revealing the significant difference between a one-incision technique and a two-incision technique.

14. Nogalski MP, Bach BR, Bush-Joseph CA, Luergans S: Trends in decreased hospitalization for ACL surgery. *Arthroscopy* 1995, 11:134–138.

15. Malek MM, DeLuca JV, Kunkle KL, Knable KR: Outpatient ACL surgery: a review of safety, practicality, and economy. Instructional course lectures. Rosemont, IL: AAOS; 1996, 45:281–286.

16. Losee GM, Troop RL, Robertson DB, Howard ME: Analysis of outpatient ACL surgery: six year results in 314 patients. Presented at 1993 Specialty Day, AOSSM. San Francisco, CA; February 21, 1993.

17. Zoellner T, Richter A: Inpatient versus outpatient anterior cruciate ligament reconstruction: a comparison of 701 cases. *Arthroscopy* 1996, 12:374.

18. Scranton PE, Pinczewski L, Auld K, Khalfayan EE: Outpatient endoscopic quadruple hamstring anterior cruciate ligament reconstruction. *Oper Tech Orthop* 1996, 6:177–180.

19. Williams J, Wexler G, Novak PJ, *et al.*: A prospective study of pain and analgesic use profiles in outpatient endoscopic ACL reconstruction [abstract]. *Arthroscopy* 1996, 12:368.

20. Felger E, Pritchard J: Outpatient ACL Reconstruction. Abstract presented at the AANA Annual Meeting. Washington, DC; April 11–14, 1996.

21. Novak P, Bach B, Bush-Joseph CA, Badrinath S: Cost containment: a charge comparison of anterior cruciate ligament reconstruction. *Arthroscopy* 1996, 12:160–164.

4

CHAPTER

Revision Anterior Cruciate Ligament Surgery

JAMES D. DALTON, JR. AND CHRISTOPHER D. HARNER

The causes of anterior cruciate ligament (ACL) graft failure include inadequate treatment of coexisting pathology, imprecise surgical technique or error, and poorly designed or noncompliant patient rehabilitation. Successful revision ACL reconstruction involves recognition and treatment of any coexisting instabilities or malalignments, precise surgical technique (which may be difficult in revision cases because normal anatomic landmarks may have been changed), and strict adherence to a well-designed revision ACL rehabilitation protocol.

Patients with failed ACL grafts comprise a heterogenous population in terms of anatomic variability, motivation, and surgical expectations. Consequently, no one ideal revision ACL surgical technique exists that is applicable to every patient. Some revision cases are more straightforward, and

others are more complex, but the general principles of ligamentous reconstruction should be adhered to during all revision cases. Because of the different problems that may be encountered during the procedure, the surgeon should have an arsenal of technique options available. This chapter covers some of the options that are useful during revision cases.

PREOPERATIVE CONSIDERATIONS

A failed ACL reconstruction is one in which the patient experiences symptomatic instability with activities of daily living or sports and the reconstructed knee shows laxity on physical examination or instrumented knee testing (KT1000 or KT2000; Medmetric, San Diego, CA) [1•]. In addition to graft failure, poor motion secondary to suboptimal graft placement is also an indication for revision surgery. The candidate should be highly motivated and have realistic goals. The history of the initial injury and operative findings should be determined if possible. A knowledge of the initial surgical technique, including graft and fixation choices, should be obtained. It is also important to determine whether the patient was able to return to a preinjury level of activity after the primary reconstruction. Graft failure may also have occurred because of a reinjury, and this should be discussed with the patient as well.

On examination, standing alignment may provide a clue as to the reason for failure. Because the ACL is a secondary restraint to valgus stress, it may be stretched in a valgus knee with an incompetent medial collateral ligament (MCL) [2]. The gait pattern also provides useful information about the reason of failure or coexisting pathology. Instability patterns, arthrofibrosis, and notch impingement may be reflected by different gait mechanics. Range of motion should be documented and compared with that of the opposite extremity. Typically, motion should be restored before revision surgery. Simultaneous ligamentous surgery with restoration of motion should be undertaken with caution. Both the primary and secondary restraints of anterior tibial translation should be assessed. Ligamentous stability testing should include Lachman's testing, pivot shift testing, posterior drawer testing, varus-valgus testing at 20° and 0°, and testing for rotational instabilities. KT1000 or KT2000 readings may be helpful in some instances. In particular, posterolateral instability has been associated with failure of ACL reconstructions [3]. Increased anteromedial rotatory instability in the setting of a previous meniscectomy may be best treated with a

concomitant medial meniscal transplantation. Although septic arthritis following ACL reconstruction is rare, it should be considered as a possible cause of failure and can usually be ruled out based on the clinical findings [4]. An important component of the examination is the documentation of previous surgical scars and skin problems, which are important when preparing for the revision procedure and may alter the location of incisions or arthroscopic portal sites.

Radiographic evaluation should include a 45° posteroanterior flexion–weight bearing, lateral, and axial patellar views. The 45° posteroanterior flexion–weight bearing view is used to assess early arthritic and degenerative changes [5]. The lateral view gives the most information about tunnel placement (Fig. 4-1). A maximum extension lateral view may be helpful in evaluating the position of the tibial tunnel with regard to the roof of the intercondylar notch. Tunnel size, bone quality, and methods of graft fixation may be determined using plain radiographs. Mechanical alignment can be determined with full-length (hips-to-ankles) views of both lower extremities. Other imaging modalities that may be helpful in selective cases include magnetic resonance imaging (MRI), computed tomography (CT), and bone scintigraphy.

STAGING OF REVISION SURGERY

The clinician should consider staging the revision reconstruction in the presence of loss of motion or significant expansion of the tibial or femoral tunnels. Preoperative motion loss is a poor prognostic indicator for postoperative motion. Alternatives to revision in some situations include manipulation under anesthesia,

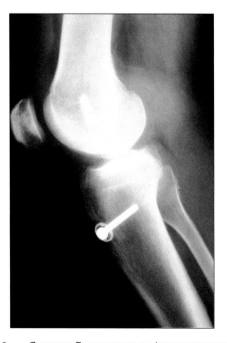

Figure 4-1. A lateral radiograph gives the most information about tunnel placement. Here, the femoral interference screw and tunnel are too anterior.

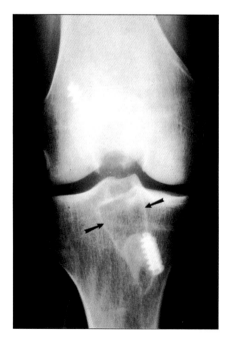

Figure 4-2. Osteolysis of the bone tunnels (*arrows*) can be seen with any type of graft. It usually occurs on the tibial side, but can be seen on the femoral side as well. Staging the revision surgery in severe cases of osteolysis is the treatment of choice. The tunnels are bone grafted during the first stage, and the anterior cruciate ligament is reconstructed during the second stage.

arthroscopic debridement, performance of a notch-plasty or enlargement of an existing one, and the use of an extension drop-out cast postoperatively. If osteolysis of the bone tunnels has occurred, the ACL graft can be debrided and the tunnels bone grafted during a first-stage procedure (Fig. 4-2). After incorporation of the bone graft, revision ACL reconstruction can be performed. An alternative to this technique can be applied if the tunnels are only minimally expanded and are in an acceptable location. In this situation, the tunnels can be slightly overreamed, and a large bone plug can be used to fill the larger tunnel. The graft must be rotated correctly so that its ligamentous attachment side is in the most anatomic location possible.

TECHNICAL CONSIDERATIONS

Skin Incisions

Preoperative consideration should be given to the placement of skin incisions relative to preexisting surgical incisions. Previous skin incisions should be used when possible to avoid devascularizing skin by disrupting its blood supply from two sites. Use of small incisions and arthroscopic portal sites are less likely to cause this problem. Use of allograft material for the revision graft allows for smaller incisions and should be strongly considered. Incisions should be made for hardware removal only if the hardware is loose, painful, or obstructing a portion of the procedure.

Hardware Removal

In general, all hardware does not necessarily need to be removed. Large bony defects may be created during its removal, which may lead to compromised graft fixation in tunnels, stress risers, and slower rehabilitation. Hardware can intentionally be avoided in some situations on the femoral side by altering the direction of the femoral tunnel or by using a form of fixation other than that which was previously used. Femoral tunnels placed arthroscopically are oriented more vertically, and femoral tunnels placed using a rear-entry guide are oriented more horizontally. Therefore, it may be advantageous to use the rear-entry method if the patient has an embedded femoral screw in an arthroscopically placed tunnel from previous surgery. If the patient already has a bicortical screw, interference screw, or staple on the anterolateral aspect of the femur, then an arthroscopically placed tunnel with an interference screw may be the best option during the revision procedure (Fig. 4-3).

If the location of the existing hardware is problematic or if the patient has pain attributed to the hardware, it should be removed. Loose hardware should likewise be removed because of its potential to migrate interarticularly and thereby cause symptoms. Arrangements should be made during preoperative planning to have all necessary equipment, including screwdrivers in appropriate sizes, staple extractors, and osteotomes, available to remove the hardware. All soft tissue should be cleared from the hardware to ensure complete seating of the extraction device or screwdriver and to be sure of the fit. Stripping the head of a screw can lead to bony defects during removal attempts. Commercially available "easy-out" devices may be useful in removing damaged screws.

Revising Prosthetic Ligaments

Because of the good results obtainable with autograft and allograft material, synthetic ligaments and augmentation devices are not commonly used and are only rarely encountered. Several points should be made about the revision of synthetic material. First, tunnel osteolysis may be present with Gore-Tex grafts (WL Gore & Associates, Inc, Flagstaff, AZ). Preoperative CT or MRI axial images of the knee may help determine if bone grafting of the enlarged tunnels is necessary [6]. Second, arthroscopic shavers are not sufficiently forceful to remove synthetic material. Therefore, prosthetic ligaments are best removed by freeing their tibial and femoral attachments and

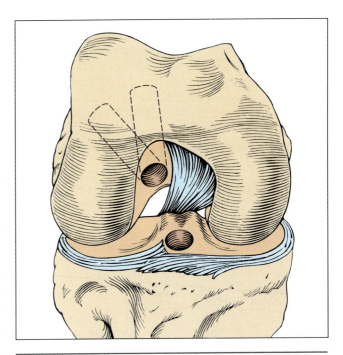

Figure 4-3. The direction of the femoral tunnel differs depending on the method of drilling. The two-incision technique creates a more horizontal tunnel, and the endoscopic technique creates a more vertical tunnel. Knowledge of both techniques is useful in order to avoid hardware placed during the primary reconstruction. (*Adapted from* Bach [15].)

totally removing them. Ligament augmentation devices, if appropriately placed, are anchored at only one end. Finally, the inner surfaces of the bone tunnels should be prepared by curetting or reaming to remove any remaining synthetic material or fibrous coating.

Notchplasty

Although not always required, arthroscopic notchplasties are useful in most revision settings for two reasons. The first is to prevent notch impingement. A revision notchplasty is necessary in cases in which graft failure occurred because of regrowth or overgrowth of a previous notchplasty. An anteriorly placed tibial tunnel can cause the graft to impinge on the roof of the notch; more clearance can be achieved with a larger notchplasty. Adequate notchplasty also allows for improved visualization of the femoral tunnel site. Complete visualization of the over-the-top position with confirmatory palpation using an arthroscopic probe is required before drilling of the femoral tunnel.

Notchplasties may be performed with arthroscopic shavers, burrs, or osteotomes, depending on the amount of bone and cartilage to be removed (Fig. 4-4). Arthroscopic burrs may leave whiskers of cartilage at the site of debridement, which may impede visualization. These whiskers can be removed easily by reversing the direction of rotation of the burr and lightly shaving the area again. Larger notchplasties can be performed more efficiently using arthroscopic osteotomes. Adequacy of the notchplasty can be assessed arthroscopically by inserting a commercially available bone tunnel expander (Instrument Makar,

Inc, Okemos, MI) through the tibial tunnel and into the joint. The knee is then brought into extension while the tunnel expander and the notch are visualized. Extension equal to that of the opposite extremity should be achieved at the point at which the tunnel expander touches the notch roof.

Tunnel Placement

The single most important aspect of primary or revision ACL reconstruction is correct placement of the tunnels. Appropriate radiographic studies should be obtained to help visualize the course of the previous tunnels. A maximum extension lateral, CT, or MRI scan may be required. The goal is anatomic placement of the tunnels within good quality bone at the proper ACL insertion sites on the tibia and femur. The tibial tunnel should be centered at an approximately equal distance between the condylar walls in the notch and in the posterior half of the native tibial footprint. The ACL graft should have some contact with the posterior cruciate ligament (PCL) once it has been placed. The femoral tunnel should be just anterior to the over-the-top position at between the 10 o'clock and 11 o'clock positions in the notch for a right knee and between the 1 o'clock and 2 o'clock positions for a left knee. Correct tunnel placement is complicated somewhat by anatomic landmarks that are distorted by bony deficiencies and previous surgery. An intraoperative lateral radiograph with a guide pin, drill, or bone tunnel expander used as a tunnel marker can verify correct positioning of the tunnel (Fig. 4-5).

Revision of femoral bone tunnels usually involves tunnels that are either anatomic, slightly anterior, far

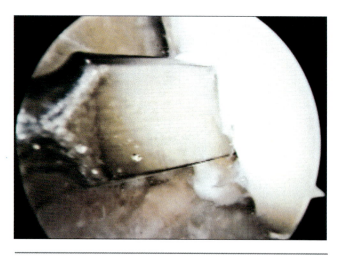

Figure 4-4. Notchplasties are usually required in revision settings to improve visualization of the "over-the-top" position and to prevent notch impingement during knee extension. Notchplasties may be performed with osteotomes, rasps, or motorized arthroscopic instruments.

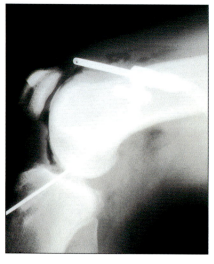

Figure 4-5. An intraoperative lateral radiograph with a guide pin or tunnel expander in place will verify correct tunnel placement.

anterior, or so posterior that the posterior cortex has broken through. Femoral tunnel expansion is less common than is tibial tunnel expansion, but it may still be encountered in ACL revision surgery (Fig. 4-6). Anatomically placed tunnels and tunnels with well-incorporated bone plugs or grafts can simply be redrilled, assuming that the fixation hardware can be removed or is not in the way.

Tunnels placed slightly anterior may be expanded to leave a 1 to 2 mm rim of bone posteriorly, then filled with an appropriately sized bone plug graft end (Fig. 4-7). If this is done using the endoscopic method, as opposed to the rear-entry two-incision technique, the tibial tunnel must also be enlarged to accommodate passage of the drills and graft. This may not be desirable in all cases. An alternate method is to place a guide pin in the desired location, drill a pilot hole with a 6-mm reamer, and then sequentially dilate the hole with tunnel expanders. In cases in which large bone defects exist, it is more appropriate to use a staged procedure first consisting of autogenous bone grafting followed in 10 to 16 weeks by revision ACL reconstruction.

Far-anterior tunnels can usually be avoided altogether. The most common site of the far-anterior tunnel is the so-called "resident's ridge," which is located on the lateral wall of the intercondylar notch. Because this site is significantly anterior to the over-the-top position, it does not represent an obstruction to correct tunnel placement. Interference screws placed in this position can also often be left in place (Fig. 4-8).

Placement of the femoral tunnel too posteriorly may result in posterior cortical blowout. This represents a problem only in that it may change the type of fixation used on the femoral side. If this situation occurs during either a primary or revision procedure, the graft should be positioned in the groove created by the reamer (the over-the-top position) and then fixed to the lateral cortex (Fig. 4-9). Many methods of fixation for over-the-top grafts exist: heavy, nonabsorbable sutures can be tied around a bicortical screw and washer; staples can be used to fix the soft tissue end of Achilles tendon allograft; and Endobuttons (Acufex Microsurgical, Andover, MA) and soft tissue washers may be used in some situations.

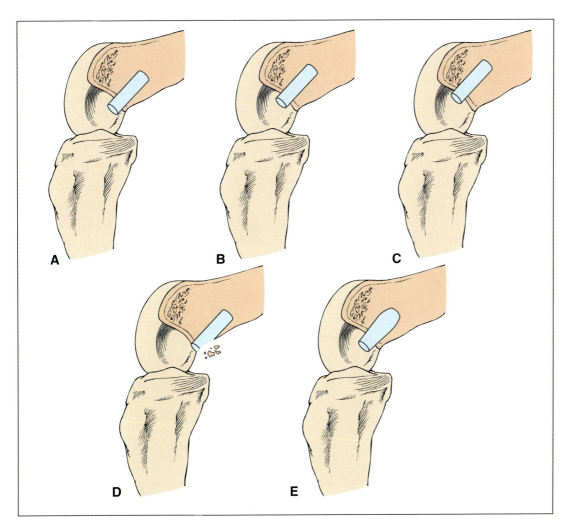

Figure 4-6. Variations in femoral tunnel placement. **A,** Ideal femoral tunnel placement with 2 mm of posterior cortical rim remaining. **B,** Slightly anterior femoral tunnel placement. **C,** Far-anterior femoral tunnel placement. **D,** Posterior cortical blowout. **E,** Tunnel expansion. (*Adapted from* Rosenberg and Graf [16]; with permission.)

Tunnel expansion can be seen with nearly every type of graft and is thought to be partially due to a windshield-wiper effect of the graft within the tunnel. Because of the amount of tunnel widening that can be seen, bone grafting is usually necessary before anatomic tunnels can be drilled. One alternative for very mild cases of tunnel expansion is to fix the femoral bone plug with two interference screws, each placed at different points around the bone plug. The biomechanical properties of this form of fixation have not been tested.

Management of the tibial tunnels is similar to that of the femoral tunnels. Tibial tunnels can be redrilled as long as large bone defects do not exist. In situations involving bone defects or tunnel expansion, the bone loss must be corrected first. Tricortical or cancellous iliac crest bone grafting can be performed if a staged procedure is necessary. Revision ACL reconstruction can be performed after both full motion is established and radiographic evidence of bone graft incorporation is present.

Graft Selection

The graft choices that are available for ACL revision cases include autograft, allograft, and synthetic graft material. Each has its own advantages and disadvantages. Autologous bone incorporates more rapidly than allograft bone without the added risk of viral disease transmission. The authors' graft preference, when available, is autologous bone–patellar tendon–bone (BPTB). In some revision settings, it is advantageous to have bone plugs on each end as opposed to soft tissue grafts, such as hamstrings or iliotibial band. However, the authors do not harvest the patellar tendon if it has been harvested previously or if there is a history of anterior knee pain. Likewise, it is not harvested from the opposite extremity because doing so may create pain in an otherwise asymptomatic knee [7].

If bone blocks are not required, autologous gracilis and semitendinosus tendons may be used. In primary reconstructions, the results of gracilis and semitendi-

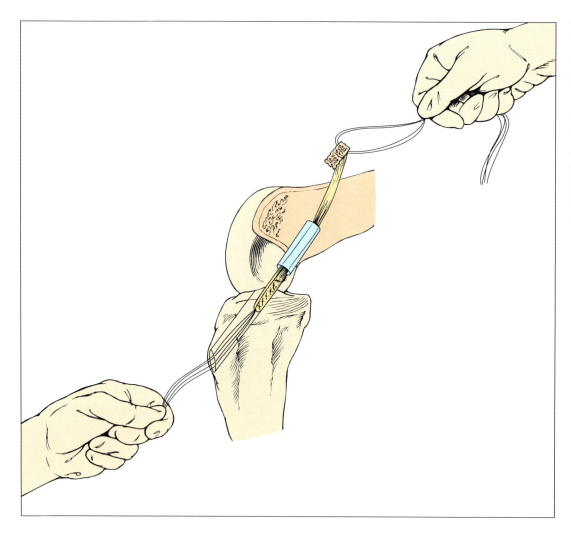

Figure 4-7. Slightly anterior femoral tunnels can be enlarged and then filled with a large bone plug. Achilles tendon allografts come with a large piece of calcaneal bone that can be trimmed to nearly any size, making them ideal for filling large bony defects.

nosus grafts are comparable with BPTB grafts. Theoretically, the initial strength of a doubled gracilis–semitendinosus graft has approximately 240% of the strength of a normal ACL [8,9•]. However, its initial fixation is not thought to be as secure as that of an interference screw with bone blocks. Ipsilateral quadriceps tendon is another possibility, but this graft is stiffer than is normal ACL tissue, and the size of the bone block is limited.

Allograft tissue has the benefits of no donor site morbidity, allowing for smaller incisions and decreased operative time. Especially useful in the revision setting are Achilles tendon and BPTB allografts. Achilles tendon allografts come with a large calcaneal bone plug that can be contoured to fill bony defects in a tunnel. The graft itself has a large cross-sectional area for added strength. BPTB allografts typically come with a complete patella on one end and a large bone block from the tibial tuberosity on the other end. They are ideal if autograft cannot be used, or if large bone plugs are needed (Fig. 4-10). Maday *et al.* [10] retrospectively reviewed 35 patients following revision ACL reconstruction with BPTB allografts. Of these, 92% had no limitations with activities of daily living, but only 57% returned to their preprimary ACL reconstruction level of activities. This is comparable with the results in other revision ACL series [11–13].

Synthetic ligaments are mentioned only for the sake of completeness. They have limited use in both primary and revision cases and have demonstrated relatively poor long-term results. With the availability and documented records of autograft and allograft, synthetic ligaments are rarely, if ever, indicated.

Ideally, it is advantageous to have a graft of first choice and a backup graft in case the unexpected occurs. The revision graft used depends on the patient, the etiology of failure, previous graft material utilized, and the surgeon's experience and comfort level with a particular type of graft.

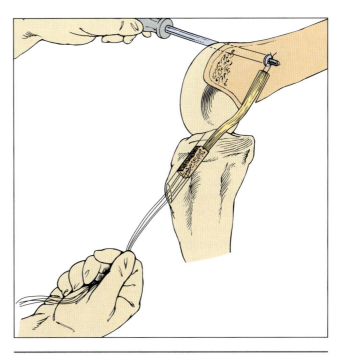

Figure 4-9. Graft placement in the presence of posterior cortical blowout is achieved by placing the graft in the "over the top" position. Graft fixation can be achieved with staples, a screw, and soft tissue washer, or by tying sutures over a bicortical screw, as shown here.

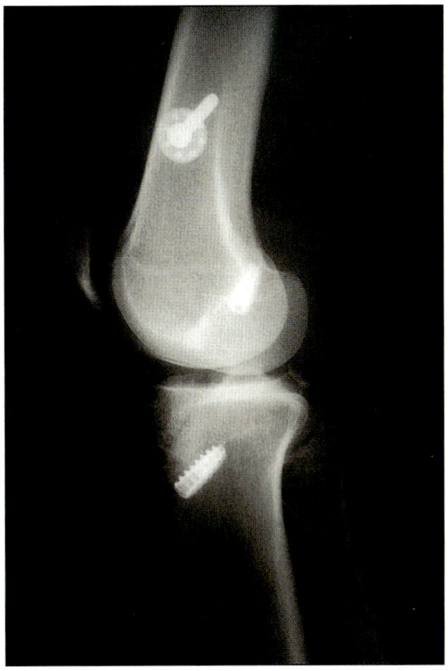

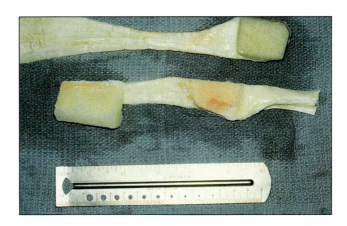

Figure 4-10. The most useful allograft materials in revision anterior cruciate ligament surgery are the Achilles tendon (*top*) and the bone–patellar tendon–bone (BPTB; *bottom*). The Achilles tendon is long and has a large piece of calcaneous attached to its bony end. The BPTB has two bony ends and is a shorter graft. The presence of bony defects, the type of graft fixation, the quality of bone, and patient and surgeon preference all play a role in graft selection.

Figure 4-8. Interference screws, if not readily found or easily removed during arthroscopic examination, may be left in place and an alternate form of fixation used. In this case, a very active gymnast ruptured his initial patellar tendon graft. A revision anterior cruciate ligament reconstruction was carried out using an Achilles tendon allograft in the "over-the-top" position. The new graft was fixed with an interference screw on the tibial side and a screw with a soft tissue, spiked washer on the femoral side.

Graft Fixation

When possible, interference screw fixation should be used because of its superior pullout strength [14]. However, because of the type of graft used, the size or condition of the tunnel and poor bone quality that is sometimes encountered in revision surgery, interference screws cannot always be used. Alternatives include tying heavy (#5) nonabsorbable sutures around a bicortical screw and washer, using a soft tissue washer (spiked washer), using an Endobutton, using a transverse intraosseous screw (SemiFix; Arthrex, Naples, FL), and using staples (single, double, or "belt-buckle"). Of all the choices listed, the weakest is thought to be the single staple, but it is not known whether this weakness is clinically relevant.

Secondary Restraints

An often-overlooked cause of ACL reconstruction failure is an injured secondary restraint to the ACL. Failure to correct the secondary restraints at the time of revision surgery leads to failure of the revision reconstruction. An arthroscopic ACL revision may need to be coupled with an open procedure. Laxity in the MCL or posterior oblique ligament (POL) may necessitate a medial reefing or MCL reconstruction. Posterolateral rotatory instability may be treated with a reconstructive procedure. Anteromedial rotatory instability in a patient with a history of a medial meniscectomy can be corrected with a medial meniscal transplantation. Malalignments should be corrected with an osteotomy, as either a single or staged procedure.

POSTOPERATIVE REHABILITATION

Rehabilitation protocols in patients with revision ACL reconstructions should be individualized based on the extent of the surgery, the goals of the patient, and the quality of tissue encountered at the time of surgery. The new graft should be protected from acute bending angles, weak fixation, inconsistent tension through healing, weak secondary restraints, and longer recovery times [1•]. The authors' current belief is to consider a revision reconstruction as a salvage operation and, therefore, use a less aggressive rehabilitation approach.

CONCLUSION

Many causes of ACL graft failure exist. Careful preoperative evaluation of the patient, involving a history, physical examination, radiographs, and supporting imaging studies, is essential to determine the cause of failure. Special attention should be made to the secondary restraints of the ACL during the physical examination. Examination with the patient under anesthesia at the time of surgery should be performed. The patient should be counseled preoperatively regarding the expected outcomes of the surgery in terms of pain, restoration of stability, and activity level.

A thorough preoperative plan should be formulated before each revision procedure. Numerous technical considerations should be addressed, including graft selection, fixation methods (with alternates), placement of incisions, hardware removal, ligament removal, notchplasty, tunnel placement, bone defects, and repair of the secondary restraints. An individualized rehabilitation program should be constructed after the procedure, keeping in mind the quality of the native bone, secondary restraints, and fixation methods used. With proper preoperative planning, patient counseling, technical execution, and rehabilitation, a successful outcome of revision ACL surgery can be achieved.

REFERENCES AND RECOMMENDED READING

Recently published papers of particular interest have been highlighted as:
• Of interest

1.• Safran MR, Harner CD: Technical considerations of revision anterior cruciate ligament surgery. *Clin Orthop* 1996, 325: 50–64.
Good overview of the technical aspects of revision ligamentous surgery, including patient selection and operative techniques.

2. Haimes JL, Wroble RR, Grood ES, Noyes FR: Role of the medial structures in the intact and ACL-deficient knee—limits of motion in the human knee. *Am J Sports Med* 1994, 22:402–409.

3. O'Brien S, Warren RF, Pavlov H, *et al.*: Reconstruction of the chronically insufficient anterior cruciate ligament with the central third of the patellar tendon. *J Bone Joint Surg* 1991, 73:278–286.

4. Williams RJ, Laurencin CT, Warren RF, *et al.*: Septic arthritis after arthroscopic anterior cruciate ligament reconstruction: diagnosis and management. *Am J Sports Med* 1997, 25:261–267.

5. Rosenberg TD, Paulos LE, Parker RD, *et al.*: The forty-five degree posteroanterior flexion weight-bearing radiograph of the knee. *J Bone Joint Surg* 1988, 70(suppl A):1479–1483.

6. Seemann MD, Steadman JR: Tibial osteolysis associated with Gore-tex grafts. *Am J Knee Surg* 1993, 6:31–38.

7. Rubinstein RA, Shelbourne KD, VanMeter CD, *et al.*: Isolated autogenous bone-patellar tendon-bone graft site morbidity. *Am J Sports Med* 1994, 22:324–327.

8. Noyes FR, Butler DL, Grood ES, *et al.*: Biomechanical analysis of human ligament grafts used in knee ligament repairs and reconstructions. *J Bone Joint Surg* 1984, 66(suppl A):344–352.

9.• Ritchie JR, Parker RD: Graft selection in anterior cruciate ligament revision surgery. *Clin Orthop* 1996, 325:65–77.

Excellent discussion of grafts that are currently available for knee ligamentous reconstructions. The authors of this paper cover the basic science, biomechanics, and clinical results of autografts, allografts, and synthetic grafts. The pros and cons for each are discussed.

10. Maday MG, Harner CD, Fu FH: Revision anterior cruciate ligament surgery: evaluation and treatment. In *The Crucial Ligaments*, edn 2. Edited by Feagin JA. New York: Churchill Livingstone; 1994:711–723.

11. Uribe JW, Hechtman KS, Zvijac JE, Tjin-A-Tsoi EW: Revision anterior cruciate ligament surgery: experience from Miami. *Clin Orthop* 1996, 325:91–99.

12. Wirth CJ, Kohn D: Revision anterior cruciate ligament surgery: experience from Germany. *Clin Orthop* 1996, 325:110–115.

13. Noyes FR, Barber-Westin SD: Revision anterior cruciate ligament surgery: experience from Cincinnati. *Clin Orthop* 1996, 325:116–129.

14. Kurosaka M, Yoshiya S, Andrish JT: A biomechanical comparison of different surgical techniques of graft fixation in anterior cruciate ligament reconstruction. *Am J Sports Med* 1987, 15:225–229.

15. Bach BR Jr: Arthroscopy-assisted patellar tendon substitution for anterior cruciate ligament insufficiency: surgical technique. *Am J Knee Surg* 1989, 12:199–203.

16. Rosenberg TD, Graf B: *Endoscopic Technique for ACL Reconstruction with Pro-Trac Tibial Guide: EndoButton Fixation.* Mansfield, MA: Acufex Microsurgical, Inc; 1991.

5

Anterior Cruciate Ligament Reconstruction in the Skeletally Immature Patient

ROGER V. LARSON AND MICHAEL H. METCALF

Complete tears of the anterior cruciate ligament (ACL) in children and adolescents were once thought to be quite rare. As recently as 1983, accepted dogma regarding ACL tears in children was that "complete ligamentous disruption occurs only after growth plate closure" [1]. This concept came from the observations of injury to the physis or long bones before ligament damage had occurred [2,3]. Several biomechanical studies have shown that the ligaments are generally stronger than is the growth plate [4,5]. In addition, Clanton et al. [3] postulated that the anatomic location of the insertion of knee ligaments in relation to the physis leads to the preferential injury to the physis.

More recently, it has been recognized that ligamentous injury can occur in the pediatric population; in fact, Cook and Leit [6] have shown that the knee is the most frequently injured site in the child athlete. Avulsion injuries from the tibial spine [3,7,8], the femoral insertion [9,10], or both tibial and femoral insertions [11] have been reported. More recently, there have been multiple reports of complete ACL tears in skeletally immature children [3,9,12–14], the youngest in a 3-year-old child [15].

As children have become more active in more dangerous sporting activities, injuries to the ACL are becoming an increasingly common clinical presentation. DeLee [16] has identified three factors that have led to increased interest in children's knee injuries: 1) a greater number of children participating in organized sports, 2) increased recognition of pediatric knee injuries by the medical community, and 3) improved methods for diagnosing ligamentous disruptions among all age groups.

Ideally, operative treatment of ACL injuries in children are postponed until physeal closure. In certain instances, however, this is not practical. Controlling the activities of children is difficult, given the immaturity of the athlete and the increasing pressure to excel at younger ages. Nationally, programs have been created to identify and support athletes with special talent. Reward for success at the professional level has pushed the age of entry into the specialized programs younger and younger. An injured athlete may miss his or her "window of opportunity" if unable to compete.

TREATMENT OPTIONS

The goal of treatment in a child with ACL insufficiency is the same as that for the adult: "You must prevent recurrent 'giving-way' episodes" [17]. Repeated "giving-way" bouts in patients with ACL insufficiency lead to meniscal tears, osteochondral damage, and premature degenerative arthritis. If repeated injuries can be prevented by non-operative means, it is desirable in any age group, but particularly in the pediatric group. The most important factor, however, in preventing repeat injuries is activity modification, particularly avoidance of high-level athletic activities that require jumping, pivoting, contact, or participation on unpredictable surfaces.

Several studies have shown a high incidence of secondary meniscal injuries, degenerative joint disease, and symptomatic instability in both sports and daily activities in conservatively treated skeletally immature patients [13,18–20]. Skeletally immature patients are, in fact, much less likely to limit their activities and adapt to ACL insufficiency than are skeletally mature counterparts. Because of this, many skeletally immature patients must be considered surgical candidates, because risk of injury from operative intervention may be much lower than the potential damage caused by repeat injury.

Several operative options have been described in the literature. Primary repair of interstitial tears of the ACL in children has been shown to be minimally successful [21,22]. As in adults, primary repair of interstitial tears alone has a high failure rate and should not be considered adequate or appropriate treatment for this injury. Primary repair with appropriate augmentation, however, may offer some advantages in this age group over those of reconstruction alone.

Primary repair of avulsion injuries has been shown to be more successful [23]. This is particularly true if a bony avulsion, which can be anatomically restored, is present. It must be cautioned, however, that pure avulsion injuries are uncommon; frequently, avulsion injuries exist in conjunction with interstitial ACL tears. Arthroscopic inspection is usually necessary to determine whether a bony avulsion is truly an isolated avulsion or whether it has occurred in conjunction with an interstitial tear.

Partial tears of the ACL in skeletally immature patients have been documented. Studies have shown that partial tears of the ACL can result in a satisfactory result when treated non-operatively [13,24]. The important factor in whether or not a good result can be anticipated with a partial tear is the presence of pathologic laxity. If a partial tear stabilizes with laxity that is less than required for the pivot-shift phenomenon, then a satisfactory result can be anticipated in some patients.

Extra-articular reconstructions have been suggested as a means of providing stability in this age group without compromising the physis. Although these procedures avoid drilling through the physis, the nonisometric position of the graft leads to increased intragraft strain and instability over time [14,19]. It is also believed that extra-articular procedures that require dissection and fixation devices near the physis may run a greater risk of interfering with growth than will careful drilling of a central transphyseal hole. Except for primary repair of torn secondary restraints, extra-articular procedures in the skeletally immature patient are generally not recommended [25].

Intra-articular reconstruction without transphyseal drill holes has been described [26,27]. These procedures generally use a groove over the front of the tibia and a groove over the top of the femur, or an "over-the-top" position on the femur, thus avoiding transphyseal drill holes. Results of these procedures have been mixed. As in extra-articular reconstructions, this type of procedure does not allow for isometric graft placement. The effect of hardware used for graft fixation near the growth plate is unclear. The anterior position of the graft on the tibia has resulted in graft impingement and persistent abnormal magnetic resonance imaging (MRI) signals within the graft tissue [27].

The most commonly accepted method for intra-articular ACL reconstruction in the skeletally immature patient uses a transphyseal tibial drill hole and an over-the-top position on the femur, as noted in Figure 5-1 [12]. It is thought that the relatively central tibial drill hole will not cause angular deformity if disturbance in growth occurs. Avoidance of a laterally extending femoral drill hole lessens the possibility of asymmetric growth arrest on the distal femur. Dissection on the distal lateral thigh, however, and use of fixation devices near the lateral femoral physis, may create some risk for growth disturbance [28].

Several studies of ACL reconstruction in skeletally immature patients using both tibial and femoral drill holes have been reported [14,19]. The reported results are generally acceptable; however, most studies are reported on patients who are very near skeletal maturity. A recent study by Matava and Siegel [29••], however, has shown subsequent symmetric growth from both the tibial and femoral physes after the creation of transphyseal drill holes.

All reported studies on ACL reconstruction in skeletally immature patients are complicated by the wide age range of patients. Most studies deal with patients who are postpubertal and near skeletal maturity. This is clearly different than a prepubescent patient. A review of available literature, however, is sufficient to allow formulation of specific important questions related to surgery in this age group, as well as data for formulating treatment guidelines (Table 5-1). The important considerations for this age group include: 1) appropriate injury classification, 2) determination of skeletal age, 3) patholaxity, 4) the effect of transphy-seal drill holes on subsequent growth, 5) special considerations in graft selection in the skeletally immature, and 6) special psychosocial issues. A discussion of each of these categories follows.

SPECIAL CONSIDERATIONS FOR ANTERIOR CRUCIATE RECONSTRUCTION WITH OPEN GROWTH PLATES

Appropriate Injury Classification

The type of ACL injury is important in formulating a treatment plan and predicting outcome. Injuries can be classified as 1) bony avulsions, 2) interstitial tears, or 3) bony avulsions with associated interstitial tears. It is generally agreed that bony avulsions have a better prognosis than do interstitial tears. Determination of injury type may require arthroscopic inspection. With true isolated bony avulsions, a good result can be expected with anatomic replacement of the avulsed fragment.

Determination of Skeletal Age

Determination of biologic skeletal age is necessary when comparing treatment methods and when

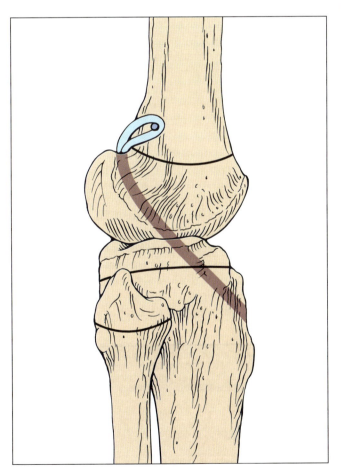

Figure 5-1. The most commonly recommended procedure for anterior cruciate ligament reconstruction in the skeletally immature patient is to use a tibial drill hole and an over-the-top position on the femur, as depicted.

Table 5-1	General Recommendations for Anterior Cruciate Ligament Reconstruction in the Skeletally Immature Patient

Bony avulsions of the ACL should be anatomically restored.

Partial tears of the ACL in this age group should normally be treated non-operatively unless significant patholaxity is present (positive pivot shift).

With the exception of the primary repair of torn secondary restraints, extra-articular reconstruction should be avoided in this age group.

Postpubertal patients who are nearly full grown and nearing skeletal maturity should be treated as adults.

Centrally placed transphyseal drill holes of the smallest possible diameter have minimal chance of interfering with future growth.

Excessive dissection near a physis or placement of fixation devices near a physis should be avoided.

Only soft-tissue grafts should be utilized in prepubescent patients. Bone blocks or fixation devices across the physis must be avoided.

A careful plan must be in place to monitor the subsequent growth of patients in this age group. In case physeal closure occurs, an intervention plan must be in place.

ACL—anterior cruciate ligament.

devising a treatment plan. The Tanner Staging of biologic age is an appropriate way to classify skeletally immature patients [30]. The Tanner classification is shown in Table 5-2. Simplification of this system would combine groups I and II into a prepubescent category and groups III and IV into a second, pubescent, category. Those in the pubescent group have developed secondary sexual characteristics and are near full growth. Patients in this group can be generally treated as adults and make up the majority of cases of most published studies. Prepubescent patients (groups I and II) constitute the group of greatest concern, because they have considerable growth remaining. Most recommendations of this chapter pertain to the treatment of prepubescent patients.

Patholaxity

Determination of the level of laxity following ACL injury in children is important in treatment decisions. Children, in general, have greater normal laxity than do adults, and a comparison with the opposite knee is vital. Absolute laxity is also important because functional disability is closely related to absolute laxity (Table 5-3). The pivot-shift phenomenon usually occurs with anterior laxity of 11 to 12 mm. Laxity less than this amount (negative pivot shift) should generally be treated nonoperatively, particularly in the prepubescent population. If anterior laxity becomes greater than 15 mm (grade IV), not only are sporting activities dangerous, but everyday activities may become impaired, making surgical intervention more necessary.

Effect of Transphyseal Drill Holes

A review of published literature reveals incomplete knowledge of the effect of drill holes on the physis. Most data on physeal closures have been extrapolated from traumatic injuries [31]. It is thought that a carefully placed drill hole is far less traumatic to the growth plate than are injuries that are included in most growth-arrest studies. Due care, however,

should be taken to minimize the trauma to the physis when creating drill holes. Several general principles regarding surgery near the physis can be made:

1. Drill holes should be as small as possible.
2. Centrally placed tunnels, if growth is affected, are less likely to cause an angular deformity than is a peripherally placed tunnel.
3. Soft-tissue grafts only should traverse the physis. Bone blocks or fixation devices that traverse the physis are much more likely to cause growth arrest.
4. Extra-articular procedures that require extensive dissection or fixation devices near the physis may potentially be more damaging than carefully placed tunnels.

Graft Selection

Soft-tissue grafts only should be considered when transphyseal drill holes are used for ACL reconstruction. Bone blocks traversing the physis have considerable risk for physeal closure at that location. Harvesting an autogenous bone–patellar tendon–bone graft also creates the risk of damaging the tibial tubercle apophysis. Use of allograft or synthetics in this age group is not widely indicated. The ideal graft for traversing the physis is one of autogenous hamstring tendons.

Psychosocial Issues

Because the potential, however small, exists for growth interference following ACL reconstruction through an open physis, understandable anxiety remains on the part of patients and parents alike. A plan must be in place to observe subsequent growth and to intervene with conventional means should growth disturbance occur. Rehabilitation also often needs to be modified to make it more fun, which increases patient cooperation and participation. Should stiffness (arthrofibrosis) develop within patients in this age group, arthroscopy and release of adhesions are preferable to manipulation

Table 5-2	Tanner Staging of Biologic Age	
Group	Tanner Stage	Age
Prepubescent	I	< 10
	II	10–13
Pubescent	III	12–14
	IV	> 14

Table 5-3	Patholaxity: Absolute Anterior Laxity
Status	Amount of laxity, mm
Normal laxity	3–7
Increase with anterior cruciate ligament tear	3–10
Pivot shift	11–12
Grade IV instability	15–17

alone because less than gentle manipulation may potentially endanger the physis.

PREFERRED TECHNIQUE FOR ANTERIOR CRUCIATE LIGAMENT RECONSTRUCTION IN THE SKELETALLY IMMATURE PATIENT

The authors' preferred technique in the skeletally immature patient is transphyseal ACL reconstruction with hamstring tendons and Endobutton (Acufex Microsurgical, Mansfield, MA) femoral fixation.

Rationale

The goal of ACL reconstruction in the skeletally immature patient is to restore normal anterior laxity of the knee joint with the lowest amount of risk to subsequent growth. The preferred technique is the use of both tibial and femoral centrally placed drill holes, hamstring tendon autografts, fixation distant from the physis, and avoidance of dissection near the physis. Use of small centrally placed tunnels and soft-tissue grafts minimizes the risk of physeal closure. Should closure occur, the centrally placed tunnels will not likely produce angular deformity. By avoiding dissection near either the tibial or femoral physis, interruption of blood supply is minimized. Keeping fixation devices distant from the physis avoids the chance of inadvertent influence. Use of an Endobutton avoids use of fixation devices, such as interference fit screws, that may traverse the physis.

Set-up

A tourniquet is normally used during this procedure and should be placed proximally on the thigh to allow exposure of considerable areas of the anterior thigh. A low-profile thigh holder can be used over the tourniquet.

Incision

Three incisions are necessary for the procedure. Anterolateral and anteromedial arthroscopy portals are created directly adjacent to the patellar tendon to facilitate access to the intercondylar notch. An incision, approximately 1 in long, is made vertically overlying the pes anserinus at the level of insertion of the semitendinosus and gracilis tendons (Fig. 5-2).

Diagnostic Arthroscopy

Before graft harvest, it is advisable to perform diagnostic arthroscopy to evaluate the status of the ACL stump and to treat associated pathology. If a tibial stump is intact, consideration may be made for primary repair with semitendinosus augmentation. Generally, the ACL stump will require debridement. It is preferable in this age group to avoid greater notch debridement than necessary to identify tibial and femoral ACL attachment sites. Notchplasty is generally not performed.

Graft Harvest

The semitendinosus and gracilis tendons are next isolated at their insertion points into the tibia. They are released, then separated; each is harvested with a tendon stripper, and care is taken to first section extraneous bands that may run to the medial head of the gastrocnemius. After harvest, the grafts are cut to approximately 22 cm long, and muscle tissue

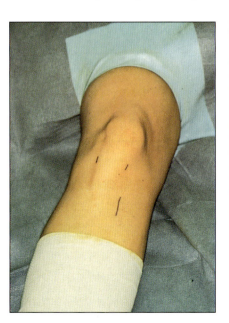

Figure 5-2. Incisions needed for the described approach are anterolateral and anteromedial arthroscopy incisions made adjacent to the patellar tendon and a small, vertical incision overlying the insertions of the semitendinosus and gracilis tendons.

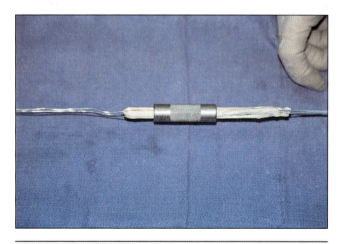

Figure 5-3. The prepared grafts are sized so the smallest possible bone tunnels can be created.

is removed from each graft. Each graft is then tagged with a Bunnell stitch of #2 nonabsorbable suture to facilitate tibial fixation. The grafts are then passed through a sizing tube so that bone tunnels as small as possible to accept the grafts can be created (Fig. 5-3). The grafts are moistened, then set aside for later use.

Creation of the Tibial Tunnel

The tibial tunnel is created by passing a guide pin into the joint from the anteromedial tibia, well medial to the tibial tubercle apophysis. The starting point is generally just above the level of the harvested semitendinosus tendon. A tibial guide with a 45° angle is used to pass the guide pin into the joint to a point corresponding to a central tibial attachment site. The guide pin's position is checked by extending the knee to be sure that the guide pin advances toward the apex of the intercondylar notch and that at terminal extension, it equals at least the radius of the desired tunnel, short of touching the superior notch. If the position is not optimal, it can be fine tuned with a parallel drill guide.

When the position of the guide pin has been optimized, it is overdrilled with a cannulated drill, creating the smallest possible tunnel that will allow passage of the hamstring grafts. The tunnel traverses the tibial physis as shown in Figure 5-4.

Creation of the Femoral Tunnel

The femoral tunnel is created through the tibial tunnel using an over-the-top referencing drill guide with a 5-mm offset. This allows placement of the femoral tunnel sufficiently deep within the notch to ensure a near isometric position [32]. The tunnel should be created so the medial edge is at the approximate 12 o'clock position high in the notch; therefore, it should be centered at approximately the 11 o'clock or 1 o'clock position. The femoral guide pin is drilled with the knee flexed at 90°, and the guide pin is advanced until it engages the anterolateral femoral cortex.

Over the guide pin, a femoral socket is created with an endoscopic cannulated drill of the predetermined diameter. It is drilled to a depth of 35 mm. A 4.2-mm drill is then used to create a passing channel for the

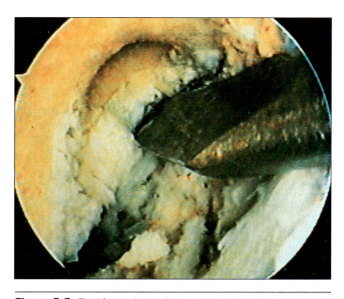

Figure 5-5. Final femoral tunnel position is high and to the extreme back of the intercondylar notch.

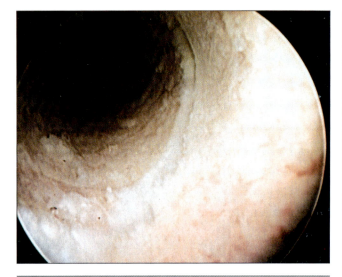

Figure 5-4. The physeal cartilage can be clearly seen in the tibial tunnel.

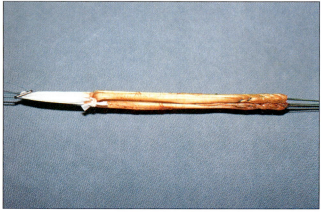

Figure 5-6. The midportion of the semitendinosus and gracilis tendons is connected to the Endobutton (Acufex Microsurgical, Mansfield, MA) with a doubled 5-mm polyester tape. The construct is adjusted to allow 25 mm of graft penetration into the femoral tunnel.

Endobutton to and through the anterolateral femoral cortex. Total depth of the femoral tunnel is then determined with a depth gauge. Final femoral tunnel position is demonstrated in Figure 5-5.

Graft Preparation

An Endobutton is next attached to the midportion of the semitendinosus and gracilis tendons, creating a four-banded graft. Attachment is done with doubled 5-mm polyester tape. The construct is adjusted to allow 25 mm of penetration of the grafts into the femoral tunnel, which is well across the femoral

physis. Passing sutures are then attached to the Endobutton. The completed construct is shown in Figure 5-6.

Graft Passage

The grafts are next inserted into the joint by passing a pin through the tibial tunnel across the joint and out the femoral tunnel to the anterolateral thigh. The passing sutures are then pulled through the anterolateral thigh, which allows the Endobutton and graft to be pulled into the joint and into the femoral socket (Fig. 5-7A). The Endobutton is pulled through the passing channel to the anterolateral femoral cortex, where it is set. The final graft position (shown in Fig. 5-7B) is adjacent to the posterior cruciate ligament (PCL), with adequate clearance of the lateral notch. The graft barely touches the superior notch at terminal extension.

Graft Tensioning and Tibial Fixation

With the knee flexed to approximately 20°, the grafts are next tensioned and fixed to the tibia. A low-profile screw and washer are placed at the end of the tendons just distal to the tibial tunnel exit point, which is well distal to the tibial physis. Sutures of each of the two tendons are then tied together around the post. Additional tension is then applied while the soft tissue washer directly fixes the grafts to the tibia (Fig. 5-8).

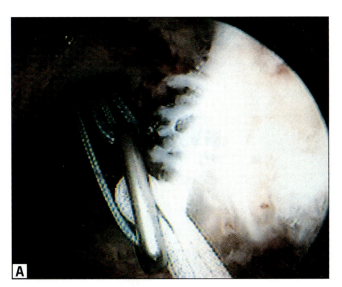

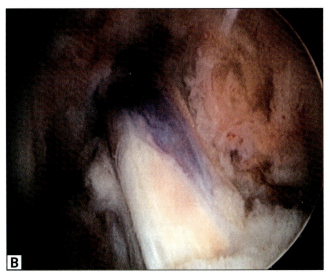

Figure 5-7. A, An Endobutton (Acufex Microsurgical, Mansfield, MA) is used for femoral fixation. **B,** The final position of the graft.

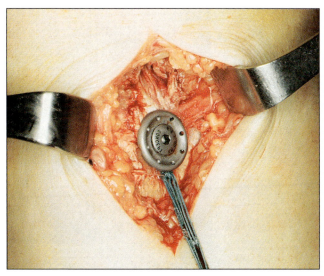

Figure 5-8. The grafts are tensioned and then fixed to the tibia by tying each graft separately around a screw post. As shown, a low-profile soft-tissue washer completes the fixation.

Knee extension to 0° should then be verified. Arthroscopic observation of the graft should reveal it to be adjacent to the PCL, with good clearance of the lateral wall of the intercondylar notch. The graft should barely touch the superior notch at terminal extension. Radiographic views of tunnels and fixation devices are shown in Figure 5-9.

Postoperative Rehabilitation

Rehabilitation following this procedure is generally quite easy. The patient is placed in a postoperative knee brace to prevent hyperextension during weight bearing. The brace can be removed when not bearing weight. The patient is allowed to bear weight as tolerated with crutches and to discontinue use of the crutches when they are no longer felt necessary. Stationary bicycling is started as soon as motion allows, usually by 10 days postoperatively. After 6 weeks, the patient no longer is required to wear the brace. Activities such as recreational bicycling, swimming, and most other activities on predictable surfaces are started 12 weeks postoperatively. Running and terminal knee extensions are not started until 6 months postoperatively, and level III jumping and pivoting sports are generally delayed until 9 months postoperatively.

CONCLUSION

The effect of surgical intervention on subsequent growth in the skeletally immature patient is a major factor influencing treatment decisions. Risks, however small, must be weighed against potential damage to the knee caused by repeated participation and giving-way bouts, which are common in this age group. It is essential to prevent repeat injuries; if this cannot be done in a non-operative manner, surgical intervention may need to be considered.

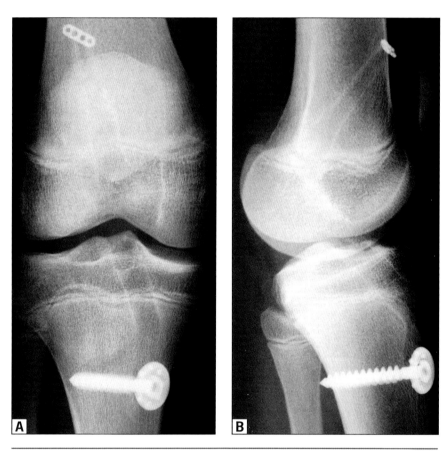

Figure 5-9. Anteroposterior (**A**) and lateral (**B**) radiographs of the tunnels reveal that they are centrally located in the frontal plane. Fixation devices are distant from the physis.

REFERENCES AND RECOMMENDED READING

Recently published papers of particular interest have been highlighted as:

••   Of outstanding interest

1. Rang M, ed. *Children's Fractures*. Philadelphia: JB Lippincott; 1983:290.

2. Bradley GW, Shives TC, Samuelson KM: Ligament injuries in the knees of children. *J Bone Joint Surg Am* 1979, 61:588–591.

3. Clanton TO, DeLee JC, Sanders B, *et al.*: Knee ligament injuries in children. *J Bone Joint Surg Am* 1979, 61:1195–1201.

4. Bright RW, Burstein AH, Elmore SM: Epiphyseal-plate cartilage: a biomechanical and histological analysis of failure modes. *J Bone Joint Surg Am* 1974, 56:688–703.

5. Noyes FR, Grood ES: The strength of the anterior cruciate ligament in humans and Rhesus monkeys. *J Bone Joint Surg Am* 1976, 58:1074–1082.

6. Cook PC, Leit ME: Issues in the pediatric athlete. *Orthop Clin North Am* 1995, 26:453–464.

7. Meyers MH, McKeever FM: Fracture of the intercondylar eminence of the tibia. *J Bone Joint Surg Am* 1970, 52:1677–1684.

8. Wiley JJ, Baxter MP: Tibial spine fractures in children. *Clin Orthop* 1990, 255:54–60.

9. Angel KR, Hall DJ: Anterior cruciate ligament injury in children and adolescents. *Arthroscopy* 1989, 5:197–200.

10. Eady JL, Cardenas CD, Sopa D: Avulsion of the femoral attachment of the anterior cruciate ligament in a seven-year-old child: a case report. *J Bone Joint Surg Am* 1982, 64:1376–1378.

11. Robinson SC, Driscoll SE: Simultaneous osteochondral avulsion of the femoral and tibial insertions of the anterior cruciate ligament: report of a case in a thirteen-year-old boy. *J Bone Joint Surg Am* 1981, 63(suppl A):1342–1343.

12. Lipscomb AB, Anderson AF: Tears of the anterior cruciate ligament in adolescents. *J Bone Joint Surg Am* 1986, 68:19–28.

13. Kannus P, Jarvinen M: Knee ligament injuries in adolescents. Eight year follow-up of conservative management. *J Bone Joint Surg Br* 1988, 70:772–776.

14. McCarroll JR, Rettig AC, Shelbourne KD: Anterior cruciate ligament injuries in the young athlete with open physes. *Am J Sports Med* 1988, 16:44–47.

15. Waldrop JI, Broussard TS: Disruption of the anterior cruciate ligament in a three-year-old child. A case report. *J Bone Joint Surg Am* 1984, 66:1113–1114.

16. DeLee JC: ACL insufficiency in children. In *The Crucial Ligaments*. Edited by Feagin JAJ. New York: Churchill-Livingstone; 1988:649–676.

17. Larson RV, Friedman MJ: Anterior cruciate ligament: injuries and treatment. *Instr Course Lect* 1996, 45:235–243.

18. Graf BK, Lange RH, Fujisaki CK, *et al.*: Anterior cruciate ligament tears in skeletally immature patients: meniscal pathology at presentation and after attempted conservative treatment. *Arthroscopy* 1992, 8:229–233.

19. McCarroll JR, Shelbourne KD, Porter DA, *et al.*: Patellar tendon graft reconstruction for midsubstance anterior cruciate ligament rupture in junior high school athletes: an algorithm for management. *Am J Sports Med* 1994, 22:478–484.

20. Mizuta H, Kubota K, Shiraishi M, *et al.*: The conservative treatment of complete tears of the anterior cruciate ligament in skeletally immature patients. *J Bone Joint Surg Br* 1995, 77:890–894.

21. DeLee JC, Curtis R: Anterior cruciate ligament insufficiency in children. *Clin Orthop* 1983, 172:112–118.

22. Engebretsen L, Svenningsen S, Benum P: Poor results of anterior cruciate ligament repair in adolescence. *Acta Orthop Scand* 1988, 59:684–686.

23. Rinaldi E, Mazzarella F: Isolated fracture-avulsions of the tibial insertions of the cruciate ligaments of the knee. *Ital J Orthop Traumatol* 1980, 6:77–83.

24. Angel KR, Hall DJ: The role of arthroscopy in children and adolescents. *Arthroscopy* 1989, 5:192–196.

25. Pearl AJ, Bergfeld JA: Extraarticular reconstruction in the anterior cruciate ligament deficient knee [monograph]. In *American Orthopaedic Society for Sports Medicine*. Champaigne, IL: Human Kinetics Publishers; 1992:5–6.

26. Brief LP: Anterior cruciate ligament reconstruction without drill holes. *Arthroscopy* 1991, 7:350–357.

27. Parker AW, Drez D Jr, Cooper JL: Anterior cruciate ligament injuries in patients with open physes. *Am J Sports Med* 1994, 22:44–47.

28. Andrews M, Noyes FR, Barber-Westin SD: Anterior cruciate ligament allograft reconstruction in the skeletally immature athlete. *Am J Sports Med* 1994, 22:48–54.

29.•• Matava MJ, Siegel MG: Arthroscopic reconstruction of the ACL with semitendinosus-gracilis autograft in skeletally immature adolescent patients. *Am J Knee Surg* 1997, 10:60–69.

   Study documenting growth at both tibial and femoral physes following anterior cruciate ligament reconstruction with transphyseal drill holes and hamstring tendon autografts.

30. Tanner JM, Whitehouse RM, Marshall WA, *et al.*: *Assessment of Skeletal Maturity and Prediction of Adult Height (TW2 method)*. London: Academic Press; 1976:1075.

31. Lombardo SJ, Harvey JP Jr: Fractures of the distal femoral epiphyses. Factors influencing prognosis: a review of thirty-four cases. *J Bone Joint Surg Am* 1977, 59:742–751.

32. Sidles JA, Larson RV, Garbini JL, *et al.*: Ligament length relationships in the moving knee. *J Orthop Res* 1988, 6:593–610.

The Use of Allograft Tissue in Knee Ligament Reconstruction

Gregory C. Fanelli and Daniel D. Feldmann

Materials used for knee ligament reconstructive surgery include autograft tissue, allograft tissue, and knee ligament prostheses. Each of these ligament-substitute materials has a distinct place in the armamentarium of the knee ligament surgeon. This chapter discusses the advantages, disadvantages, preparation, indications, and results with the use of allograft tissue for knee ligament reconstructive surgery.

The most common types of allograft tissue are bone–patellar tendon–bone (BPTB), Achilles tendon, fascia lata, semitendinosus tendon, and gracilis tendon (Fig. 6-1, Table 6-1). The most common use for these tissues in knee ligament reconstructive surgery are reconstructions of the anterior cruciate ligament (ACL), posterior cruciate ligament (PCL), posterolateral complex (PLC), fibular collateral ligament (FCL), and medial collateral ligament (MCL).

Preservation methods for allograft tissue include fresh freezing, freeze drying, and cryopreservation. These allografts can be harvested under sterile conditions or in a "clean," nonsterile fashion using secondary sterilization.

ALLOGRAFT CONSIDERATIONS

Allograft tissue is readily available, eliminates donor-site morbidity, and allows for smaller incisions that enhance the cosmetic result. Because host tissue is not compromised, larger grafts with increased cross-sectional area can be used, which increases the strength of the ligament substitute. Other advantages include reduced postoperative stiffness, decreased operating and tourniquet time, and increased strength at time zero [1,2].

Disadvantages associated with the use of allograft tissue include greater expense, risk of disease transmission, immunogenetic behavior with possible tissue rejection, slower healing rates, local bone resorption, and the development of bone cysts [1,2].

ALLOGRAFT HARVESTING

The American Association of Tissue Banks (AATB) has established standards and guidelines for tissue procurement and tissue banking [1,3,4]. These guidelines were established to ensure the highest quality of allograft tissue possible and to reduce or eliminate the risk of disease transmission during grafting. The AATB emphasizes donor screening, paying particular attention to the medical and social history, laboratory blood testing, autopsy results, bacterial and fungal cultures of the graft at harvest and before implantation, and lymph node examination. The donor's family is also interviewed before surgical donation, and a thorough review of the patient's medical records is performed. Table 6-2 lists the steps in allograft procurement and processing.

After the donor has passed the initial screening, the allograft tissue is harvested 2 to 6 hours after death under either "clean" (nonsterile) or sterile conditions. Nonsterile procurement requires secondary sterilization treatment of the harvested tissue before implantation. Sterilization of allograft tissue is commonly done using gamma irradiation or ethylene gas. Both are discussed in the next section.

ALLOGRAFT PRESERVATION AND STERILIZATION METHODS

Four basic types of implantable allograft tissue exist: fresh (recently harvested tissue), fresh frozen, freeze dried, and cryopreserved. Each type of graft tissue varies in its preservation technique, immunogenicity potential, preimplantation preparation, survivability of the native cells of the tissue, biomechanical characteristics following implantation, and the storage shelf life of the tissue after it has been processed (Table 6-3). Before or after preservation, the graft may be sterilized secondarily.

Fresh allografts preserve living ligament or tendon cells. These allograft tissues must be transplanted within hours of death and do not undergo any preservation techniques. These grafts require the coordinated activities of donor and recipient services such that donor and recipient graft sizing and tissue human lymphocyte antigen matching occur before implantation. Potential immune response reaction and rejection seem to be higher than with processed allograft tissue. This may be caused by the allograft's (ie, fibroblasts' and ground substance's) ability to incite a marked

Table 6-1	Commonly Used Allograft Materials for Knee Ligament Reconstruction

Bone–patellar tendon–bone
Achilles tendon
Fascia lata
Semitendinosus tendon
Gracilis tendon

Table 6-2	Steps in Allograft Procurement and Processing

1. Donor physical examination, medical record review, family interview
2. Serologic testing
3. Sterile tissue recovery
4. Autopsy with lymph node examination
5. Cultures of tissues and grafts
6. Graft processing (freeze dried, deep frozen)
7. Graft selection (size match-up)
8. Preimplantation preparation (reconstitution, thawing)
9. Graft implantation

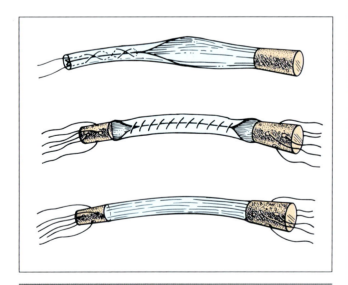

Figure 6-1. Some of the most commonly used grafts and their preparations. Achilles tendon allograft (*top*), bone–patellar tendon–bone allograft (*middle*), and patellar tendon autograft (*bottom*). Patellar tendon autografts can also be made for press-fit in the femur, with the larger of the bone plugs harvested from the tibial side. (*Adapted from* Port and Jackson [46].)

inflammatory response characterized by the infiltration of lymphocytes and plasma cells. The antigens responsible for this immune response are thought to be the major histocompatibility complex (MHC) antigens on the surface of the native cells of the tissue.

The fresh-frozen method of allograft preservation consists of sterile procurement followed by sterile wrapping and deep freezing of the allograft tissue to -70°C to -80°C. Fresh-frozen allograft tissues can be stored up to 5 years at -70°C, and for up to 6 months at -20°C. Deep freezing does not preserve living ligament or tendon cells and therefore reduces, but does not eliminate, the tissue's immunogenicity. Although this process remains not fully understood, it is believed that deep freezing denatures viable cells, which disrupts surface MHC antigens. The resulting inflammatory response to the implanted allograft is therefore greatly reduced. Before use, frozen allograft tissue must be slowly thawed, which may take up to 1 hour [5•]. Freezing seems to have no adverse effect on the mechanical properties of the tendon tissue, and deep freezing to -80°C may prevent bacterial infection [6–8].

Freeze drying (lyophilization) is a preservation process whereby deep-frozen allograft tissue is dried to between 3% and 5% residual moisture and packaged in a vacuum-sealed container. Freeze-dried tissue can be stored without refrigeration and is usable for at least 5 years. Preimplantation preparation is limited to reconstitution (rehydration) of the graft with saline solution [5]. Freeze drying also does not preserve living ligament or tendon cells. As with deep freezing, freeze drying reduces (by disruption of the MHC), but does not eliminate, the immunogenicity of allograft tissue. No difference seems to be present in ultimate strength between fresh-frozen and freeze-dried allograft tissue [9].

Cryopreservation is the latest preservation method developed. It entails controlled-rate freezing of donor tissue in the presence of "cryoprotective agents" (dimethyl sulfoxide and a nutrient media) to prevent formation of ice crystals within the cellular structure [10]. This procedure maintains between approximately 45% and 80% of cellular viability of allograft tissue and preserves protein structure. It is believed that the maintenance of native cells in the graft allows for a "smoother" transition through the graft remodeling process. The tissue is stored in liquid nitrogen or vapor phase nitrogen, which inhibits water migration seen with conventional storage of fresh-frozen allografts at -70°C to -80°C. Before use, the cryopreserved graft must be thawed. Shelf life is reported to be up to 10 years (personal communication, Cryolife, Malietta, GA). Immunogenicity is reportedly low, with no apparent migration of lymphocytes into the allografts 6 months postoperatively, despite the maintenance of native cellular structure [8]. Strength comparison between cryopreserved allograft tissue and autograft tissue indicates no difference 6 months after implantation [8]. DNA studies indicate that host cells completely replace the donor cells by 24 months in cryopreserved allograft tissue, indicating that the preservation of living cells in allograft tissue may be of no significant benefit [10].

If allograft tissue has been harvested under nonsterile conditions, secondary sterilization procedures must be employed to eradicate bacterial and viral infection. Currently, most tissue banks harvest their allograft tissue under sterile conditions and then process the tissue either by deep freezing or freeze drying the tissue. These techniques effectively eradicate bacterial contamination. However, concern remains among surgeons and tissue-bank personnel that these processing techniques do not eradicate viral (eg, HIV) contamination. For this reason, many tissue banks offer allograft tissue that has undergone secondary sterilization despite sterile harvesting and processing techniques. The two most common secondary sterilization

		Fresh	Fresh Frozen	Freeze Dried	Cryopreserved
Table 6-3	**Allograft Characteristics**				
Preservation technique		None	Freezing	Freezing and drying in a vacuum	Controlled-time freezing
Immunogenicity potential		High	Low	Low	Low
Preimplantation preparation		Tissue matching	Thawing	Reconstitution	Thawing
Survivability of native cells at transplantation, %		100	0	0	45–80
Biomechanical characteristics		?	No effect of freezing	No effect of drying	No effect of freezing
Shelf life		N/A	5 y at -70°C	5 y without refrigeration	10 y

procedures used include gamma irradiation and ethylene oxide gas sterilization.

Gamma irradiation is the more promising method. Current recommendations to sterilize allograft tissue are 1.5 to 2.5 Mrad [3,4,11]. Although this dose effectively eradicates bacterial contamination, controversy continues as to the effective dose to prevent viral contamination. This dosing regimen may not be adequate to inactivate HIV in infected BPTB allografts, and larger doses may be required [12]. Some authors recommend doses as high as 3.6 Mrad to inactivate HIV [11]. Increasing doses of gamma irradiation is not without complication. Irradiation of graft tissue negatively alters the biomechanical properties in a dose-dependent fashion. In general, doses below 3 Mrad are thought to be well tolerated by the allograft, with insignificant changes in the compression and torsional or bending strength of the graft [5•]. However, in the most recent study to date, Fideler et al. [12] found that doses as low as 2 Mrad significantly altered maximum force and strain energy (structural properties) and modulus and maximum stress (material properties) tolerated by the graft. At 3 and 4 Mrad of irradiation, all parameters measuring structural and material properties were significantly affected in a dose-dependent fashion. Some studies indicate that freezing of allograft tissue after irradiation seems to improve the biomechanical characteristics such that 3 Mrad of irradiation is well tolerated without affecting compression or torsional or bending strength [5•]. Currently, it seems that a dose somewhere between 2 and 3 Mrad is best and beneficial for use of frozen tissue. It is clear that the deleterious (biomechanical alteration) and beneficial effects (sterilization) of irradiating allograft tissue are dose dependent. A need for further study certainly exists in this area.

Ethylene oxide gas sterilization is an older technique of sterilization and is falling out of favor with tissue banks and surgeons [13]. It has been shown that the byproducts of ethylene oxide (ethylene chlorohydrin and ethylene glycol) have a deleterious effect on the graft, necessitating its removal. Clinical complications of note include persistent joint effusions, loss of osteoinductive potential, bone tunnel resorption with cyst formation, and the "applesauce reaction" associated with graft dissolution over time [14–16]. At present, use of ethylene oxide–sterilized allograft is not recommended.

DISEASE TRANSMISSION

The risk of acquiring viral disease (eg, HIV or hepatitis) from allograft tissue is a major concern for the potential recipient of the tissue [17]. To reduce risk, steps are taken prior to graft procurement to ensure disease-free donation (see Table 6-2). A thorough history and physical examination of the donor are performed with specific attention to evidence of drug abuse, chronic illness, and overall physical condition. A detailed history is obtained from the donor's family regarding lifestyle and possible exposure to infectious diseases. A thorough review of the donor's medical records is also performed.

Before surgical donation, thorough blood-work screening for disease is also performed. Serologic tests for HIV-I/II antibodies, HIV antigen, polymerase chain reaction–HIV, hepatitis B surface antigen, hepatitis B surface antibodies, hepatitis B core antibodies, hepatitis C virus antibodies, and human T-cell lymphotrophic virus-I/II antibodies, and rapid plasma reagin test for syphilis are performed. Cultures of tissue are taken during harvest as well as before implantation. Following surgical donation, a complete autopsy is also performed with specific attention to lymph nodes. Any indication of disease is an indication for rejection of the donor [18–20].

If the donor's history and physical examination results are negative, as well as those of the blood work, tissue cultures, and autopsy, the probability of obtaining an HIV-infected allograft is approximately one in 1.6 million [18]. If any of the steps are omitted, the risk rises significantly. A thorough and complete donor screening process seems to be the critical phase of allograft procurement and processing because no sterilization methods exist that effectively eliminate the HIV virus without compromising the structural integrity of the allograft tissue.

ALLOGRAFT HISTOLOGY

The remodeling process of allograft following implantation has been well-studied and described by various authors [21•,22] (Table 6-4). Regardless of whether the graft is an allograft or autograft, fresh frozen, freeze

Table 6-4	Allograft Remodeling

1. Cellular in-growth of fibroblasts
2. Existing collagen degradation and avascular necrosis coupled with new collagen synthesis
3. Realignment of new collagen along lines of stress
4. By 6 mo, histologic appearance as normal connective tissue (graft is weakest at this time)
5. By 12 mo, graft maturity and increase in cross-sectional area
6. By 18 mo, histologic maturity

dried, or cryopreserved, the graft is avascular at the time of implantation. This graft must be revascularized if it is to survive. Initially, the graft is revascularized or revitalized through vascular tissues from the infra-patellar fat pad, synovium, and the endosteal vasculature of the bone tunnels in the femur and tibia. This occurs during the first 4 to 6 weeks following implantation. DNA studies also indicate that by 4 weeks, no native DNA remains in the implanted graft. Ischemic necrosis of the central portion of the graft also occurs during this time, leaving behind a connective tissue "scaffold" of collagen. As the graft revascularizes, cellular proliferation occurs, aiding in the cellular repopulation of the graft. Vascularization occurs on the surface of the tissue by 6 to 8 weeks, and complete revascularization occurs by 12 to 16 weeks.

The cellular in-growth consists primarily of fibroblasts. As these cells mature, the existing collagen scaffold is degraded, and new collagen synthesis occurs. As new collagen is laid down and matures, realignment of fibers occurs along the lines of stress of the graft. This process occurs over a period of 5 months; by 6 months, the histologic appearance is that of normal, regularly oriented connective tissue. Over the next 12 months, the graft increases in cross-sectional area as it matures; however, the graft matures with smaller-diameter collagen fibers. An initial period of decreased allograft strength is present at 6 months, but by 18 months the allograft reaches histologic maturity through the remodeling process. The allograft appears to act as a viable ACL 6 months after implantation. The rate of avascular necrosis, revascularization, and remodeling compared with autograft tissue is not known, but seems to take more time with allograft tissue.

BIOMECHANICS

Normal properties of the ACL have been evaluated by several authors. Noyes and Grood [23] determined the linear stiffness and load of the ACL to be 182 N/mm and 1730 N, respectively. Woo et al. [24,25] have determined through a different experimental protocol that ACL stiffness is 242 N/mm, and the ultimate load is 2160 N. Noyes had determined that a 14-mm wide

Table 6-5	Indications for Allograft Use

Multiple ligament injuries

Posterior cruciate ligament reconstruction with Achilles tendon allograft

Revision surgery when autogenous tissue is not available

Preference for avoiding donor-site morbidity

strip of BPTB had an ultimate load of 2900 N (jack 81), which is approximately the same strength as normal ACL, as determined by Woo et al. France et al. [26] proposed that allograft tissues used to replace the ACL should be approximately twice as strong as the ACL at time zero because 50% of the allograft's strength is lost during healing.

Jackson et al. [6,7] compared fresh-frozen allograft and patellar tendon autograft (see Fig. 6-1) in an animal model. Their findings indicated that at 6 months postimplantation, the strength of the autografts was 62% of normal control ACL strength, whereas allograft strength was 27% of the control ACL. Autografts were significantly stronger than the allografts 6 months after surgery. However, apparently the level of functioning did not decrease. The implication is that allograft tissue has a slower period of maturation than does autograft tissue.

INDICATIONS FOR ALLOGRAFT USE

Autogenous tissue is the most common graft source in knee ligament reconstructive surgery; however, the use of allograft tissue can be advantageous in specific situations (Table 6-5). Perhaps the most common indication for the use of allograft tissue is multiple ligament injuries of one or both knees. Such knees are severely compromised, and the morbidity associated with autogenous tissue harvest may further increase trauma to the involved lower extremity. PCL surgery is a reasonable situation for the use of allograft tissue for primary reconstruction. PCL reconstruction is exposed to high mechanical forces, and the larger cross-sectional area and increased strength that an Achilles tendon allograft (Fig. 6-2) offers may be beneficial.

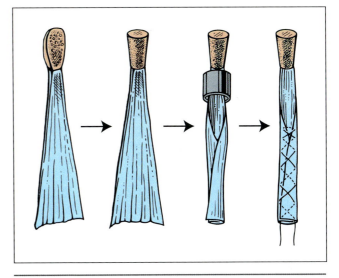

Figure 6-2. Sizing and preparation of an Achilles tendon allograft. (*Adapted from* Port and Jackson [46].)

Revision single- or multiple-ligament reconstructive surgery if autogenous tissue is not available, is already compromised, or is of poor tissue quality is an indication for the use of allograft tissue. Given the graft tissue options, some patients choose allograft tissue to completely avoid donor-site morbidity.

ALLOGRAFT TISSUE SELECTION

The ideal allograft provides strength, a natural scaffold to allow host tissue in-growth, and should possess biomechanical properties to the tissue it replaces. Autografts and allografts are not perfect ligament substitutes. They are collagen struts that serve as a check-rein to instability. Allografts have less tensile strength after remodeling than do their time-zero implantation strength, so their ideal initial maximum strength should be twice as strong as that of the ligament they are used to replace. This is because approximately 50% of the allograft's strength is lost during healing [26]. As mentioned previously, Noyes and Grood [23] demonstrated the strength of the ACL to be 1730 N to failure, and Woo et al. [24,25] demonstrated the ACL strength to failure to be 2160 N. It seems that the ideal allograft used for ACL reconstruction should be twice as strong as these values. The larger the cross-sectional area of the allograft, the stronger it is. This would make the bone–Achilles tendon and bone-quadriceps tendon allografts very favorable for reconstructions.

The ideal allograft should be one obtained from a reputable tissue bank that strictly adheres to the AATB's standards for donor screening, harvesting, and preparation of allograft tissue. The graft should be sterilely harvested so that no secondary sterilization, which could compromise graft strength, is required. The allograft should have the largest cross-sectional area possible for maximum strength, and there should be a bone plug on at least one end for fixation strength and bone-to-bone healing.

RESULTS USING ALLOGRAFT TISSUE

Results using allogenic tissue for ACL reconstruction are comparable to those of reconstructions using autogenous tissue. BPTB is the most common allograft tissue used for ACL reconstruction. Stringham et al. [27] compared autograft with allograft ACL reconstructions using BPTB. At mean follow-up of 34 months, values for Lysholm and Tegner knee ligament rating scales, physical examination findings, instrumented laxity measurements, and isokinetic strength results were not of a statistically significant difference between the two groups. Levitt et al. [28] reported on 181 allograft ACL reconstructions using

BPTB with 4 years follow-up. Using fresh-frozen or freeze-dried BPTB, they found 79% excellent or good results, which allowed return to preinjury levels of activity. Valenti et al. [29] found at 35 months follow-up that overall functional results were satisfactory in 85% of their series using fresh-frozen BPTB allografts. Furthermore, no reported infections, disease transmission, or tissue rejection were reported. Indelicato et al. [30] used fresh-frozen BPTB allografts in 41 patients and reported good and excellent results in 73% of patients at 27 months follow-up using a modified Hughston knee score. Subjectively, 90% of their patients felt their knee was normal. Harner et al. [31•] reported on 64 patients 3 to 5 years after ACL reconstruction using nonirradiated fresh-frozen BPTB allograft. When compared with autograft control subjects, essentially no difference was present between the groups. In the longest-term published series to date, Noyes and Barber-Westin [32] demonstrated satisfactory results 5 to 9 years postoperatively using BPTB and fascia lata allografts. Tierney et al. [33] reported on 227 ACL reconstructions using 58 allografts successfully on an outpatient basis. From recent data available, it appears that a properly placed BPTB allograft yields satisfactory results at least 75% of the time.

Research focusing on cryopreserved allograft tissue remains sparse. Kirkpatrick et al. [10] reported on the use of cryopreserved tissue for ACL reconstruction in the canine model. In comparing cryopreserved allograft with traditional autograft, they found allograft tissue to have poorer biomechanical properties (decreased strength) at time intervals 3, 6, 9, and 24 months after transplantation. The most promising study supporting the use of cryopreserved tissue was reported by McCarthy et al. [8]. They compared cryopreserved BPTB allograft, fresh autograft and fresh-frozen allograft ACL reconstructions in primates. At 6 months postoperative, the strength of fresh autograft and cryopreserved allograft were similar (approximately 50% of native ACL), whereas the strength of fresh frozen allograft was only 35% that of native ACL.

Freeze-dried fascia lata allografts have been very successful. Pritchard et al. [34] used freeze-dried fascia lata allografts to reconstruct 79 ACL-deficient knees. At average follow-up of 134.5 months, 75% displayed less than 3 mm of anterior-posterior tibial translation when compared with the contralateral knee when measured with the KT1000 arthrometer (Medmetric, San Diego, CA). Furthermore, 77% were able to return to sporting activities. No patients displayed evidence of graft rejection. Defrere and Franckart [35] reported the results of 70 ACL reconstructions with freeze-dried fascia lata allografts and found 82% good and excellent results subjectively, and 95% excellent and good results objectively, 1 to 5 years after surgery. They also concluded that measurements made 1 year postoperatively correlate with measurements made during the ensuing years, which may have prognostic value for the graft. They also performed second-look arthroscopy in 47 of their patients and were able to correlate objective findings with a visual evaluation of the allograft. Fascia lata allografts have also been used with success in skeletally immature athletes with ACL insufficiency. Andrews et al. [36] reconstructed eight such patients with either fascia lata or Achilles tendon allografts. After a mean follow-up of 54 months, they report six excellent, one good, and one fair result. No growth-plate disturbances were noted.

Allograft use in PCL reconstruction has produced favorable clinical results, with no statistically significant differences between autograft and allograft reconstructions evaluated with knee ligament rating scales and arthrometer testing. Fanelli et al. [37,38] have reported on the use of allograft Achilles tendon for PCL in two separate patient populations. The first group consisted of 21 patients with PCL and posterolateral complex reconstructions with 24 to 54 months follow-up. Patients were evaluated with physical examination, KT1000 arthrometer, Lysholm, Tegner, and Hospital for Special Surgery–knee ligament rating scales. Of the patients, 48% were restored to normal posterior drawer and normal tibial step-off, and 48% were restored to a grade 1 posterior drawer and decreased tibial step-off of less than 5 mm. There was no statistically significant difference between allograft Achilles tendon and autogenous BPTB for PCL reconstruction. The second group consisted of 20 arthroscopically assisted combined ACL-PCL reconstructions using allograft Achilles tendon and autogenous BPTB for the PCL reconstructions with 24 to 48 month follow-up. These patients were also evaluated with physical examination, KT1000 arthrometer, Lysholm, Tegner, and Hospital for Special Surgery–knee ligament rating scales. Whereas nine patients were restored to a normal posterior drawer and normal tibial step-off, 11 patients achieved a grade 1 posterior drawer and decreased tibial step-off of 5 mm or less. No statistically significant difference existed between autograft BPTB and allograft Achilles tendon in PCL reconstruction in this group of patients.

Allografts have also been used successfully in surgery for ACL revision. Decreased operative time, tissue availability, smaller incisions, no donor-site morbidity, a variety of available graft sizes, and the ability to fashion bone plugs corresponding to large tunnel sizes secondary to tunnel osteolysis are all advantages of using allograft tissue under revision circumstances. Harner and Safran [39] reported revision results with allograft tissue on 35 failed ACL reconstructions. The most common cause of graft failure cited in this series was surgical technique. Postrevision, all patients objectively showed improvement (ie, on arthrometer, pivot shift, Lachman tests). Subjectively, 70% were able to return to their desired preprimary reconstruction level of activity. Serial radiographic follow-up failed to reveal any cystic enlargement of bony tunnels. Furthermore, no disease transmission or graft rejection were reported [39]. Other authors [16,40–42] have also found that allograft tissue produces favorable results for ACL revision surgery.

Animal studies [43,44] indicate that allograft tendon material can be successfully used for extra-articular ligament reconstruction in the knee. These studies demonstrated revascularization, collagen reorganization and maturation, and equivalent stiffness and ultimate load compared with controls when allogenic tendon was used to reconstruct the medial collateral ligament [43]. Allograft tissue has also been used for successful reconstruction of the posterolateral corner [44].

COMPLICATIONS

Complications with the use of allograft tissue can occur. Inadequate donor screening and selection can lead to disease transmission. Improper graft preparation, sterilization, and packaging can lead to biomechanical deficiencies in allograft tissue, and can lead to allograft contamination preoperatively due to faulty packaging techniques from the manufacturer. Both compromise the surgical result. ACL reconstruction using freeze-dried ethylene oxide–sterilized BPTB allografts has been associated with a high failure rate and adverse reactions from the sterilization method [15,16]. Complications can occur from donor-recipient size mismatch, for example, a tall donor, and a short recipient. Such size mismatch may lead to compromised allograft fixation and poor postoperative results.

Several definitions of graft failure exist. Failure occurs when the patient complains of functional instability with activities of daily living or sports activity and shows evidence of increased knee laxity on physical examination [39]. Failure may also be defined as an increase of anterior-posterior displacement of 5.5 to 6.0 mm greater than the contralateral knee with arthrometer testing, or of a pivot shift of grade 2 (gross subluxation) or grade 3 (gross subluxation with impingement of the posterior aspect of the lateral tibial plateau against the femoral condyle) [40].

Biomechanical inadequacy of the allograft, improper tunnel and allograft placement, allograft impingement, improper allograft tensioning, and inadequate fixation can all lead to surgical failure [41]. Increased shelf life has also been correlated with graft failure [45].

CONCLUSION

Allograft tissue is a useful tool in knee ligament reconstruction. Results of clinical and animal studies indicate that allograft tissue is able to stabilize knees effectively in ACL and PCL reconstructive procedures. Less objective information is available concerning collateral ligament reconstruction. Risks associated with allograft tissue use include disease transmission and possible rejection phenomenon, although these decrease with current screening and processing standards.

REFERENCES AND RECOMMENDED READING

Recently published papers of particular interest have been highlighted as:

• Of interest

1. Fu FH, Jackson DW, Jamison J, *et al.*: Allograft reconstruction of the anterior cruciate ligament. In *The Anterior Cruciate Ligament. Current and Future Concepts.* Edited by Jackson DW. New York: Raven Press; 1993.

2. Harner CD, Olson EJ, Fu FH, *et al.*: The use of fresh frozen allograft tissue in knee ligament reconstruction: indications, techniques, results and controversies. Scientific Exhibit #1410. Washington, DC: American Academy of Orthopaedic Surgeons; 1992.

3. American Association of Tissue Banks: *Standards for Tissue Banking.* McLean, VA: American Association of Tissue Banks; 1996.

4. American Association of Tissue Banks: *Technical Manual of Musculoskeletal Tissues.* McLean, VA: American Association of Tissue Banks; 1992.

5.• Seltzer DG, Lombardo SJ: Allografts in knee ligament surgery. In *The Knee.* Edited by Scott WN. St. Louis: Mosby; 1994:865–894.

Comprehensive text on the use of allografts in knee ligament reconstruction.

6. Jackson DW, Grood EW, Golistein J, *et al.*: A comparison of patellar tendon autograft and allograft used for anterior cruciate ligament reconstruction in the goat model. *Am J Sports Med* 1993, 21:176–185.

7. Jackson DW, Grood ES, Goldstein J, *et al.*: Anterior cruciate ligament reconstruction using patella tendon autograft and allograft an experimental study in goats. *Trans Orthop Res Soc* 1991, 16:208.

8. McCarthy J, Blomstrom G, Steadman J, *et al.*: ACL reconstruction using cryopreserved patellar tendon allografts. Paper presented at the 17th annual meeting of the Society for Biomaterials. Scottsdale, AZ. May 1–5, 1991.

9. Paulos L, France E, Rosenberg T, *et al.*: Comparative material properties of allograft tissues for ligament replacement: effects of type, age, sterilization, and preservation. *Trans Orthop Res Soc* 1987, 12:129.

10. Kirkpatrick JS, Seaber AV, Glisson RR, Bassett FH: Cryopreserved anterior cruciate ligament allografts in a canine model. *J South Orthop Assoc* 1996, 5:20–29.

11. Conway B, Tomford WW, Hirsch MS, *et al.*: Effects of gamma irradiation on HIV-1 in a bone allograft model. *Trans Orthop Res* 1990, 15:225.

12. Fideler BM, Vangsness CT, Moore T, *et al.*: Effects of gamma irradiation on the human immunodeficiency virus (HIV): a study in frozen human bone-patellar ligament-bone grafts obtained from infected cadavers. *J Bone Joint Surg* 1994, 76(suppl A):1032–1035.

13. Bechtold JE, Eastlund DT, Butts MK, *et al.*: The effects of freeze-drying and ethylene oxide sterilization on the mechanical properties of human patellar tendon. *Am J Sports Med* 1994, 22:562–566.

14. Herron LD, Newman MH: The failure of ethylene oxide gas-sterilized freeze-dried bone graft for thoracic and lumbar spinal fusion. *Spine* 1989, 14:496–500.

15. Jackson DW, Windler GE, Simon TM: Intraarticular reaction associated with the use of freeze-dried ethylene oxide-sterilized bone-patellar tendon-bone allografts in the reconstruction of the anterior cruciate ligament. *Am J Sports Med* 1990, 18:1–10.

16. Roberts TS, Drez D, McCarthy W, Paine R: Anterior cruciate ligament reconstruction using freeze-dried, ethylene oxide-sterilized, bone-patellar tendon-bone allografts: two year results in thirty-six patients. *Am J Sports Med* 1991, 19:35–41.

17. Simmonds RJ, Holmberg SJ, Hurwitz R, *et al.*: Transmission of human immunodeficiency virus type 1 from a seronegative organ and tissue donor. *N Engl J Med* 1992, 326:726–732.

18. Buck BE, Malinin TI, Brown MD: Bone transplantation and human immunodeficiency virus: an estimate of risk of acquired immunodeficiency syndrome (AIDS). *Clin Orthop* 1989, 240:129.

19. Buck BE, Malinin TI: Human bone and tissue allografts: preparation and safety. *Clin Orthop* 1994, 303:8–17.

20. Olson EJ, Harner CD, Fu F, Silbey MB: Clinical use of fresh, frozen soft tissue allografts. *Orthopaedics* 1992, 15:1225–1232.

21.• Arnoczky SP: Biology of ACL reconstructions: what happens to the graft? In *Instructional Course Lectures in Orthopaedics.* Edited by Pritchard DJ. Park Ridge, IL: American Acadamy of Orthopaedic Surgeons; 1996:229–233.

Thorough review of allograft basic science.

22. Jackson DW, Corsetti J, Simon TM: Biologic incorporation of allograft anterior cruciate ligament replacements. *Clin Orthop* 1996, 324:126–133.

23. Noyes FR, Grood ES: The strength of the anterior cruciate ligament in humans and rhesus monkeys: age-related and species-related changes. *J Bone Joint Surg* 1976, 58(suppl A):1074–1082.

24. Woo S L-Y, Buckwalter J: Ligament and tendon autografts and allografts. In *Bone and Cartilage Allografts: Biology and Clinical Applications*. Edited by Friedlander G, Goldberg V. Park Ridge, IL: American Academy of Orthopaedic Surgeons; 1991:103–121.

25. Woo S L-Y, Hollis J, Adams D, *et al.*: Tensile properties of the human femur-anterior cruciate ligament-tibia complex: the effects of specimen age and orientation. *Am J Sports Med* 1991, 19:217–225.

26. France E, Paulos L, Rosenberg T, Harner C: The biomechanics of anterior cruciate allografts. In *Prosthetic Ligament Reconstruction of the Knee*. Edited by Friedman M, Ferkel R. Philadelphia: WB Saunders; 1988:180–185.

27. Stringham DR, Pelmas CJ, Burks RT, *et al.*: Comparison of anterior cruciate ligament reconstructions using patellar tendon autograft and allograft. *Arthroscopy* 1996, 12:414–421.

28. Levitt RL, Malinin T, Posada A, Michalow A: Reconstruction of anterior cruciate ligaments with bone-patellar tendon-bone and Achilles tendon allografts. *Clin Orthop* 1994, 303:67–78.

29. Valenti JR, Sala D, Schweitzer D: Anterior cruciate ligament reconstruction with fresh frozen patellar tendon allografts. *Int Orthop* 1994, 18:210–214.

30. Indelicato PA, Linton RC, Huegel M: The results of fresh-frozen patellar tendon allografts for chronic anterior cruciate ligament deficiency of the knee. *Am J Sports Med* 1992, 20:118–121.

31.• Harner CD, Olson E, Irrgang JJ, *et al.*: Allograft versus autograft anterior cruciate ligament reconstruction. *Clin Orthop* 1996, 324:134–144.

Comparative clinical results of autograft and allograft anterior cruciate ligament reconstruction.

32. Noyes FR, Barber-Westin SD: Reconstruction of the anterior cruciate ligament with human allograft: comparison of early and late results. *J Bone Joint Surg* 1996, 78(suppl A):524–537.

33. Tierney GS, Wright RW, Smith JP, Fischer DA: Anterior cruciate ligament reconstruction as an outpatient procedure. *Am J Sports Med* 1995, 23:755–756.

34. Pritchard JC, Drez D, Moss M, Heck S: Long-term followup of anterior cruciate ligament reconstruction using freeze-dried fascia lata allografts. *Am J Sports Med* 1995, 23:593–596.

35. Defrere J, Franckart A: Freeze-dried fascia lata allografts in the reconstruction of anterior cruciate ligament defects. *Clin Orthop* 1994, 303:56–66.

36. Andrews M, Noyes FR, Barber-Westin SD: Anterior cruciate ligament allograft reconstruction in the skeletally immature athlete. *Am J Sports Med* 1994, 22:48–54.

37. Fanelli GC, Giannotti BF, Edson CJ: Arthroscopically assisted combined posterior cruciate ligament/posterior lateral complex reconstruction. *Arthroscopy* 1996, 12:521–530.

38. Fanelli GC, Giannotti BF, Edson CJ: Arthroscopically assisted combined anterior and posterior cruciate ligament reconstruction. *Arthroscopy* 1996, 12:5–14.

39. Harner CD, Safran MR: Revision ACL surgery: technique and results utilizing allografts. In *Instructional Course Lectures* 1996:407–415.

40. Noyes FR, Barber-Westin SD: Revision anterior cruciate ligament surgery: experience from Cincinnati. *Clin Orthop* 1996, 325:116–129.

41. Noyes FR, Barber-Westin SD, Roberts CS: Use of allografts after failed treatment of rupture of the anterior cruciate ligament. *J Bone Joint Surg* 1994, 76(suppl A):1019–1031.

42. Uribe JW, Hechtman KS, Zvijac JE, Tjin-A-Tsoi EW: Revision anterior cruciate ligament surgery: experience from Miami. *Clin Orthop* 1996, 325:91–99.

43. Horibe S, Shino K, Nagano J, *et al.*: Replacing the medial collateral ligament with an allogenic tendon graft: an experimental canine study. *J Bone Joint Surg* 1990, 72(suppl B):1044–1049.

44. Veltri DM, Warren RF: AAOS instructional course lecture: posterolateral instability of the knee. *J Bone Joint Surg* 1994, 76(suppl A):460–472.

45. Sterling JC, Meyers MC, Calvo RD: Allograft failure in cruciate ligament reconstruction: follow-up evaluation of eighteen patients. *Am J Sports Med* 1995, 23:173–178.

46. Port J, Jackson DW: Posterior cruciate ligement arthroscopic techniques. In *Current Techniques in Arthroscopy*, edn 2. Philadelphia: Current Medicine; 1996:89–106.

7
CHAPTER

Arthroscopic Rotator Cuff Repair Using the Giant-Needle Technique

Basim A. Fleega

Neer's [1,2] technique of subacromial decompression and the rotator cuff repair as described by Mc Laughlin [3] have proven successful in decreasing pain and restoring function [4–6], becoming the standard open surgical treatment for repair of rotator cuff tears. Despite the reported high success rate, this technique does have limitations, such as deltoid function deficits [7–9], rehabilitation problems, and some function restrictions. These are all disadvantages to the approach, but not to the repair itself.

Limiting invasiveness of the surgical procedure can solve particular problems in treating rotator cuff tears in athletes and elderly patients [10]. Ellman [11] popularized arthroscopic subacromial decompression, which has proven to be successful in treating the most common cause of cuff tear. One inherent diffi-

culty is assessing the amount of bone to be removed using decompression.

Arthroscopic stapling of small rotator cuff tears has been described recently [12,13], but staple impingement problems and poor fixation remain major problems [14,15]. The use of a suture anchor for arthroscopic repair of small tears was popularized by some authors [16]. Considerations of anchor fixation in a cancellous bony trough [17] and technical difficulty [18] are other disadvantages of using the suture anchor. None of these techniques has dealt with large rotator cuff tears.

The limitations of open procedures include a somewhat difficult rehabilitation, some functional restriction, advanced age as a contraindication because of possible surgical trauma, the low percentage of athletic patients who return to the preinjury level of performance, and the absence of an arthroscopic procedure dealing with all sizes of cuff tears. These limitations compelled the author to develop the arthroscopic giant-needle technique of rotator cuff repair in 1989. A report discussing it was published in 1993 [19].

The goal was to establish a guideline for the amount of bone to be removed by subacromial decompression and to create an arthroscopic technique that allows the same type of repair to be performed as that used in open procedures. In addition, the goal was to achieve the same success rate as that in open repair while adding the advantages inherent in minimally invasive surgery and the results of many years of previous experience with open repair [20–22].

IDENTIFICATION OF THE CAUSE OF TEAR

Before operating on the shoulder for rotator cuff lesions, it is important to understand the cause of the tear that will be treated. In the literature [23] and in the author's experience [6], 95% of rotator cuff tears are caused by outlet impingement, and fewer than 5% result from trauma.

Most of the confusion in the literature regarding the amount of bone to be removed arthroscopically in treating impingement through decompression is due to the fact that all studies [24,25] have dealt with the acromion geometry in work on cadavers and in radiologic studies. No consideration was given to the narrowing that exists between the anterior acromion and the cuff, where the actual pathology of impingement takes place (ie, the impingement space), regardless of the type or shape of the acromion. Moreover, there was no attention paid to the great possibilities of arthroscopy in establishing standards for the classification of the impingement-space narrowing.

In 1993, arthroscopic classification of the causes and stages of outlet impingement was first divided into superior and inferior causes that lead to narrowing of the impingement space, that is, the space between the anterior acromion and the rotator cuff (the anterior acromion cuff [AAC] space) [26].

The main superior causes of impingement-space narrowing leading to cuff tear are anterior acromial spur, hooked acromion, increased slope of the acromion, prominences of the acromioclavicular (AC) joint and, rarely, impaired scapular rotation, unfused anterior acromial epiphysis, and malunion and nonunion of the acromion. Inferior causes leading to impingement-space narrowing are mainly instability impingement leading to mechanical narrowing on

elevation [27] and hypertrophy of the rotator cuff, mainly in athletes. Other rare causes of tears are single injury, repetitive microtrauma, and glenohumeral dislocation in patients older than 40 years of age [28].

IDENTIFICATION OF THE STAGE OF SUBACROMIAL NARROWING (ANTERIOR ACROMION CUFF CLASSIFICATION)

A system based on measuring the distance between the anterior acromion and the rotator cuff in 410 cases of subacromial arthroscopy using a special measuring needle, with the patient in an 80° sitting position, was used to develop an arthroscopic classification of the impingement space [29]. No impingement pathology was found in an AAC space of more than 1.2 cm, except in cases of instability impingement. Type I narrowing has a space greater than 0.5 cm and less than 1.2 cm, and type II, less than 0.5 cm. In type III narrowing, the anterior acromion lies immediately on the cuff so that the measuring needle cannot be seen.

A total of 75% of rotator cuff tears presented in stage III narrowing, 20% in stage II, and 5% in stage I. No tear was found in type 0 narrowing (ie, more than 1.2 cm). The goal of decompression is to remove bone from the undersurface of the anterior acromion to produce a space without impingement, which is greater than 1.2 cm.

TEAR CLASSIFICATION (INVOLVED TENDON AND SIZE SYSTEM)

Several classification systems have been used to describe rotator cuff disease. They are mainly based on the pathologic anatomy [3,30], size of the defect [31], configuration of the defect [32], and arthroscopic appearance of the cuff tear [12,33]. The classification used by the author depends on evaluating the size of the defect, with relation to shoulder size and the nature of tendinous involvement (involved tendon and size [ITS]). The author classifies tears as follows: small tears involve one tendon alone without retraction; medium-sized tears involve one or two tendons with retraction of one tendon (usually the supraspinatus in the case of impingement cuff tear); and large or massive tears involve two or more tendons with a retraction reaching the glenoid rim [6].

This classification system takes into account the size of the shoulder. In a classification system determined by measurement only, whereas a tear larger than 2 cm can involve two tendons in a small shoulder, it can be localized in only one tendon in a larger shoulder.

SET-UP
Patient Positioning

The patient is placed in an 80° sitting position with the acromion approximately parallel to the floor and the arm hanging freely (Fig. 7-1). This position allows the greatest possible manipulation of the shoulder in all directions in order to bring the involved tendon under the instrumentation portal for the repair as external rotation and flexion for repair of the subscapularis, internal rotation and extension for the infraspinatus, and neutral rotation for the supraspinatus. In addition, it has the advantage of providing a comparable view to that of the supraspinatus outlet radiographic view, which is a great help during surgery for decompression.

Portals

Three standard portals are used for shoulder arthroscopy (*see* Fig. 7-1): 1) the posterior lateral portal is placed 1 cm inferior and 1 cm anterior to the posterior angle of the acromion for the arthroscope; 2) the posterior portal is placed 1.5 cm medial and 1.5 cm inferior to the posterior angle of the acromion and is used for an accessory inflow cannula, as well as for evaluation of the glenohumeral joint; and 3) the anterior lateral portal is placed 3 to 4 cm inferior and lateral to the acromion at the same level as the

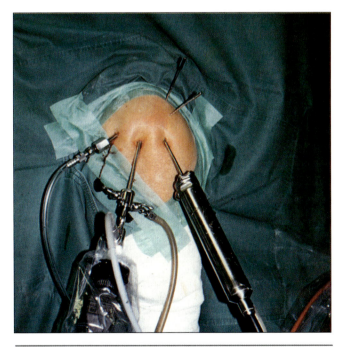

Figure 7-1. Subacromial arthroscopy with the arm hanging free in the sitting position. The portals shown are, from anterior to posterior, the lateral anterior portal for instrumentation, the lateral posterior portal for the arthroscope, and the posterior portal for the water inflow cannula. Two measuring needles are placed as guides for decompression of the anterior acromion cuff space.

supraspinatus (*ie*, important for tying the knots). This portal is used for surgical instrumentation.

Instrumentation

The instruments used for this technique are the standard 30° arthroscope; an infusion pump; an electrosurgical pencil; a shaver with a 4.5-mm full-radius blade and a 4-mm abrader; a needle that measures the impingement space; and the author's Rotator Cuff Repair Systems Instrumentation (Aeratec, Uniondale, NY) (Fig. 7-2). The latter includes a giant-needle special holder; a bone-cutting giant needle with #2 absorbable sutures (two different colors); soft-tissue giant needles with #2 absorbable sutures (two different colors); chop-needles set; punch needle with #2 absorbable suture for subscapularis repair; giant-needle guide; punch-needle guide; concave knot-pushing device; and convex knot-pushing device. Additional instruments include an arthroscopy punch, a standard arthroscopic hook, a small sharp elevator, and a giant-needle holder.

TREATMENT OF TEAR ETIOLOGY
Standarized Arthroscopic Subacromial Decompression

The patient is placed in a sitting position, as previously described. First, an arthroscopic evaluation of the glenohumeral joint through the posterior portal is made. The arthroscope is then reinserted through the posterior lateral portal. Two impingement-space special measuring needles are placed under arthroscopic visualization, outlining the acromial attachment of the coracoacromial ligament (CAL), and measuring the impingement space. The medial needle is inserted in front of the acromion, just anterior and 1 mm lateral to the AC joint; the lateral needle is inserted at the anterolateral angle of the acromion (*see* Fig. 7-1). Any debris or bursal tissue that obstructs viewing is removed with a 4.5-mm shaver inserted through the instrumentation portal.

The impingement space (*ie*, space between the anterior acromion and cuff) is measured and documented. An electrosurgical cutting tool is used to resect the CAL, beginning at the medial pin and continuing in a straight line toward the lateral pin. A sharp-cutting shaver blade inserted through the lateral instrumentation portal is used to remove all soft tissue and periosteum from the undersurface of the anterior acromion. The bony resection is begun with a high-speed acromionizer or ball burr. The burring is started laterally approximately 1.5 cm posterior to the anterior edge of the acromion, moving anteriorly with parallel lines to resect the lower surface of the anterior acromion in a wedge-shaped form with the base positioned anteriorly. The burring proceeds to reach a complete flat surface with a type 0 impingement-space narrowing, which is a space greater than 1.2 mm, as measured with the measuring needles.

If there is an increased slope of the acromion or rotator cuff hypertrophy causing narrowing of the impingement subacromial space, decompression to produce type 0 space can affect the anterior deltoid, such that a gap is formed between it and the remainder of the anterior acromion. In this case, a reconstruction of the anterior deltoid with the soft-tissue giant needle (as described later in this chapter) is needed.

Treatment of Concomitant Pathology

Prominence of the undersurface of the AC joint may encroach on the supraspinatus tendon and must be removed with the burr so that it is beveled with the undersurface of the anterior acromion. In the presence of painful arthritis of the AC joint (determined preoperatively), 1.5 cm of the distal clavicle is resected arthroscopically with a burr approached through an anterior medial portal [34]. If instability is present, an arthroscopic inferior capsular shift is made to stabilize the glenohumeral joint [35], with postoperative immobilization for 3 weeks.

ARTHROSCOPIC REPAIR OF THE ROTATOR CUFF
Mobilization

The pattern of rotator cuff tears depends on determining forces. As the subscapularis pulls part of the supraspinatus remains anteriorly, the infraspinatus and teres minor pull the posterior part of the supraspinatus tendon posteriorly, and the supraspinatus muscle exerts a medial force on the apex of the tear. Understanding this concept helps greatly when mobilizing a tendon for repair.

After removal of adhesions around the cuff, as described previously, most primary tears of the cuff can be closed using the giant-needle technique. In some cases, dividing the coracohumeral ligament from the base of the coracoid and, when necessary, dividing the capsule inside the joint to allow displacement of the tendon and capsule laterally and cephalad, may be necessary to achieve a closure of the tear. For mobilization purposes, an arthroscopy scissor or punch and a small arthroscopic rasp may be required.

Techniques of Repair

The giant-needle technique is mainly used in cuff repair. In some cases, other tools, such as chop needles or punch needle, are needed. The rationale of the giant-needle technique is to use special needles (giant

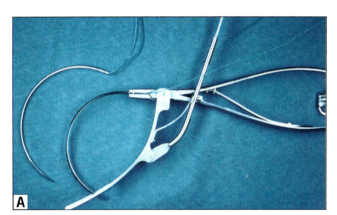

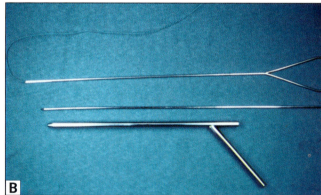

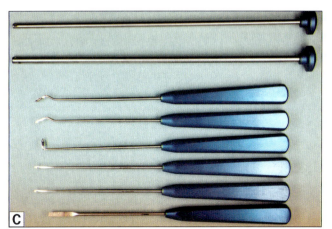

Figure 7-2. Instruments used for rotator cuff repair (Aeratec Co, Uniondale, NY). **A,** Giant needles. **B,** The punch needle (*top*), the Kirschner wire (*middle*), and the punch-needle guide (*bottom*). **C,** The knot-pushing device (*top*), the convex knot-pushing device (*second from top*), the chop-needle set (*middle five devices*), and the sharp elevator (*bottom*). (*Courtesy of* Aeratec Co.)

needles) with sutures to pass through tendon and bone or from tendon to tendon. The needle is not restricted by any portal and simply passes through skin, tendon, and bone in one step. Tying the knots is achieved in another step. No hardware implants are used, and the technique is relatively simple.

Giant-Needle Technique for Tendon-to-Bone Repair

Depending on the size of the tear, a 0.5-cm wide bone trough is made on the greater tuberosity, where the tendons have been detached, using a 4-mm burr.

Punctures are made in the trough with an arthroscopy hook to mark the point of entry of the giant needle, usually at 5-cm intervals.

With slight abduction of the arm, the tendon stump is brought in contact with the trough (Fig. 7-3). In this position, using the special needle holder, the bone-cutting giant needle is passed through the skin in front of the acromion, through the tendon, through the trough, and out through the lateral cortical surface (Fig. 7-4). If there is an infraspinatus tear, the needle is passed medial to the acromion.

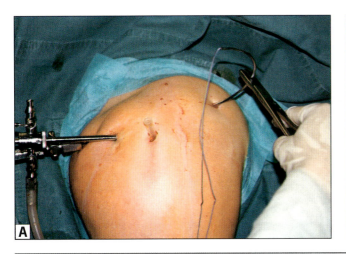
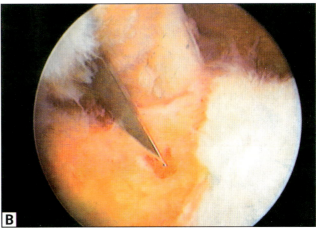

Figure 7-3. Outside (**A**) and arthroscopic (**B**) views of the giant needle being passed through the skin in front of the acromion, through the tendon, and through the trough.

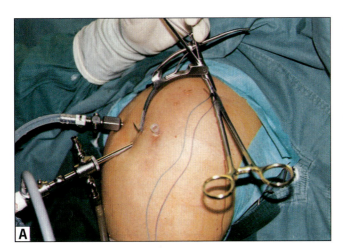
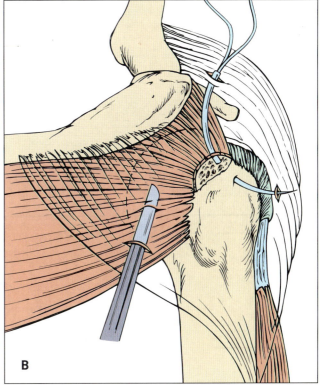

Figure 7-4. Outside (**A**) and schematic (**B**) views of the needle being pulled out through the shaft and skin. The needle tip is pointed with the needle guide.

In most cases, the needle passes through the deltoid to be visualized through the skin. The needle is pulled out, and the sutures are cut from their attachment to the needle outside the shoulder. If the tip of the needle is not visualized through the skin, the needle guide is fixed to the proximal end of the giant needle, and the skin pusher arm is brought down, pushing the skin medially so the tip can be visualized (*see* Fig. 7-4).

When the tear is small, the lower and upper limbs of the suture are pulled out through the instrumentation portal, and a sliding Niky knot is created to close the defect (Fig. 7-5).

When the tear is large, a second bone-cutting giant needle is placed through the tendon as well as through the bony trough 5 mm posterior to the first one (Fig. 7-6) to prepare for creating a "giant-needle complex" (one mattress suture and two simple

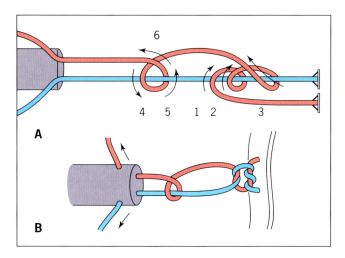

Figure 7-5. Technique of tying the arthroscopic Niky knot. **A,** Two overhand half hitches are made on the primary post. 1) and 2), Two overhand hitches are made by moving over up, over down, under up, and through. 3) to 6) The knot is pushed inside. **B,** Using the initial post for security, a second step creates a half hitch.

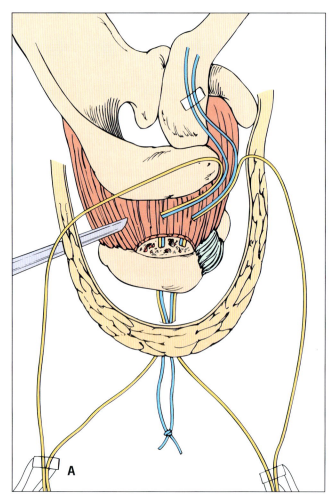

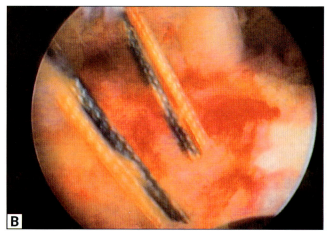

Figure 7-6. The second needle is placed through the trough (**A**) and the lower limbs of the two suture pairs are pulled out through the instrumentation portal from the space between the shaft and the deltoid. A knot is then made outside the joint for the lower part of the mattress suture (**B**).

sutures). Two different-colored sutures are passed with each needle. The lower limbs of the suture are pulled out through the instrumentation portal with a hook. The lower ends are held under tension to help in locating them with the hook.

To create the lower part of the mattress suture, two lower limb sutures of the same color (one from each pair of sutures) are tied together tightly with a secure square knot, followed by several additional throws. The knot is then approximated to the cortical surface of the humeral shaft by placing tension on the upper limbs of the sutures (*see* Fig. 7-6).

The upper strand of the anterior simple suture is pulled out superior to the tendon through the instrumentation portal with a hook. Using the small concave knot pusher, a Niky sliding knot is used to tie the anterior simple suture in slight abduction (Fig. 7-7). The second upper strand of the posterior simple suture is then tied after taking a similar course. Two simple sutures (anterior and posterior) are then created. The upper strands of the mattress suture are then pulled out from the subacromial space through the instrumentation portal and tied, using the convex knot pusher to

produce a square knot on the tendon to complete the circle of the mattress suture and firmly embed the cuff in the trough (Fig. 7-8).

The two simple sutures are used to coapt the tendon to the head while the mattress suture firmly affixes the tendon to the bleeding bony trough (Fig. 7-9).

Punch-Needle Technique for Subscapularis Repair

The punch-needle technique (*see* Fig. 7-2*B*) is used only in very rare cases of subscapularis repair. A 4-mm trough is made at the place of insertion of the tendon on the humerus. A 2.4-mm Kirschner wire is passed through the punch guide, through the upper part of the tendon, through the head, and out posteriorly through the skin.

The guide is removed, and a second Kirschner wire is passed in the same manner, approximately 1.5 cm below the first. The lower wire is removed, and a punch needle with a suture is passed through posteriorly; the other suture is then passed in the same way. The posterior limbs are then pulled out through the instrumentation portal, and a knot is made and pulled

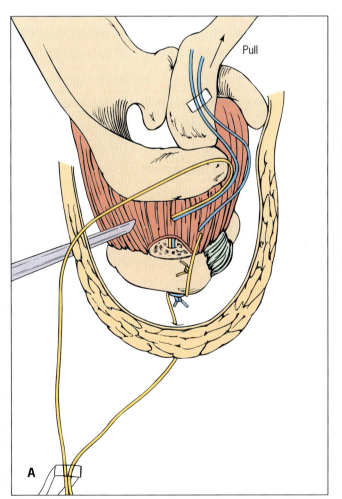

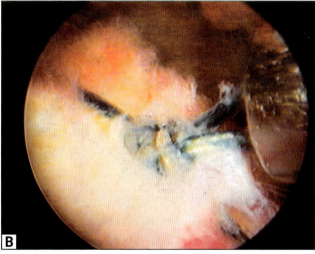

Figure 7-7. Schematic (**A**) and arthroscopic (**B**) views of the upper limbs of the mattress suture being pulled up to place the knot on the shaft. With a probe, the upper limb of the anterior simple suture is pulled out through the instrumentation portal, and the anterior simple suture is tied with a Niky knot.

through the anterior limbs to lie on the infraspinatus or shaft. Next, the anterior limbs are tied to form a mattress suture in the same fashion as that used in the giant-needle mattress repair.

Soft-Tissue Giant-Needle Technique for End-to-End Repair

The soft-tissue giant needle is used to repair small longitudinal tears lying medial to the insertion of the tendon on the humeral head or to close open rotator cuff intervals. The giant needle is passed through the skin and deltoid anterior to the acromion. Then, under arthroscopic visualization, it is passed through one end of the tendon defect and up through the other end, coming out through the deltoid and skin posteriorly. The suture limbs are then retrieved from the subacromial space through the instrumentation portal, and a tied knot is tightened using a knot pusher.

If a defect is created at the origin of the anterior deltoid from the acromion after decompression, repair is done using one or two soft-tissue giant needles. The needles are passed through the skin and deltoid under arthroscopic view about 2 cm distal to the proximal deltoid edge and up through the periosteum at its junction with the upper edge of the residual anterior acromion, and out through the skin cephalad. Next, an arthroscopy hook is passed anteriorly through this latter needle outlet deep to the subcutaneous tissue to reach the inferior suture limb at its passage between the subcutaneous tissue and the deltoid, and the suture limb is pulled out through the skin needle exit. The two strands are then tied using the Niky sliding knot to reattach the deltoid and close the gap.

Chop-Needle Technique

Chop-needle repair is used for tears that cannot be reached with the giant needle, such as medial tears above the upper glenoid rim and low infraspinatus or subscapularis tears. It is also used for placing stay sutures for tendon mobilization in some patients.

The chop-needle technique is applied in rare cases of massive tears in order to pass the suture through both ends of the tendon. This is done by using the suture pusher to pass the suture through one side of one tendon (eg, subscapularis and remainder of the supraspinatus), and then with the suture catcher, pulling the suture through the other tendon (eg, infraspinatus). After passing the suture through both sides, the two strands are pulled out through the instrumentation portal, at which point a knot is made and pushed to tie the two ends of the cuff together (Fig. 7-10).

Large and Massive Tears
Medial Closure

When there is a massive tear, the tendons usually can be brought together through mobilization as described previously. In medially extended tears, sutures are

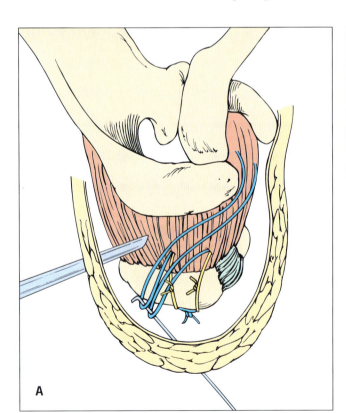

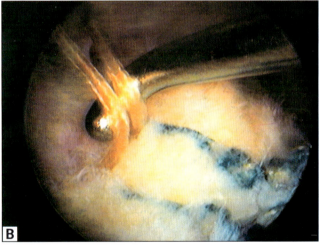

Figure 7-8. After the two simple sutures are tied, the upper limbs of the mattress sutures are pulled out through the instrumentation portal. Schematic (**A**) and arthroscopic (**B**) views.

created using tendon end-to-end chop-needle repair and then pulled laterally and tied to the greater tuberosity using the giant-needle technique (*see* Fig. 7-10).

Subscapularis Transfer

In rare cases, a transfer of the upper part of the subscapularis tendon and realignment and incorporation of the long head of the biceps may be neces-

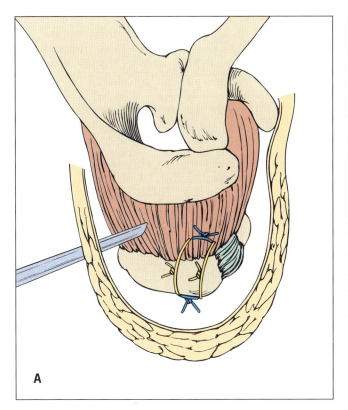

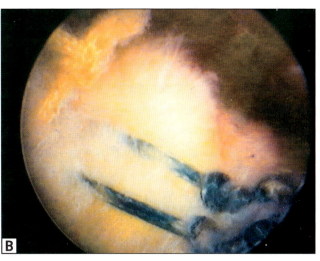

Figure 7-9. Using a square knot and several additional throws, a Niky knot is made to complete the tying of the mattress suture. The giant-needle complex is now completed with one mattress and two simple sutures. Schematic (**A**) and arthroscopic (**B**) views.

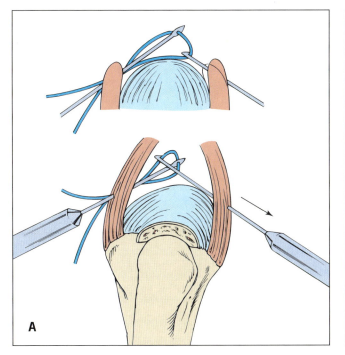

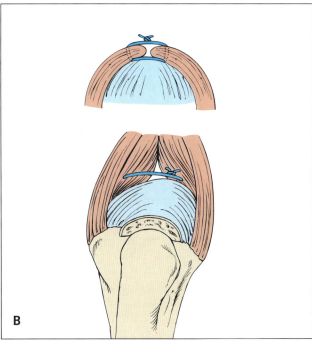

Figure 7-10. Chop-needle repair technique. The suture pusher passes the suture through one end of the tendon, and the puller pulls the suture through the other end (**A**) after the Niky knot is tied (**B**).

sary. At approximately 30° abduction and external rotation, the upper third of the subscapularis is cut from its insertion with a punch or electrocautery device, held with a stay suture placed with the chop needles, and brought cephalad over the biceps tendon (if present) to a trough made at the insertion of the supraspinatus posterior to the biceps sulcus. There, it is attached to the greater tuberosity with the bone-cutting giant needle using the giant-needle complex repair process, and then to the infraspinatus or the remains of supraspinatus using the soft-tissue giant needle or chop needles. Repair is then completed by tying the supraspinatus and infraspinatus remains to the bony trough using the giant-needle complex tendon-to-bone repair (Fig. 7-11).

Biceps Incorporation

If transfer of the subscapularis and infraspinatus is insufficient to close the defect, the long head of the biceps may be incorporated into the repair process. Using the giant-needle complex technique for fixation, the long head of the biceps is tenodesed in a slot prepared with a ball burr about 1 cm posterior to the bicipital groove. The subscapularis and infraspinatus tendons are then sewn to it using the soft-tissue giant needle (Fig. 7-12).

Biceps Rupture

In acute proximal biceps tendon ruptures, some patients want to have a rotator cuff and biceps repair during the same procedure. The stump of the biceps is palpated, and a 3-cm incision is made longitudinally. The stump is freed from adhesion, and stay sutures are placed. An arthroscopic hook is passed under arthroscopic visualization through the bicipital sulcus in the joint down to the incision. The stay sutures are pulled up to bring the tendon to the sulcus, which has been previously roughened with a burr. The stump is then fixed to the head using the giant-needle complex repair.

Incomplete Partial Tear

Partial tears are detected with the use of a blunt cuff-thickness detector instrument to palpate small holes in the continuity of the tendon. When more than half of the thickness of the tendon is torn, the partially torn area of the cuff is resected with a shaver, and the defect is then closed using the giant-needle technique.

Niky Knot

The Niky knot is a one-step sliding knot with two half-hitches and one hitch in the opposite direction. It is formed outside the shoulder and advanced down

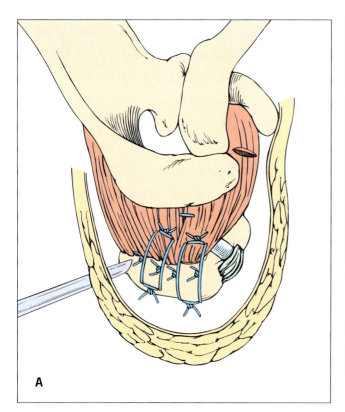

A

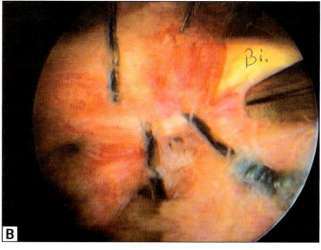

B

Figure 7-11. Transfer of the subscapularis. The upper third of the subscapularis is resected from its insertion and pulled up with the stay sutures. Using the giant needle, the subscapularis is fixed posteriorly to the biceps tendon (**A**). Using the giant-needle complex technique, the subscapularis is tied to the bony trough on the greater tuberosity as well as the remains of the supraspinatus and infraspinatus (**B**).

the post with the knot pusher and securely placed on the bone or tendon. (*see* Fig. 7-5). Using the initial post, a second half hitch is used for security. The upper limb is used as a post. The knots are created by making two overhand half hitches and moving over up, over down, under up, and through so that a half hitch is formed outside and moved down using the concave knot pusher while the post is pulled to slide in the knot. Through this one-step action, the knot cannot be loosened; the second-step half hitch provides additional security.

THE AUTHOR'S SYSTEM OF ARTHROSCOPIC ROTATOR CUFF REPAIR

In summary, the author uses the following system for arthroscopic repair of the rotator cuff: First, decompression is done to obtain type 0 impingement space. Then the undersurface of the AC joint is beveled if needed. When there is painful arthritis, AC joint resection is performed. Next, the cuff is mobilized, and its superficial surface is freed. The glenohumeral ligament and joint capsule are incised, if needed for mobilization.

Next, the cuff is closed. For small medial tears, the giant-needle end-to-end technique is used to close the cuff. For small insertional tears, the tendon-to-bone simple suture technique is used. For medium and large tears, the giant-needle complex repair (one mattress suture and two simple sutures) is used to close the cuff. For massive tears, the cuff is closed by using the chop-needle technique for medial side-to-side closure; the giant-needle technique for tendon-to-bone fixation; the giant-needle and chop-needle techniques for subscapularis transfer (if needed); the giant-needle complex technique for biceps realignment and incorporation; and the punch-needle mattress-repair technique for subscapularis repair.

After the cuff is closed, the anterior deltoid is repaired, if necessary. Use of an abduction brace is needed for 3 to 6 weeks in 10% of patients with this type of tendon repair.

RESULTS

A review was done of the clinical results at the Godesberger Orthopedic Hospital (GOC; Bonn, Germany). There were 307 consecutive cases of rotator cuff tear in 304 patients, with 6 years' follow-up with an average of 50 months. Of these, 42% were small, 29% were medium, and 29% were large and massive tears. A tendinous side-to-side repair was done in 124 shoulders, and tendon-to-bone fixation in 183. The average age of the patients was 56 years. No significant difference was found between the range of forward elevation in the operative and contralateral shoulders. Weakness was detectable by physical examination in an average of 15% of patients at time of final examination. Three patients required further

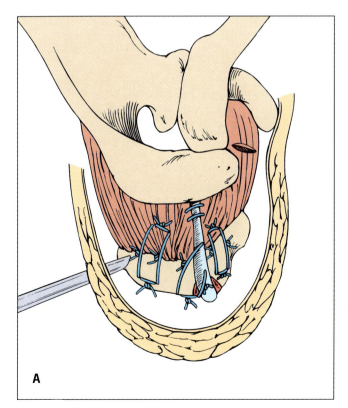

A

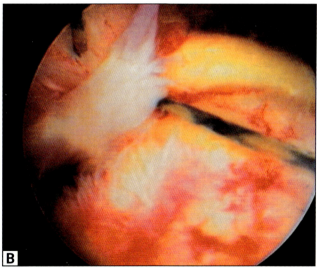

B

Figure 7-12. A, Suturing the cuff remains to the tendon. **B,** Tenodesis of the biceps tendon that will be incorporated in the repair about 1 cm posterior to the sulcus during repair of the massive tear to the tendon and tuberosity.

shoulder surgery, one for traumatic rerupture, and two for subsequent calcifications. No other significant complications were noted.

In another two patients, reconstruction was not possible because 80% of the cuff was absent. A total of 68% of the 31 active athletes in this series returned to their preinjury levels of performance. A total of 76% of the patients were very satisfied with the surgery, 21% were satisfied, and only 3% were not satisfied. Age was not a contraindication for surgery, since 9% of the patients were older than 70 years of age.

CONCLUSION

Arthroscopic rotator cuff repair using the giant chop-needle system enables the same reconstruction to be done as with the open technique, with similarly good results. The technique is simple and quick, providing good tendon-to-bone stable fixation without the types of complications found with the use of implants. It can be used to repair large tears, and in an experienced surgeon's hand, the surgery takes approximately 10 minutes to repair a medium-sized tear.

In the 1154 arthroscopic rotator cuff repairs using giant needles conducted in the GOC hospital for the period ending in December, 1996, a burr was needed in only three instances to enlarge the exit hole through the humeral shaft in order to pass the bone-cutting needle [36].

Compared with the open technique of cuff repair, a higher percentage of patients have been able to return to their previous competitive athletic levels. Age is not a contraindication using the arthroscopic giant-needle technique.

REFERENCES

1. Neer CS II: Anterior acromioplasty for the chronic impingement syndrome in the shoulder: a preliminary report. *J Bone Joint Surg* 1972, 54(suppl A):41–50.

2. Neer CS II: Impingement lesions.*ClinOrthop* 1983, 173:70.

3. McLaughlin HL: Lesions of musculotendinous cuff of the shoulder. I The exposure and treatment of tears with retraction. *J Bone Joint Surg Am* 1944, 26:31–49.

4. Stuart MJ, Azevedo AJ, Cofield RH: Anterior acromioplasty for treatment of the shoulder impingement syndrome. *Clin Orthop* 1990, 260:195–200.

5. Ellman H: Diagnosis and treatment of incomplete rotator cuff tears.*Clin Orthop* 1990, 254:64–74.

6. Fleega B: Late results of reconstruction of large and massive rotator cuff tears. A 10 years follow-up. Paper presented at the American Shoulder and Elbow Surgeons Tenth Open Meeting. New Orleans, LA; 1994.

7. Neer CS: Reoperations of failed cuff repairs. Paper presented at the Closed Meeting of the American Shoulder and Elbow Surgeons; October, 1987.

8. Adamson GJ, Tibone JE: Ten-year assessment of primary rotator cuff repairs. *Shoulder Elbow Surg* 1993, 2:57–63.

9. Post MN, Silver R, Manmohan S: Rotator cuff tear: diagnosis and treatment. *Clin Orthop Rel Res* 1983, 173:78–91.

10. Gachter A, Sellig W: Arthroscopy of the shoulder joint. *Arthroscopy* 1992, 8:89–97.

11. Ellman H. Arthroscopic subacromial decompression. *Arthroscopy* 1987, 3:173.

12. Snyder SJ, Petee GA: Shoulder arthroscopy in the evaluation and treatment of rotator cuff lesions.*Techniques Orthop* 1988, 3:47–58.

13. Johnson LL: *Arthroscopy Surgery: Principles and Practice*. St. Louis: Mosby; 1986:1301–1445.

14. France EP, Paulos LE, Harner CD, Straight CB: Biomechanical evaluation of rotator cuff fixation methods. *Am J Sports Med* 1989, 17:176–181.

15. Paulos LE, France EP, Harner CD, Straight CB: Biomechanical evaluation of rotator cuff fixation methods. Paper presented at the 34th Annual meeting of the Orthopedic Research Society. Atlanta, GA; 1988.

16. Bartlett E: Arthroscopic evaluation and treatment of rotator cuff pathology. Paper presented at Arthroscopy Association of North America Annual Meeting Instructional Course. Palm Desert, CA; April, 1993.

17. Wolf EM: Arthroscopic rotator cuff repair. Paper presented at Arthroscopy Association of North America Annual Meeting. San Francisco, CA; 1997.

18. Matthews LS: Arthroscopic assisted rotator cuff repair. Paper presented at Arthroscopy Association of North America Annual Meeting. San Francisco, CA; 1997.

19. Fleega BA: A new method of arthroscopic reconstruction of full thickness rotator cuff ruptures. Proceedings of the 7th Congress of the European Society for Surgery of the Shoulder and Elbow. Aarhus, Denmark; 1993.

20. Fleega BA: Arthroscopic translation of open reconstruction of rotator cuff ruptures: 2-5 years follow-up. *J Shoulder Elbow Surg* 1996, 5(suppl):100.

21. Fleega BA: Arthroscopic closing of massive tears of the rotator cuff. *J Shoulder Elbow Surg* 1996, 5(suppl):72–73.

22. Fleega BA: Comparison of arthroscopic reconstruction with open surgical closing of massive tears of the rotator cuff. *J Shoulder Elbow Surg* 1996, 5(suppl):63–64.

23. Neer CS, Flatow EL, Lech O: Tears of the rotator cuff: long term results of anterior acromioplasty and repair. Paper presented at the American Shoulder and Elbow Surgeons Society Open Meeting. Atlanta, GA; 1988.

24. Morrison DS, Bigliani LU: The clinical significance of variation in acromial morphology. Paper presented at the AAOS Specialty Day Meeting, American Shoulder and Elbow Surgeons. San Francisco, CA; January, 1987.

25. Aoki M, Ishi S, Usui M, *et al*.: The slope of the acromion and rotator cuff tear. Anatomical Study by cadaver specimens. Proceedings of the Third International Conference on Surgery of the Shoulder. Fukuoka, Japan; 1986.

26. Fleega BA: Arthroscopic classification of impingement syndrome. Proceedings of the 7th Congress of the European Society for Surgery of the Shoulder and Elbow. Aarhus, Denmark; June, 1993.

27. Fleega BA: Treatment of secondary impingement due to anterior instability and results of surgical treatment in athletes: new arthroscopic classification. Paper presented at the 6th International Congress on Surgery of the Shoulder (ICSS). Helsinki, Finland and Stockholm, Sweden; 1995.

28. Fleega BA: Glenohumeral joint instability, anatomical classification and comparative study of the surgical repair. Paper presented at the Combined Meeting of the Third International Conference on Surgery of the Shoulder and 13th Annual Meeting of Japan Shoulder Society; October, 1986.

29. Fleega BA: Pathology of the subacromial space and its relation to impingement syndrome. *J Bone Joint Surg* 1996, 5(suppl):104.

30. Bosworth DM: An analysis of twenty-eight consecutive cases of incapacitating shoulder lesions, radically explored and repaired. *J Bone Joint Surg* 1940, 22:369–392.

31. Cofield RH: Subscapular muscle transportation for repair of chronic rotator cuff tears. *Surg Gynecol Obstet* 1982, 154:667–672.

32. Leffert RD, Rowe CR: Tendon rupture. In *The Shoulder*. Edited by Rowe CR. New York: Churchill Livingstone; 1988:131–154.

33. Snyder SJ: Evaluation and treatment of the rotator cuff. *Orthop Clin North Am* 1993, 24:173–192.

34. Fleega BA: Arthroscopic resection of the lateral end of the clavicle for osteoarthritis: 5 years follow-up. Paper presented at the 6th International Congress on Surgery of the Shoulder (ICSS). Helsinki, Finland and Stockholm, Sweden; 1995.

35. Fleega BA: T-arthroscopic t-shaped inferior capsular shift of the shoulder for recurrent anterior instability. Paper presented at the ISAKOS Biennial Congress. Buenos Aires, Argentina; May, 1997.

36. Fleega BA: The giant needle rotator cuff repair system technique and results. Paper presented at EFORT, III Congress. Barcelona, Spain; April, 1997.

8

Suture Anchors: An Update

KEVIN P. SHEA

The surgical attachment of soft tissue to bone is one of the most important surgical techniques practiced by the orthopedic surgeon. Traditionally, soft tissue has been surgically attached to bone by drilling one or more holes through bone, passing sutures through these holes, and passing the free ends of suture through soft tissue. Although this method was largely successful, several difficulties are associated with it. It is well accepted that drilling holes in the anterior aspect of the glenoid to reattach the labrum (the modified Bankart procedure) added 45 minutes to 1 hour to the procedure. In many other procedures, widening of the surgical exposure was necessary in order to drill holes through bone. The quality of bone can be poor, and the drilling of holes can irreparably damage the bone, such as in the repair of some massive rotator cuff

tears, thus weakening the repair. Finally, if the suture pulled out of the bone tunnel or broke during knot tying, the surgeon had to remove all previously tied sutures and begin again.

Metallic staples and screws, placed either arthroscopically or open, were developed to improve the ease with which soft tissue could be attached to bone [1,2]. In theory, less surgical exposure was required to insert staples and screws compared with drilling transosseous holes, and suture breakage was not an issue. The soft tissue was simply placed over the bony attachment site, and the screw or staple inserted through the tissue and imbedded into bone. However, Matthews *et al.* [3] and others noted that metallic staples had a high rate of loosening, becoming intra-articular bodies resulting in articular damage. Additionally, Shea *et al.* [4] documented that staple repairs had a significantly decreased initial pull-out strength when compared with suture repairs in a Bankart repair model.

A new class of surgical implants, suture anchors, were developed in response to the difficulties with suture passage through bone tunnels and to the failures of metallic screws and staples [5]. In general, a suture anchor consists of an implant (with an attached suture), which is secured into bone by some means. The suture is then passed through the soft tissue, and the knot is tied. In theory, suture anchors eliminate the need for large surgical exposure for the drilling of transosseous holes and are implanted entirely in bone, greatly lessening the possibility of their loosening and becoming free in the joint. Many of the newer arthroscopic reconstructive procedures, in particular arthroscopic shoulder stabilization and arthroscopic rotator cuff repair, are now possible only with the use of suture anchors.

At present, with more than 30 suture anchors available to the orthopedic surgeon, this chapter aims not to advocate one design over another, but instead to give the surgeon a framework on which to base his or her choice in selecting a suture anchor for surgical implantation.

MECHANICAL DESIGN

Suture anchors come in a variety of designs and are made of several different materials. Although no optimal suture anchor design exists, an understanding of the advantages and disadvantages of each of these design considerations should assist the surgeon in selecting the optimal suture anchor for implantation during a given surgery. Most of the suture anchors available to the surgeon today are of two general types: pound-in anchors and screw-in anchors. Each design characteristic has it own inherent good and bad characteristics.

Pound-in Anchors

It is estimated that more than 70% of the anchors in use today are of the "pound-in" type. These anchors are designed to be inserted into either cortical or cancellous bone, usually after a pilot hole of a small diameter has been drilled. Each anchor has some design feature that, after being pounded into the pilot hole, resists pullout. The design features are typically external ribs or barbs on the outside of the anchor, which interdigitate with the bone after insertion (Fig. 8-1). Other anchors "deploy" or expand by some mechanism after insertion into the pilot hole. The expanded portion of the anchor then provides resistance to pulling out of bone. Each anchor has an eyelet through which the suture is passed before insertion. Every eyelet accommodates a single #1 or #2 suture, although some accommodate two or more sutures. The suture should easily slide back and forth through the eyelet after being inserted. If it does not, the suture is more likely to break during knot tying, particularly when knots are tied arthroscopically.

Pound-in anchors have several advantages. They are relatively simple to use. A pilot hole is drilled, and then the suture anchor is gently impacted into the bone. Probably the most important advantage, however, may be that the suture can be passed once through the soft tissue and then passed through a suture anchor before implantation. Although this technical consideration is not of great value in performing open surgery, it can be of distinct advantage in arthroscopic reconstruction. After the pilot hole has been drilled in the desired location in bone, many instruments are available that can easily pass a monofilament suture, either absorbable or nonabsorbable, through a desired location in soft tissue. The suture can then be brought back out through an arthroscopic cannula and passed through the eyelet of the suture anchor. The anchor is placed into the hole, and the knot is tied using various techniques, securing the tissue to bone. Even though many techniques of arthroscopically passing sutures through soft tissue exist, it remains quite complicated to pass sutures through soft tissue after the anchor has been seated in bone arthroscopically (*see* further discussion later in this chapter). Newer techniques may make passing sutures through tissue easier (Fig. 8-2).

The major drawback of pound-in anchors is the inability to remove them after the anchor has been seated. Although this is usually not a problem, occasionally the suture breaks or pulls out of the eyelet, or the anchor is in the wrong place. The suture breakage

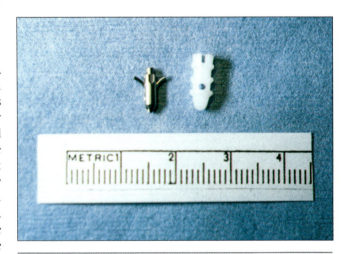

Figure 8-1. Examples of pound-in suture anchors. *Left,* TAG rod II (Smith & Nephew Endoscopy, Andover, MA) and *right,* Mitek G2 (Mitek Surgical Products, Norwood, MA). (*Courtesy of* Smith & Nephew Endoscopy and Mitek Surgical Products.)

problem is easily addressed by using an anchor that allows two sutures through its eyelet. If one breaks, one suture remains useful. Additionally, if both sutures are used, the initial failure strength of the anchor-suture-tissue repair is increased by 50% [6].

The problem of difficult removal greatly complicates the treatment of postsurgical infection. Principles of the treatment of infection require that all foreign materials, including suture and anchors, be removed at the time of initial debridement. Large defects in bone may be created when removing pound-in anchors from bone. Fortunately, postsurgical infections are rare, occurring in less than 0.3% of arthroscopic shoulder surgeries.

The pull-out strength of pound-in anchors has been extensively studied [6–8,9••,10••]. The pull-out strengths of each anchor vary widely and are determined by the type of bone in which the anchor is inserted. Barber *et al.* [7] has noted that pound-in anchors have a higher pull-out strength in cortical bone compared with cancellous bone, and the pull-out strength tends to increase inversely with the pilot

hole's diameter. Although the pull-out strength is the measure by which anchors are usually compared, it must be remembered that in attaching soft tissue to bone, the surgeon is creating a system composed of the anchor, the suture, the knot, and the soft tissue. The pull-out strength on the anchor needs only to be stronger than the other components. In fact, the system should be designed so that the tissue (the only component that the surgeon cannot completely control) is the weak link. Pull-out strength will be discussed in more detail later in this chapter.

Screw-in Anchors

The original suture anchor design was a screw-in type. It was a self-tapping, drill-in anchor with swedged-on suture [5]. Since the development of that original anchor, many other screw-in anchors have been designed (Fig. 8-3). Each has an eyelet through which sutures are passed that can accommodate one or more sutures, just like the pound-in types do. All anchors have external screw threads that resist pull-out by interdigitating with the bone after insertion. Most require a pilot hole to be drilled first; several, however, are drilled directly into bone. Although most pound-in anchors are designed for use in both cancellous or cortical bone, many screw-in anchors are intended for just one type of bone. In particular, screw-in anchors designed for use in Bankart repairs are smaller and have more threads per inch. Those used primarily for rotator cuff repairs are larger with fewer but wider threads, which provide greater resistance to pull-out in the weaker bone of the greater tuberosity of the humerus.

Screw-in anchors possess several advantages. First and foremost, screw-in suture anchors are easily removable. If the suture pulls out of the eyelet, or if the suture breaks during knot tying, the screw-in

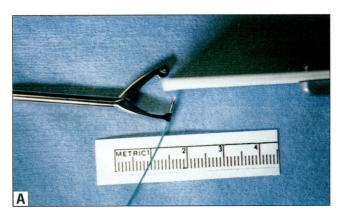

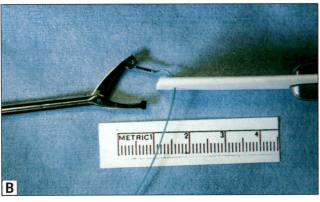

Figure 8-2. Newer suturing devices such as the Suture Punch (Smith & Nephew Endoscopy, Andover, MA) have made arthroscopic tissue repair more easily accomplished, particularly when using screw-in suture anchors. A nonabsorbable braided suture with a swedged-on needle (**A**) can easily be passed arthroscopically through tissue (**B**) after the anchor has been inserted into bone. (*Courtesy of* Smith & Nephew Endoscopy.)

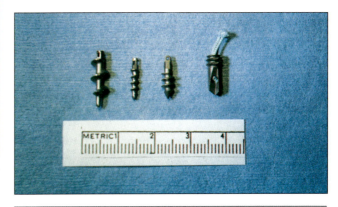

Figure 8-3. Examples of screw-in suture anchors. From *left to right*, the Corkscrew (Arthrex, Naples, FL), the Fast tack (Arthrex), the Revo (Linvatec, Largo, FL), and the Statak (Zimmer, Warsaw, IN). (*Courtesy of* Arthrex, Linvatec, and Zimmer.)

anchor can be removed, the suture rethreaded in the eyelet, and the anchor screwed back into place. Easy removal is also helpful in the event of postoperative infection.

Screw-in anchors also have disadvantages, however, particularly in arthroscopic techniques. After the pilot hole has been drilled, the screw-in suture anchor must be inserted into bone before the suture is passed through the soft tissue. After the suture anchor has been inserted, the limbs of this suture are then passed through soft tissue. If the suture is passed through the soft tissue first, the two suture limbs will twist and knot while the anchor is being screwed into place. Although this is of little consequence in open procedures, complex suturing techniques are required in order to pass the suture through soft tissue secondarily. The arthroscopic surgeon should be confident in his or her ability to pass sutures through soft tissue and to tie an arthroscopic knot before selecting a screw-in type anchor for arthroscopic use. As already stated, newer techniques of suture passage may make this technique more easily achieved for the arthroscopic surgeon (*see* Fig. 8-2).

The pull-out strength of screw-in anchors has also been studied and found to vary widely, as with the pound-in types [6–8,9••,10••]. Of some concern, when screw-in anchors pull out of bone, large holes are created at the juncture where the screw threads had engaged the bone. However, clinically, pull-out of anchors after implantation is rarely seen.

MATERIALS

Currently, suture anchors are made out of three different types of material: metals, plastics, and bioabsorbables. The pull-out strength of identical anchors of all three types of material was found to be similar in laboratory models. As with mechanical design, each material has its own advantages and disadvantages.

Metal

Most anchors on the market today are made of metal. This material gives the anchor both rigidity and flexibility, which are particularly important in pound-in anchors. The barbs on these anchors must deform and conform to the shape of the pilot hole. The metal must then have memory to spring back to its original shape to create purchase in bone. Although it was originally assumed that metal anchors would have a greater pull-out strength than anchors made out of other types of material, this has not proven to be the case. The pull-out strength of metal anchors has been shown to be statistically equal to that of plastic anchors and those made from bioabsorbable materials.

However, the breaking strength of the eyelet appears to be stronger in the metal anchors as compared with the plastic and bioabsorbable styles.

The main advantage of metal anchors is clinical. After a Bankart-type operation or rotator cuff repair, the anchors are easily visible on postoperative radiographs. If a circumstance arises in which anchor loosening is suspected, the anchor position can always be confirmed by radiographs. It appears equally likely that metallic anchors and anchors made of other materials may pull out of their bony settings.

The disadvantage of metal anchors is that if the anchor loosens and becomes an intra-articular free foreign object, damage to the articular surface of the joint can be extensive, compared with that done by loose plastic in the joint. This remains a theoretical disadvantage and has not been proven. Fortunately, loosening of anchors is rare. In addition, should tissue failure be suspected postoperatively, the metal anchor may obscure imaging studies, in particular, magnetic resonance imaging (MRI) scans, rendering decision making more difficult.

Plastic

The second largest category of suture anchors are made of high molecular weight plastics. The advantages and disadvantages of plastic anchors are the reverse of those found in metal anchors. Plastic anchors cannot be seen on a postoperative imaging study. If symptoms of grating and catching are noted postoperatively, the surgeon cannot use standard radiographic techniques to document whether the anchors have become dislodged. On the other hand, the plastic anchors may theoretically cause much less damage if they become loose in the joint.

Barber *et al.* [7] have observed that plastic anchors can be brittle and can break when being placed into the pilot hole. If anchor breakage occurs, the broken anchor should be removed and a new anchor reinserted into the pilot hole.

Bioabsorbable

The newest suture anchor materials are bioabsorbable. These anchors are composed of polymers of either polyglyconate (PGA) or polylactate (PLA) and are designed to absorb slowly over time by hydrolysis. Few clinical data are available on the performance of these anchors. Theoretically, problems related to late anchor loosening and postoperative imaging are minimized after the anchor has dissolved. However, it remains to be proven whether these anchors will maintain their holding strength long enough for soft tissue to heal. It remains uncertain how long it takes the glenoid labrum to heal back to the bony glenoid and how long it takes the rotator cuff to reliably heal back to the greater tuberosity of the humerus. Particularly in rotator cuff repair, it is unknown whether the anchor can resist inherent tension in the rotator cuff tendon long enough for the tendon to heal back to bone.

Biopolymers are even more brittle than are plastics and are easily fractured on insertion. When using pound-in bioabsorbable anchors, it is critical to exactly align the insertion tool and the anchor with the pilot hole. Any deviation of the anchor with the axis of the hole may cause breakage when inserting the anchor into bone. The threads of bioabsorbable screw-in anchors are not strong enough to be self-tapping, and most require the hole to be tapped before insertion, adding another step to the insertion technique. If the hole has not been tapped, the anchor may crack on insertion.

Other Types of Fixation Devices

Although suture anchors are by far the most popular devices for fixating tissue to bone, other devices are also available (Fig. 8-4). A bioabsorbable tack, Suretac (Smith and Nephew Endoscopy, Andover, MA), is a bioabsorbable tack intended for arthroscopic fixation of Bankart-type lesions. It is composed of a co-polymer of PGA that bioabsorbs in over a 4-week period. The tack is cannulated and put in over a guidewire into a predrilled pilot hole. The head of the tack is used to affix the soft tissue to bone. Although it is not a suture anchor in the truest sense, it is another choice for the surgeon in the treatment of Bankart-type lesions.

Biomechanically, this device has been shown to be equivalent in initial failure strength to several popular types of suture anchors [6,7]. However, as with other bioabsorbable anchors, it is not known whether or not the fixation strength lasts long enough for the labrum to heal back to the glenoid or how much strain it will resist if the labrum is put back to the glenoid under tension.

OTHER CONSIDERATIONS

Suture anchors are only one component of the soft tissue–to–bone system of fixation. In addition to the pull-out strength of the anchor, the quality of the bone into which the anchor is inserted, the technique with which the anchor is inserted, the strength of the suture and knot, and the quality of the tissue and the tension under which the tissue is attached to bone are also key factors in the success of tissue attach-

ment to bone. All components, except the fractures inherent in the quality of the tissue, are under the surgeon's control. The goal when using anchors to surgically repair tissue to bone is to optimize the strength of all controllable components, making soft tissue the weak link in the system.

Pull-out Strength

Initial pull-out strength has traditionally been the standard by which suture anchors have been compared [4–8,9••,10••]. In these studies and in other unpublished studies, the anchor or anchors being studied are inserted into bone according to the manufacturers' recommended technique, using a steel wire instead of suture. Specimens are mounted into a materials-testing machine in which the steel wire is pulled until either the eyelet of the anchor breaks or the anchor pulls out of bone. The average of several tests determines what is then termed the "pull-out strength" of the anchor. From these studies, it could be concluded that the "best" anchor is the one with the greatest pull-out strength.

Several factors should be understood when making these types of comparisons. First, the material into which the anchor is implanted varies from study to study. Ideally, the anchor should be compared in the same bone that it will be used in clinically, *ie*, the glenoid rim and greater tuberosity of the humerus, among other examples. Most studies do compare anchors in some comparable material, (*ie*, cancellous bone, cortical bone). If the "bone" or other material in which the studied anchor or anchors are compared is not directly applicable to the clinical situation, the results of the study should be ignored. Second, the failure strength in these studies represents the worst-case

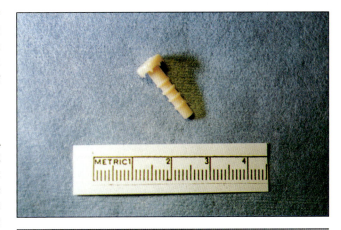

Figure 8-4. Suretac (Smith & Nephew Endoscopy, Andover, MA), a bioabsorbable device used to repair a displaced Bankart lesion to bone. (*Courtesy of* Smith & Nephew Endoscopy.)

scenario. Anchors are almost never inserted in the direct line of pull. Instead, in clinical application the direction of force in the tissue is at some angle to the long axis of the anchor. Thus, pull-out strength as noted in the studies is usually lower than that achieved in surgery. Finally, the pull-out strength is "initial" and does not represent what happens to pull-out strength with time.

When synthesizing all available data and understanding that the anchor is only one link in the system, the author recommends that an anchor should have a pull-out strength of at least 30 lbs in the type of bone in which it will be inserted clinically, that is, cancellous bone for the humerus, cortical or cortical-cancellous for the glenoid. With more than 30 lbs, some other part of the fixation system (suture or soft tissue) will fail. If the pull-out strength is at least 30 lbs under the worst-case scenario testing, the author recommends that anchors be chosen according to other criteria, such as cost or ease of insertion.

Anchor Insertion

Burkhart [10••] has studied the technique of anchor insertion extensively. He compares the soft tissue–to–bone system of fixation to a south Texas fence line. He observed that if an anchor is inserted into bone at a right angle to the repaired tissue and then tied with a vertical knot, the tissue will displace away from the anchor and the bony site intended for tissue repair (Fig. 8-5). If, however, the anchor is inserted so that the angle formed between the anchor and the suture

is less than 45°, the "deadman" angle will be optimized, and the repaired tissue will remain in the intended site for attachment.

Understanding this important principle is of vital concern when repairing a rotator cuff tear. The rotator cuff tendon has an inherent tension that tends to displace it medially. Using the "deadman" principle, if the anchor is inserted at the proper angle into bone, the edge of the tendon will remain over the debrided bony trough, and it will heal into bone. However, if the suture and anchor are vertical to the tendon, the tendon will displace medial to the bony repair site, and healing may not occur.

Suture and Knot

The ideal size and makeup of the ideal suture are largely determined by surgeon preference. Either a #1 or #2 suture is strong enough to adequately repair rotator cuff tendon or glenoid labrum to bone. As previously mentioned, if the anchor eyelet is large enough to accept two sutures, problems related to suture breakage can be minimized. Additionally, if both sutures are used, the initial failure strength of the fixation system increases by 50% [4].

Knots are more easily tied securely when a braided suture is used, in both arthroscopic and open procedures. However, most arthroscopic suture-passing devices are only capable of passing monofilament. The surgeon is again cautioned to practice arthroscopic knot tying, especially if monofilament is being used, before surgery in order to avoid complication with tissue repair techniques.

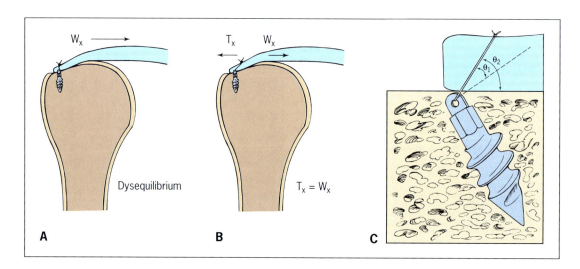

Figure 8-5. The "deadman theory" of suture anchors. If the anchor is placed directly under the repaired tissue, the inherent force (Wx) will not be balanced (**A**), causing the tissue to displace away from the anchor until the tension in the suture (Tx) exactly balances Wx (**B**). When equilibrium occurs, the tissue may be so displaced that it will no longer heal to bone **C,** If the anchor is inserted with the angle θ1° less than 45°, the tissue will stay in place because the forces on the system are balanced. (*Adapted from* Burkhart [10••].)

Soft Tissue

If all the factors above are optimized, soft-tissue failure strength will be less than the anchor-bone interface, the suture, and the knot. Theoretically, if failure in the system is to occur, it should occur at the suture-tissue interface. Obviously, the surgeon can do little to improve the tissue quality. The tissue can be inspected and the sutures placed through the most robust portion of the tissue. Tissue-weave techniques to improve the pull-out strength on the suture through the tissue are difficult to perform when an anchor is also used. It is unknown whether passing one limb of the suture is stronger than passing both limbs of the suture through the tendon. Reed *et al.* [11] noted in a cadaveric model that suture anchor repairs that passed both limbs of the suture through the tendon were stronger than suture passed through bone tunnels. At this time, the author recommends that the surgeon perform whichever technique is more familiar, with a preference for passing both limbs of suture through the tissue before tying the knot. When performing repairs in this manner, tissue failure causes problems more than 90% of the time in laboratory testing.

Performance

Despite the great body of literature [4–8,9••, 10••,12] available on the biomechanical performance of suture anchors, very few studies in the literature document long-term results of procedures using suture anchors. Snyder and Heath [13] have documented good results using suture anchors in conjunction with arthroscopic rotator cuff repairs. Bacilla *et al.* [14] have noted the 92% success rate in the treatment of Bankart lesions using arthroscopically placed suture anchors. No anchors were noted to have pulled out in either study.

No studies or literature document the percentage of anchors that pull out of bone and ultimately become loose intra-articular bodies. Further clinical studies are needed to document the efficacy of the use of suture anchors in both arthroscopic and open surgery.

Cost

Although the use of suture anchors has increased the ease with which soft tissue is attached to bone and has decreased operating time in certain procedures such as the modified Bankart procedure, it has also raised the cost of performing these procedures.

Drilling holes in bone with reusable drill bits and passing sutures through those holes adds only time to the procedure, not cost. On the other hand, using three suture anchors in an arthroscopic repair in a Bankart lesion can add a significant cost to the total cost of the procedure. In today's world where economics plays an important role in deciding how health care is provided to patients, every additional expenditure must be justified. However, the cost of suture anchors should not prohibit their use. Instead, cost of the implanted suture anchors should more than balance the decreased operative time in any given procedure. Each surgeon then has to determine whether the increased cost of using suture anchors is balanced by decreased operative time and the ease with which surgery is performed.

CONCLUSION

Each of the more than 30 suture anchors available for use in attaching soft tissue to bone has distinct advantages and disadvantages. Pound-in anchors are easy to use and make arthroscopic tissue repair more easily performed, but they cannot be easily removed if the suture breaks or infection occurs. Screw-in anchors are also easy to use, and they are easy to remove if necessary, but because the anchor must be inserted *before* the suture is passed through tissue, arthroscopic tissue repair is more complicated when compared with techniques using pound-in anchor techniques. Metal anchors are popular because they can be seen on radiographs, but they interfere with postoperative MRI scanning. Plastic anchors are not seen on radiographs but interfere less with MRI. Bioabsorbable anchors do not interfere with MRI and dissolve with time, but long-term clinical studies have not yet been published that document that these anchors retain their strength long enough for soft tissue–to–bone healing and satisfactory results to occur.

Suture anchors are only one link in the soft tissue–to–bone system of fixation. The quality of bone, the insertion technique (the deadman theory), the type of suture, and the quality of soft tissue all play a role in the strength of the system. Although the initial pull-out strength of the anchor remains the traditional measure to compare anchors, most anchors attain adequate purchase in bone to resist pull-out. The goal of all soft tissue–to–bone repair is to make the anchor-bone interface, the suture, and the knot, all of which are under the surgeon's control, stronger than the soft tissue itself.

REFERENCES AND RECOMMENDED READING

Recently published papers of particular interest have been highlighted as:

•• Of outstanding interest

1. DuToit GT, Roux D: Recurrent dislocation of the shoulder, modified Bankart capsulorraphy. *J Bone Joint Surg Am* 1956, 38:1–12.

2. Boyd HB, Hunt A: Recurrent dislocation of the shoulder: the staple capsulorraphy. *J Bone Joint Surg Am* 1965, 47:1514.

3. Matthews LS, Vetter WL, Oweida SJ, *et al*.: Arthroscopic staple capsulorraphy for recurrent shoulder instability. *Arthroscopy* 1988, 4:106–111.

4. Shea KP, O'Keefe RM, Fulkerson JP: Comparison of initial pull-out strength of arthroscopic suture and staple Bankart repair techniques. *Arthroscopy* 1992, 8:179–182.

5. Goble EM, Somers WK, Clark R, Olsen RE: The development of suture anchors for use in soft tissue fixation to bone. *Am J Sports Med* 1994, 22:236–239.

6. McEleny ET, Donovan MJ, Shea KP, Nowak MD: Initial failure strength of open and arthroscopic Bankart repairs. *Arthroscopy* 1995, 11:426–431.

7. Barber FA, Herbert MA, Click JN: The ultimate strength of suture anchors. *Arthroscopy* 1995, 11:21–28.

8. Carpenter JE, Fish DN, Huston LJ, Goldstein SA: Pull-out strength of five suture anchors. *Arthroscopy* 1993, 9:109–113.

9.•• Barber FA, Herbert MA, Click JN: Internal fixation strength of suture anchors: update 1997. *Arthroscopy* 1997, 13:355–362.

An authoritative review of the current methods used to mechanically evaluate suture anchors.

10.•• Burkhart SS: The deadman theory of suture anchors: observations along a south Texas fence line. *Arthroscopy* 1995, 11:119–123.

An extremely valuable technical note on the proper methods of suture anchor use.

11. Reed SC, Glossop N, Oglivie-Harris DJ: Full-thickness rotator cuff tears: a biomechanical comparison of suture versus bone anchor techniques. *Am J Sports Med* 1996, 24:46–48.

12. Hecker AT, Shea M, Hayhurst JO, *et al*.: Pull-out strength of suture anchors for rotator cuff and Bankart lesion repairs. *Am J Sports Med* 1993, 21:874–879.

13. Snyder SJ, Heath DD: Arthroscopic repair of rotator cuff tears with miniature suture screw anchors and permanent mattress sutures. Paper presented at the Annual Meeting of the Arthroscopy Association of North America. Orlando, FL; April 28–May 1, 1994.

14. Bacilla P, Field LD, Savoie FH: Arthroscopic Bankart repair in a high demand patient population. *Arthroscopy* 1997, 13:51–60.

9
CHAPTER

Purely Arthroscopic Rotator Cuff Repair

EUGENE M. WOLF

Arthroscopy of the shoulder has progressed and expanded rapidly during the past 15 years. Diagnostic arthroscopy has become a standard procedure for use prior to most reconstructive procedures. Operative arthroscopic procedures, such as subacromial decompression, labral repairs, and a variety of stabilization procedures, are now routinely performed. Arthroscopic surgeons have been capable of diagnosing, debriding, and decompressing rotator cuff tears, but repairing the rotator cuff with a purely arthroscopic technique is a more difficult challenge.

Although there have been reports of arthroscopically assisted rotator cuff repairs [1,2], there are no reports in the literature of purely arthroscopic repairs. The first arthroscopic cuff repairs were reported by Johnson [3], who used a staple technique. Although remarkably successful, this technique had the disadvantage of placing a metal staple in the greater tuberosity and subacromial space. It required a second operation for staple removal but had the advantage of allowing a second look at almost all the repairs. This approach was used in cases of nonretracted rotator cuff tears, in which the edge of the torn cuff could be stapled down to the underlying abraded tuberosity. This approach had obvious technical limitations since rotator cuff tears are extremely variable with respect to size, complexity, and chronicity.

With the introduction of Mitek suture anchors (Mitek Surgical, Westwood, MA) in 1989, the author began the development of an arthroscopic approach that would parallel the standard suturing techniques of rotator cuff repair [4,5]. The first clinical procedures were performed in February, 1990, on patients with small nonretracted tears. The improvement and development of "task-specific" suturing devices and suture anchors have expanded the indications for this technique to include larger and more complex tears. The advent of the Crescent Suture Hooks (Linvatec, Largo, FL), which are slightly curved needles 15, 20, and 25 mm in length, permit the placement of simple or mattress sutures with relative ease. The development of the specialized Rotator Cuff Anchor (Mitek Surgical) has made this technically demanding arthroscopic procedure more feasible. It is now possible to repair a majority of rotator cuff tears with a purely arthroscopic approach. However, the technical demands of these repairs will limit their use to surgeons with a practice primarily devoted to arthroscopy and, in particular, to shoulder arthroscopy. The mini-open deltoid-splitting approach in the anterior raphe, combined with an arthroscopic subacromial decompression, is a very attractive, accessible, and less-demanding surgical alternative.

The ability to judge the feasibility of repair of cuff tears—when using open, mini-open, arthroscopically assisted, or purely arthroscopic procedures—has become part of the process for learning how to repair rotator cuff tears arthroscopically. The ability to arthroscopically determine the feasibility of any kind of repair is an important step in the treatment of rotator cuff tears. If that determination can be made by arthroscopic evaluation, unnecessary and frustrating attempts at repairs of chronic, fixed, retracted tears, which involve significant substance loss, can be avoided. If the tear is deemed irreparable, an arthroscopic cuff debridement and decompression can be carried out with minimal morbidity and without the risk of coracoacromial (CA) arch compromise and proximal humeral migration. Use of this approach can avoid heroic attempts at open repair of large retracted tears. Such attempts can lead to a greater loss of function and more pain when compared with preoperative status. This "failed rotator cuff syndrome" is the result of an attempted open rotator cuff repair in which the repair itself fails or alters rotator cuff mechanics enough to produce a less functional cuff. Combined with a compromised CA arch, this leads to proximal humeral subluxation, increased pain, further loss of function, and a disastrous situation that has no good solution.

The author's experience with more than 100 cases of arthroscopic rotator cuff repairs has yielded results equal to or better than those in most open series, based on a modified UCLA scale [6–9]. Above all, no patients developed any loss of function as a result of the procedure. In cases in which the cuff was estimated to be retracted, fixed, and irreparable, no aggressive attempt was made to make a repair because

of the degeneration and substance loss. This ability to arthroscopically evaluate the reparability of cuff tears avoids heroic surgical attempts at repair and the negative results that can ensue.

In this unique series, patients were asked to submit to an office arthroscopy for a second look. Office arthroscopy, with its minimal morbidity, has given us insight into the healing potential of cuff repairs. A total of 70% of the patients who underwent a second-look arthroscopy procedure had a completely healed cuff as viewed from the glenohumeral joint. A total of 30% who underwent a second-look procedure had varying degrees of communication between the joint and the subacromial space. This compares favorably with reports of postoperative evaluation of open cuff repairs [2,8].

OPERATIVE TECHNIQUE

A posterior portal is created 2 cm distally and medially to the posterolateral corner of the acromion. A systematic diagnostic arthroscopy of the glenohumeral joint is carried out. This allows an evaluation of the articular aspect of the rotator cuff, glenoid and humeral surfaces, biceps tendon, labrum, and synovium. If a rotator cuff tear is noted, the surgeon should begin with a debridement and freshening of the articular surface and edges of the rotator cuff tear.

The instruments are then reconfigured into the subacromial space. Debridement, coracoacromial ligament (CAL) resection, and acromioplasty must be carried out efficiently and rapidly, producing minimal fluid extravasation.

Arthroscopic debridement and abrasion of the tuberosity is the next step. It is performed in such a way as to not compromise too much of the bony surfaces of the tuberosity. A large bony trough is unnecessary and is contraindicated when suture anchors are used. The remnants of soft tissues are removed from the tuberosity, and the surface is abraded with a full-radius resector or a 4-mm burr. On occasion, if there is enough of a stump of tendon present on the tuberosity, it is preserved to effectuate a tendon-to-tendon repair.

Cuff evaluation, mobilization, and decisions regarding the type of repair are similar to those used in open techniques. Every cuff tear is unique and requires individual planning. Decisions regarding additional portals are made depending on the size, shape, and location of the tear.

Arthroscopic suture placement is made possible with Crescent Suture Hooks in side-to-side, V-Y, or L-type repairs. The Rotator Cuff Anchors are inserted with sutures to fix the free edge to bone.

Patient Positioning

The patient is placed in the lateral decubitus position. A traction and positioning device (the Bazooka; Orthopedic Systems Inc., Union City, CA) is used. It is designed to permit easy manipulation and changes in abduction and flexion to meet the individual needs of each patient. The patient is placed on a beanbag and rolled onto the uninvolved side. The torso is positioned so that the patient is leaning back about 25°. The Bazooka is initially positioned so that the arm is in about 45° of abduction and 20° of forward flexion, but can be changed at will during the procedure.

The headrest of the operating table is elevated to decrease the tension on the brachial plexus. A total of 15 lbs of traction is applied.

Portal Placement

The margins of the acromion and coracoid are delineated with a marking pen. The placement of the posterior portal is about 1 cm medial and 2 cm distal to the posterolateral corner of the acromion but varies with the size of the patient. The arthroscope sheath and blunt obturator are inserted into the glenohumeral joint through a 5-mm incision. The humeral head and posterior glenoid margin are first identified by palpation with the tip of the obturator. The sheath and obturator are then pushed through the posterior capsule at a level that is approximately between the infraspinatus and the teres minor. The palpation continues in the joint, using the blunt obturator to palpate the articular surfaces and rotator cuff interval, through which the coracoid and CAL are palpated. The anterior portal is then created with an inside-out approach by pushing the sheath and obturator out through the rotator cuff interval just above the subscapularis tendon and below the CAL. An outflow cannula is then retrograded back into the joint by maintaining it in contact with the tip of the obturator as the sheath is withdrawn back into the joint. This anterior inferior portal is just lateral and inferior to the tip of the coracoid. The entire glenohumeral joint is then explored, and the cuff tear is evaluated. It is through this posterior portal that most of the suturing is eventually accomplished. The Crescent Suture Hooks pass through a cannula that has a 5-mm inside diameter.

Cuff Evaluation

The initial configuration uses the arthroscope in the posterior portal and a working cannula in the anterior inferior portal. The appearance of the tears varies dramatically depending on their size, shape, age, and location. Some small, complete-thickness tears are difficult to visualize from the articular surface but easy to see from the bursal surface. This is due to a tear configuration that has a larger opening on the bursal surface and only a minor opening on the articular side. The inverse may be found if the tear has a larger surface on the articular aspect. Thus, it is important to evaluate tears from both the articular and bursal aspects.

The problem of recognizing the presence of a complete-thickness tear becomes moot when the tear is large enough to allow visualization of the subacromial bursa from the articular side of the cuff. The use of a full-radius resector is often necessary to clear away fronds of torn cuff to visualize the bursa through the cuff. The debridement is carried out to remove all frayed tendon back to a firm, healthy edge. With the full-radius resector still on the articular side, remnants of cuff attachment on the tuberosity lateral to the articular margin are removed. Some cuff tears have significant tendon substance still firmly attached to the tuberosity and can be used in a tendon-to-tendon repair mode.

The arthroscope configuration is then changed to the bursal surface of the tear. This change of configuration is accomplished by first withdrawing the arthroscope and combination outflow cannula completely from the joint and then entering through the posterior portal above the cuff. After passing through the posterior bursal curtain, the sheath and obturator are directed out of the same anterior portal.

The presence of a chronic rotator cuff tear that allows leakage of synovial fluid from the glenohumeral joint produces a large bursa with a thickened wall. As opposed to what is done in open techniques, this wall is preserved, and it is worked within to perform the arthroscopic repair. There are often synovial bands within the bursa that have to be removed to completely visualize the tear and gain access to healthy cuff tissue for repair.

A lateral portal is created in the skin approximately 4 to 5 cm from the anterolateral corner of the acromion. It is first localized with a spinal needle that is directed medially and cephalad toward the subacromial space and away from the axillary nerve. After the space is entered with the needle tip, an incision is made immediately adjacent to it. A plastic cannula is then directed into the space. An aggressive shaver blade and electrocautery device are used to strip the bursal surface of the acromion of bursa, periosteum, and CAL. The acromioplasty is performed after switching the arthroscope to the lateral portal and placing the burr in the posterior portal. This lateral view of the acromion is essential to an accurate acromioplasty. It also permits evaluation of the different cuff tendons as they emerge from under the CA arch. Removal of the fibro-fatty tissue medially allows visualization and palpation of the base of the scapula spine, with the infraspinatus and supraspinatus muscles emerging from either side. The suprascapular nerve is at risk as it passes around the base of the scapular spine. With experience, each musculotendon unit, as well as its relative involvement in the tear, can be delineated

As is the case with open procedures, visualization is improved after the acromioplasty. The cutting-block technique is used with the burr in the posterior portal and the arthroscope in the lateral portal. The acromioplasty completed, a probe or grasper is brought through the posterior portal. The tendon edges are mobilized toward each other and toward the tuberosity to determine the type of repair. The evaluation is completed with the arthroscope switched back to the posterior portal and the cannula in the lateral portal. A grasper is used to advance and evaluate the cuff to determine the best possible repair configuration.

Types of Repair

Arthroscopic repairs mimic open repairs. There are four basic repair types: 1) side-to-side, 2) end-to-bone, 3) V-Y configuration, and 4) L-type configuration.

Side-to-Side Repair

Side-to-side repair is indicated in chronic tears that have rounded edges and a degree of retraction. The best example is the more longitudinal defect, whose long axis runs parallel to the fibers of the cuff. The arthroscope is in the lateral portal, and the Crescent Suture Hook is in the posterior portal. The tip of the hook crosses the tear perpendicularly, allowing multiple side-to-side sutures (#1 PDS). The significant technical advantage of #1 PDS sutures are their ease of insertion when suture hooks are used. The Crescent Suture Hook is advanced across the tear in the same way a curved needle bridges the tear in an open repair. The suture is then advanced through the hook into the subacromial space (Fig. 9-1A). The hook is withdrawn, leaving the suture across the tear. The loose end of the suture is pulled out of the same posterior portal with a suture grasper. A fisherman's slip knot is then tied outside the joint and pushed into the joint while the slack is pulled out of the loop (Figs. 9-1B and 9-1C). Two square knots are then tied over the slip knot to prevent it from backing off. The size of the tear dictates the number of sutures, which generally ranges from two to six (Fig. 9-1D).

End-to-Bone Repair

The end-to-bone approach is used in cases in which there is a nonretracted avulsion of tendon from bone. Task-specific Rotator Cuff Anchors are used to reattach the tendon to bone. The insertion of these anchors needs to be close to perpendicular to the tuberosity surface. These are inserted through an 11-mm cannula that is placed immediately lateral (juxtacromial portal) to the acromion. A spinal needle is used to localize the portal position prior to its creation. The #1 PDS sutures can be placed in the cuff edge in a mattress or simple fashion from the posterior portal (Fig. 9-2A). The suture end that is inserted into the space is retrieved through the juxtacromial portal. This end of the suture is threaded through the Rotator Cuff Anchor (Fig. 9-2B). The sharp-tipped anchor is then passed down the cannula in the juxtacromial portal and inserted into bone by malleting it into the prepared tuberosity (Fig. 9-2C). The other end of the suture is then pulled from the posterior portal out through the juxtacromial portal and tied using a slip knot (Fig. 9-2D).

V-Y and L-type Configuration Repair

The V-Y and L-type repairs are more complicated but allow repairs of larger, chronic, and more retracted tears. Mobilization and different attempts at approximation of the tear dictate the type of repair to be used.

In the L-type repair, the supraspinatus or remnant thereof is brought to the tuberosities by an initial suture that is passed through the tendon and then through the transverse ligament over the bicipital groove. This creates the L configuration, and is a combined side-to-side and end-to-bone repair (Fig. 9-3). The V-Y repair is for the most chronic retracted tears. In this case, the defect is closed side-to-side until a final end-to-bone stitch is used (Fig. 9-4).

POSTOPERATIVE REHABILITATION

The patient is immobilized for 3 weeks. Rehabilitation is then carried out with a home exercise kit that includes a pulley, bar, and elastic resistance bands, as well as a comprehensive instruction booklet. Passive range-of-motion exercises, consisting of pulley, pendulum, and bar exercises, are begun at 3 weeks postoperatively. Active range-of-motion exercises, consisting of rotator cuff, deltoid, and scapular stabilization exercises using elastic tubing, are begun slowly at 6 weeks. A return to normal activities is allowed depending on the level and type of participation.

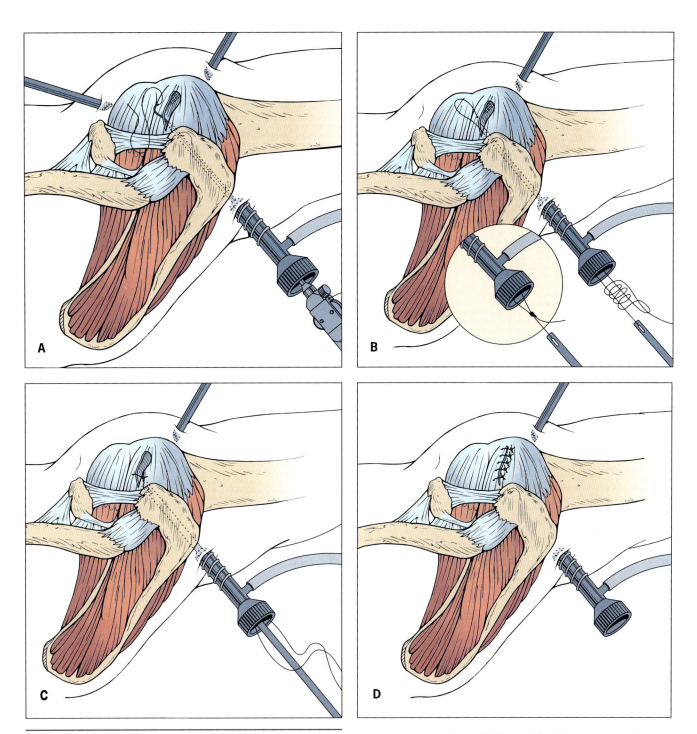

Figure 9-1. Side-to-side repair. **A,** An example of a longitudinal defect whose long axis runs parallel to the fibers of the cuff. The arthroscope is in the lateral portal, and the Crescent Suture Hook (Linvatec, Largo, FL) is in the posterior portal. The tip of the hook crosses the tear perpendicularly, allowing placement of multiple #1 PDS side-to-side sutures. The Crescent Hook is advanced across the tear in the same way a curved needle bridges the tear in an open repair. The suture is then advanced through the hook into the subacromial space. **B** and **C,** The hook is withdrawn, leaving the sutures across the tear. Using a suture grasper, the loose end of the suture is pulled out of the same posterior portal. A fisherman's slip knot is then tied outside the joint and pushed into the joint while the slack is pulled out. Two square knots are then tied over the slip knot to prevent it from backing off. **D,** The size of the tear dictates the number of sutures, which generally ranges from two to six. (*Adapted from* Wolf [10]; with permission.)

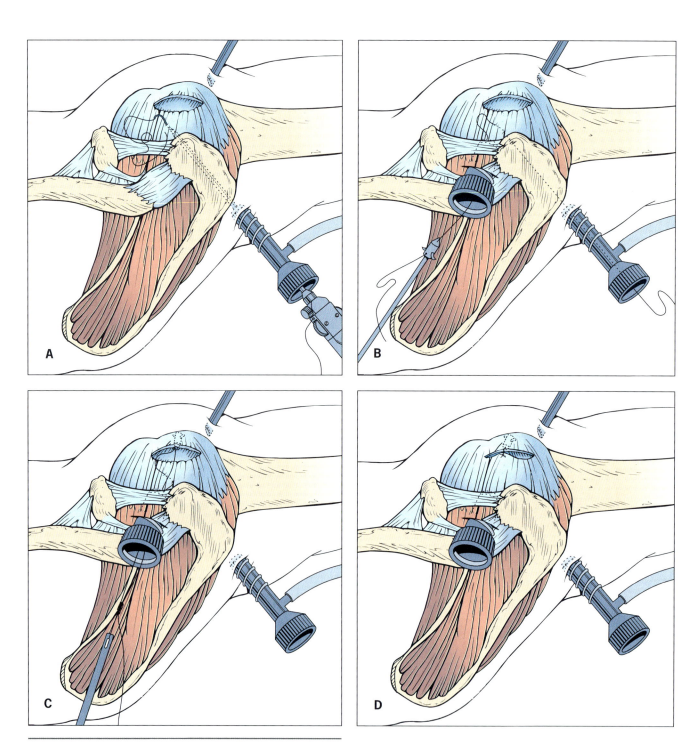

Figure 9-2. End-to-bone repair is used in cases in which there is a nonretracted avulsion of tendon from bone. **A,** The insertion of these anchors needs to be as close as possible to perpendicular to the tuberosity surface. These are inserted through a cannula that is placed immediately lateral (juxtacromial portal) to the acromion. A spinal needle is used to localize the portal position prior to its creation. The #1 PDS sutures can be placed from the posterior portal in the cuff edge in a mattress or simple fashion. **B,** The suture end inserted into the space is retrieved through the juxtacromial portal. This end of the suture is threaded through the Rotator Cuff Anchor (Mitek Surgical, Westwood, MA). **C,** The sharp-tipped anchor is then passed down the cannula in the juxtacromial portal and inserted into bone by malleting it into the prepared tuberosity. **D,** The other end of the suture is then pulled from the posterior portal out the juxtacromial portal and tied using a slip knot. (*Adapted from* Wolf [10]; with permission.)

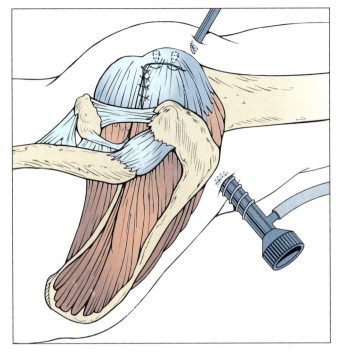

Figure 9-3. In the L-type repair, the supraspinatus or remnant thereof is brought to the tuberosities by an initial suture that is passed through the tendon and then through the transverse ligament over the bicipital groove. This creates the L configuration and is a combined side-to-side, end-to-bone repair. (*Adapted from* Wolf [10]; with permission.)

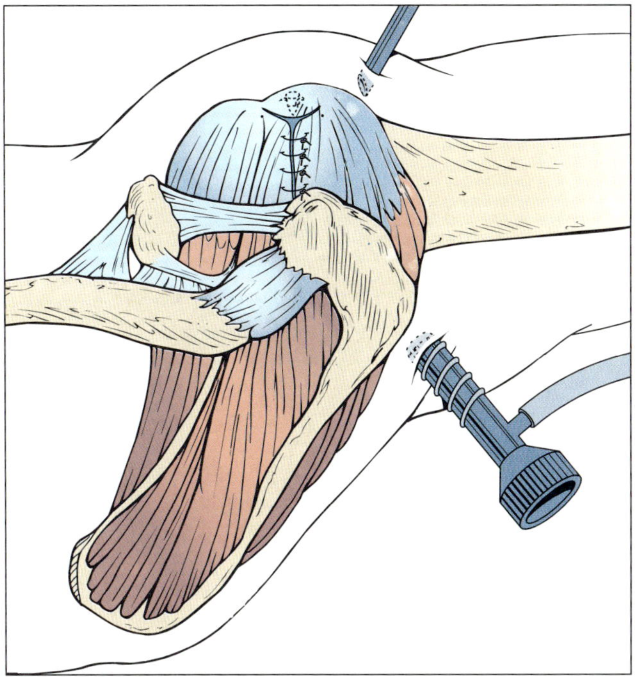

Figure 9-4. The V-Y repair is used for the most chronic retracted tears. In this case, the defect is closed with side-to-side repair, and then a final end-to-bone stitch is used. (*Adapted from* Wolf [10]; with permission.)

REFERENCES

1. Levy HJ, Uribe JW, Delaney LG: Arthroscopically assisted rotator cuff repair: preliminary results. *Arthroscopy* 1990, 6:55–60.

2. Liu SH, Baker CL: Arthroscopically assisted rotator cuff repair correlation of functional results with integrity of the cuff. *Arthroscopy* 1994, 10:54–60.

3. Johnson L: Arthroscopic rotator cuff repair. Paper presented at the UCLA Arthroscopy Seminar. Maui, Hawaii; 1991.

4. Neer CS: *Shoulder Reconstruction*. Philadelphia: WB Saunders; 1990.

5. Matsen FA, Arntz CT: Rotator Cuff Tendon Failure. In *The Shoulder*. Edited by Rockwood CA and Matsen F. Philadelphia: WB Saunders; 1990:

6. Essman JA, Bell RH, Askew M: Full thickness rotator cuff tears: an analysis of results. *Clin Orthop* 1991, 265:170–177.

7. Wolfgang GL: Surgical repair of tears of the rotator cuff of the shoulder: factors influencing the result. *J Bone Joint Surg Am* 1974, 56:14–26.

8. Gazielly DF, Gleze P, Montagnon C: Functional and anatomic results after rotator cuff repair. *Clin Orthop* 1994, 304:43–53.

9. Baylis RV, Wolf EM: Arthroscopic rotator cuff repair: clinical and second look assessment. Paper presented at the annual meeting of the Arthroscopy Association of North America. San Francisco, CA; May, 1995.

10. Wolf EM: Arthroscopic rotator cuff repair. In *Atlas of Shoulder Surgery* Edited by Fu F. London: Martin Duritz; in press.

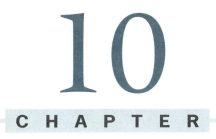

10
CHAPTER

Arthroscopically Assisted Rotator Cuff Evaluation and Repair Using Threaded Anchors

STEPHEN J. SNYDER AND MARK H. GETELMAN

Pathology of the rotator cuff is a common occurrence in people middle aged and older. Although the list of potential etiologies is long, the most commonly accepted causes are intrinsic tendon degeneration, subacromial impingement, and acute trauma. Because any or all of these factors may be involved in any given case, differentiation by cause is not attempted in this chapter. Instead, the authors offer their thoughts for evaluation of the existing pathology and present general treatment concepts designed to repair the damaged tendon and to prevent future recurrence.

ARTHROSCOPIC EVALUATION AND DECISION MAKING

A comprehensive arthroscopic evaluation is an essential step in information gathering to aid the surgeon in rendering an accurate and meaningful plan to treat a damaged rotator cuff. As with all arthroscopic evaluations, the examination should begin with a systematic point-by-point video-recorded anatomic review [1••]. For this important review, the arthroscope should be positioned in both the anterior and posterior portals in the glenohumeral joint and the bursa. Because many of the techniques used for arthroscopic cuff repair require that the surgeon be comfortable visualizing the anatomy from these alternative portals, it is advisable that surgeons routinely practice this skill on all patients with shoulder problems who come for arthroscopic surgery.

The examination is performed with the patient in the lateral decubitus position and the arm supported in 70° of abduction. A helpful supporting device for safe positioning of the arm is the two-point shoulder traction system called the STaR Sleeve (Arthrex, Inc, Naples, FL). This unit uses a sterilized foam sleeve secured with five 2-in Velcro straps that cradle the entire arm, thus minimizing the risk of localized compression injury to the soft tissues. By shifting the weights from one traction hook to another, the arm can easily move between the bursa and arthroscopy positions, and by adjusting the rotation strap, the arm can be repositioned in any desired degree of rotation (Fig. 10-1).

When an injury to the cuff is visualized, the first step is to debride the loose edges carefully. Not only does this alleviate the irritation caused by this fibrous debris, but it permits more careful and accurate evaluation of the cuff's pathology. Placing a suture marker in the cuff in the area of the articular side tear permits the surgeon to correlate that specific location with the corresponding area on the bursal side of the cuff. The marker suture is inserted while the involved area is viewed with the arthroscope in the posterior portal. A 17-gauge spinal needle is inserted percutaneously, adjacent to the lateral acromial edge so it passes through the tendon near its insertion point into the bone. A #1 absorbable monofilament suture is inserted through the needle until approximately 5 inches of material are in the joint. The needle is removed and the suture tails are cut, leaving 4 inches outside the skin. During the bursoscopy portion of the procedure, the suture marker serves as a handy visual guide to indicate the point at which the cuff is known to be damaged on the underside (Fig. 10-2).

To indicate the location of the tear on a cuff surface, our classification method for rotator cuff pathology uses the simple ABC scheme, where A is articular, B is bursal, and C is complete [2]. The severity of the injury is recorded in the classification as well. A stage 1 injury is an *insignificant* area of superficial cuff or capsule inflammation with corresponding bursal or synovial irritation. Stage 2 injury has associated fraying of the tendon in an area smaller than 2 cm. Stages 3 and 4 include *significant* partial cuff injuries: a cuff tear that is more severe and includes fragmentation of the fibers or severe fraying involving more than 2 cm is considered stage 3; when the tear is such that there is a flap on either the bursal or articular side, the tear is considered stage 4.

The classification system for complete tears is also designated 1 to 4. A stage 1 complete tear is a small puncture, usually located in the center of the rotator crescent. It is often associated with fraying (A-2 or A-3), but with only a small complete perforation. A stage 2 tear is larger, encompassing an entire tendon. A stage 3 lesion is even larger, includes more than one tendon or has a complex tear pattern, such as an L- or V-shaped tear that is not fixed in the contracted position and can be pulled to the reattachment position with no significant tension. A stage 4 tear is massive and includes two complete tendons or an L- or V-shaped pattern that can be mobilized only with significant capsular releases but still can be replaced with some difficulty in a proper position for reattachment near the anatomic neck of the humerus. Finally, massive tears that usually involve three tendons that cannot be mobilized adequately for repair may be present.

This classification system allows the surgeon to systematically assess and succinctly record the location and degree of tendon damage using a consistent scheme. It simplifies reporting and communication of information about rotator cuff injuries, ensuring that when cases are presented, an accurate portrayal of the severity and degree of damage of both complete and partial tears is possible. For example, if a patient has a small full-thickness puncture tear (~1 cm) with

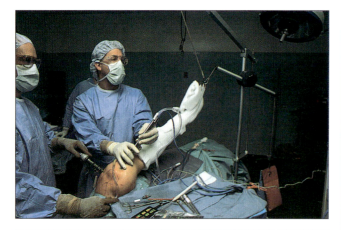

Figure 10-1. The STaR Sleeve (Arthrex, Inc, Naples, FL) is a sterile foam traction sleeve that holds the arm in both the desired abduction and rotation positions during shoulder arthroscopy.

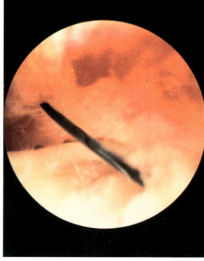

Figure 10-2. The marker suture exits a bursal side tear in the rotator cuff.

moderately severe fraying and fragmentation around it on the articular side along with minimal bursal side irritation, the entire injury could be recorded as A3B1C1.

SUBACROMIAL DECOMPRESSION

When the rotator cuff is damaged, it is often necessary to perform arthroscopic subacromial decompression and sometimes a partial distal clavicle resection (mini-Mumford). The decision to perform either procedure is influenced by the nature of the tendon damage and the anatomy of the acromion and the acromioclavicular (AC) joint. It is crucial to have a very clear AC joint view and a radiograph from the supraspinatus outlet (arch view) to determine whether a decompression should be considered and how much bone should be resected in individual cases. The AC joint view is made using a standard anterior-posterior exposure of the joint, but with the beam tilted cephalad 15°. The proper exposure shows the AC joint clearly so that the joint space and the inferior border can be evaluated for spurs and arthritis.

The technique for taking the arch view and the radiographic appearance of a good-quality exposure should be understood by the technician and the surgeon. The patient stands at a 45° angle to the beam with the posterior side of the involved shoulder against the cassette. The beam is angled 15° caudal to project the acromial arch in lateral relief. The perfect arch view is a true lateral of the acromion without rotation or tilt. Three visual checks are used to assess the acceptability of the radiograph (Fig. 10-3). First, the spine of the scapular must project as an upright column. If the film is rotated, the outline of the spine appears widened and the cortical margins are indistinct. Second, a small portion of the posterior acromion should project behind the acromial spine. Third, the bursal border of the anterior acromion should be clearly seen. If the x-ray is tilted and not a true lateral, the inferior border outline cannot be clearly seen. If the film is properly positioned, the arch can be classified.

The South California Orthopedic Institute (SCOI) classification of the acromial arch describes both the shape and the thickness of the acromion as seen in the arch view. The shape is classified according to the scheme of Bigliani and Morrison [3]. Type I has a perfectly flat bursal acromial surface, type II is smoothly curved, and type III has a hooked projection under the anterior lip. The thickness of the anterior third of the acromion is also important. There have been many cases of inadvertent acromial fracture in which the surgeon has not realized preoperatively that a particular acromion is thin and subsequently removes too

much bone. The measured thickness of the acromion at the junction of the anterior third and the posterior two thirds is classified as follows: 1 to 8 mm is A, 8 to 12 mm is B, and greater than 12 mm is C. In a study at SCOI, more than 30% of the female patients with type III arches had an "A" thickness and would be at risk for fracture if significant bone were removed from under the acromion during decompression [4].

Arthroscopic subacromial decompression is performed in four steps: 1) removing the coracoacromial ligament (CAL); 2) cutting the two orientation troughs; 3) thinning the bone and removing the anterior edge; and 4) flattening the inferior clavicle. The patient is placed in the lateral decubitus position, and the arm is held in the bursal position of 15° of abduction with 10 to 15 lbs of traction weight on the STaR Sleeve. Surgical irrigation fluid can be changed to nonconductive glycine for the first portion of the procedure, during which electrosurgery is used. An arthroscopic pump is extremely beneficial; fluid pressure should be kept as low as possible to ensure a clear field.

Removing the Coracoacromial Ligament

The surgeon must first completely remove the CAL from the undersurface of the anterior half of the acromion. The arthroscope is in the posterior portal, and a 6-mm plastic cannula is inserted into the lateral acromial portal. This portal is developed on a line that begins at the posterior edge of the AC joint and runs in a lateral direction perpendicular to the lateral border of the acromion. The blunt-tipped obturator is inserted in a perpendicular

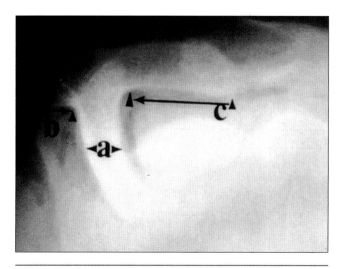

Figure 10-3. The subacromial arch outlet x-ray must be properly aligned to allow accurate evaluation of the shape and thickness of the acromion. a—spine of scapula; b—posterior edge of acromion; c—anterior edge of acromion.

orientation through a small skin puncture approximately 4 cm from the acromial edge and passed through the deltoid muscle to puncture the underlying bursa. The cannula is then directed medial and slightly anterior to enter the bursal space below the anterior third of the acromion. If the bursa has not been punctured well lateral to the acromial edge, the cannula will push the lateral bursal flap into the field, obstructing the view for the remainder of the procedure.

The shaver is used to remove any inflamed or frayed tissues that obstruct visualization. The electrosurgical tool is inserted through the lateral portal. The probe tip used is the Subacromial Electrode (Linvatec, Largo, FL). The electrode is used to remove the soft tissue in two steps. The first cut is made with the electrode across the CAL beginning at the posterior AC joint and extending to the lateral border of the acromion. The electrode is then passed three or four more times, making parallel cuts posterior and anterior to the original one. The next series of cuts are made perpendicular to the original cuts, thus creating a checkerboard pattern under the anterior acromion. No attempt should be made during the first series of cuts to amputate the CAL from the front of the bone; instead, the soft tissues should be debulked, and the gross bony outline should be defined. The shaver is then inserted through the lateral portal to remove the shreds of CAL and bursa resulting from movement of the electrode. The electrode is reinserted, the CAL is amputated carefully from the front of the acromion, and the capsule under the AC joint is opened. The shaver is used again to remove the debris until the entire undersurface of the acromion is clearly visualized.

Cutting the Two Orientation Troughs

The 4-mm barrel-shaped burr is used next to create two orientation troughs. It is helpful to insert a 5-mm drainage cannula connected to a gravity outflow tube into the anterior portal just below the detached CAL. This drain permits the controlled removal of bone dust and blood from the bursa while still maintaining sufficient positive pressure to control capillary oozing from the bone and soft tissues.

The first trough is made along the lateral border of the acromion. The burr is always used on its highest speed. The cut begins at the anterior lateral corner and extends posteriorly to the level of the lateral portal. The cut should be beveled from lateral to medial, removing only 2 or 3 mm of the undersurface lateral bone edge. The second cut connects the lateral trough to the medial border of the acromion near the back of

the AC joint. This trough is only 1 mm deep and serves to orient the surgeon for the bone removal step.

Thinning the Bone and Removing the Anterior Edge

The arthroscope is moved to the lateral portal, and the shaver is inserted into the posterior portal. The shaver is used to remove any remaining bursa that may block the view. By studying the radiograph of the acromial arch, the surgeon must plan the exact amount of bone he or she wishes to remove from the anterior edge of the acromion. It is advisable to remove no more than 50% of the thickness of the anterior edge, thereby ensuring that the deltoid muscle has ample bone stock for support and lessening the possibility of postoperative fracture.

The burr is inserted posteriorly, and the back of the trough is smoothed to remove any stepoff. The burr is then worked from the acromial facet of the AC joint on the medial side to the lateral acromial edge, beginning anterior to the trough, thus removing only the outer layer of bone, up to, but not including, the anterior edge of the acromion. The anterior edge is preserved to serve as a measuring guide comparing the width of the remaining lip with that of the 4-mm burr. The burr is moved back to the trough and additional cuts are made, each time removing only 1 mm of bone, beginning anterior to the trough and continuing up to the anterior lip of the acromion, leaving the edge still intact. It is helpful to "square" the anterior medial edge of the acromion by passing the burr along the acromial facet of the AC joint up to the anterior edge. This maneuver helps the surgeon to visualize the depth of the lip and to estimate the amount of bone resected. When the remaining anterior lip measures the predetermined thickness, the burr is passed under it to carefully remove the bone until it is coplanar with the rest of the resected bone.

Flattening the Inferior Clavicle

The final step is to inspect, and if necessary, to flatten the inferior facet of the AC joint. The subacromial electrode helps to release the capsule from under the joint. Care must be taken to avoid damaging the coracoclavicular ligaments (C-CL), which often begin only 2 cm medial to the end of the clavicle. The shaver removes any remaining soft tissue debris, and the burr flattens the distal clavicle until it is coplanar with the resected acromion. The entire clavicle facet is resected only when evidence of painful arthrosis exists on the preoperative examination and radiograph.

ROTATOR CUFF REPAIR

After the surgeon has determined that a rotator cuff tear appears repairable with arthroscopic techniques, he or she should formulate a plan of action to follow during the operation. The plan should include all the necessary steps for completing the repair in the most time-efficient manner, while never compromising on the quality of the refixation. The steps of the repair are: 1) selectively debriding the bursa and edges of the tear; 2) preparing the implantation site on the anatomic neck; 3) performing side-to-side sutures; and 4) inserting suture anchors and refixing the cuff to bone.

Selective Bursal and Cuff Debridement

To repair the rotator cuff, or for that matter, to perform any type of subacromial surgery, it is extremely helpful to selectively debride any bursal tissue that may tend to obstruct the arthroscopic view. This important step begins when the arthroscope is viewing from the anterior portal and the shaver is entering through the posterior portal. The surgeon should imagine that the tip of the shaver is the end of the arthroscope entering the posterior portal. Any bursal tissue seen near the tip of the shaver is likely to obstruct the arthroscope or possibly entangle the sutures entering that position; therefore, the tissue should be removed. Likewise, when the arthroscope is viewing from the posterior portal, any obstructing anterior bursa should also be debrided. The CAL should be left intact below the deltoid muscle, and the lateral subdeltoid bursa should not be removed except as needed for visualization.

The edges of the cuff tendon must also be cleanly debrided of nonviable fragments of tissue, and any overlying thickened bursa on the edge of the cuff must be removed. It is not necessary to perform a complete bursectomy but rather to remove any material that may compromise the view of the tendon to be repaired.

Preparation of the Implantation Site on the Anatomic Neck of the Humerus

The remaining soft tissues on the greater tuberosity and along the anatomic neck of the humerus must be debrided. The 4.2-mm full-radius shaver is inserted through the anterior, posterior, and lateral portals, as needed to effect this step. Adequate soft tissue should be removed from the greater tuberosity so that the bone is clean and clearly exposed. A 4.0-mm burr is used to decorticate the bone lightly along the edge of

the articular cartilage at the level of the anatomic neck. This action creates a shallow trough less than 1 mm deep that is the point at which the tendon will be reattached. This site on the anatomic neck is not the original point of attachment of the rotator cuff, which is farther lateral on the greater tuberosity. During the process of cuff degeneration, tearing, and debridement, some tendon length is lost. Thus, it would require that the remaining muscle and tendon be overtightened if they are replaced into the original anatomic position.

Side-to-Side Cuff Repair

Two 6-mm operating cannulae with diaphragms are placed in the anterior and posterior portals of the bursa. One of these must always have an outflow drain attached to the side port to guard against overpressurization from the pump.

An apex stitch is placed first. Usually a suture hook with a gentle crescent-shaped curve is used. Before passing the needle, it should be determined which of the two portals gives better access to the target area. This can be assessed by inserting a probe into each portal and by visually evaluating the projected direction it makes as it approaches the surgical site. The suture needle is then inserted. The point of the needle is positioned about 1 cm from the edge of the tear and worked through the tendon. The surgeon must take care not to damage the humeral articular cartilage. When the tip is seen in the gap, the needle is redirected so the point is passed below the opposite side of the tear and up and through the top of the cuff. Usually the first stitch can be passed using the medium-sized (25-mm) hook, but sometimes if the gap is wide, the larger (30-mm) hook is needed. Either a monofilament absorbable suture or a suture Shuttle Relay (Linvatec) is passed through the needle and retrieved out through the other cannula with a small grasping clamp (Fig. 10-4). A #2 braided suture is loaded in the eyelet of the Shuttle and carried back down the cannula by pulling on the opposite end of the Shuttle, located in the original operating cannula (Fig. 10-5). The suture is pulled back out through the initial cannula using a crochet hook or a suture-grasping clamp (Fig. 10-6). The suture ends are tied together using a sliding or Revo Knot with the aid of a loop-handled knot pusher (Figs. 10-7 to 10-9).

After the suture tails have been cut, additional sutures are placed as needed to complete the side-to-side repair. Usually only two or three sutures are necessary (Figs. 10-10 and 10-11). By placing and tying the side-to-side sutures first, the remaining edge

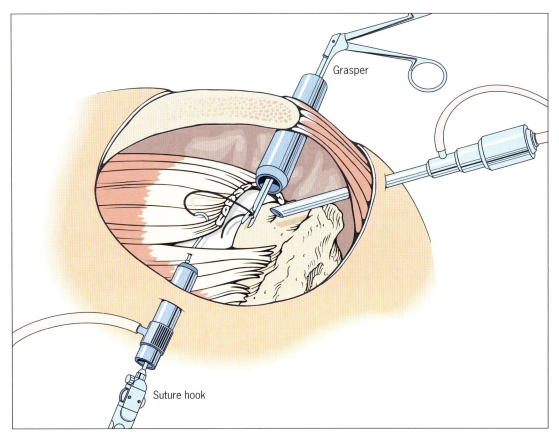

Figure 10-4. A curved crescent-shaped suture hook is inserted through a 6.0-mm operating cannula to pass across the cuff tear. A suture Shuttle Relay (Linvatec, Largo, FL) is passed through the needle and retrieved with a grasper tool out another cannula.

Grasper

Suture hook

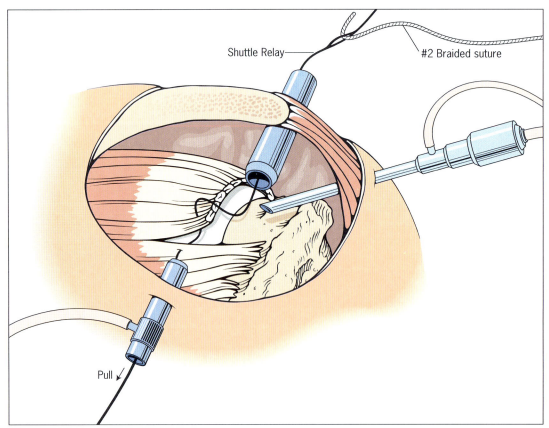

Figure 10-5. A suture is loaded in the eyelet of the Shuttle Relay.

Shuttle Relay

#2 Braided suture

Pull

of the tear, which had been pulled off bone, is reduced into better position for reattachment without as much tension.

Insertion of Suture Anchors and Refixation of the Cuff to Bone

Many good suture materials are available that can adequately refixate the torn cuff tendon to bone. The surgeon must choose the one with which he or she is most comfortable. The authors prefer to use a suture that ensures at least 3 months of holding time to permit secure healing of the cuff to the bone when anchors are used. In addition, the ease and security of knot tying must be considered, as well as the possibility of placing complex stitches, such as mattress stitches, figure eights, or over-end loop stitches. At the present time, the authors' preference is to use a lightly coated braided #2 nonabsorbable suture that facilitates ease of knot tying, causes minimal trauma when pulling through tissues, and yet still permits strong, secure knots to be laid using arthroscopic techniques. The Ethibond #2 suture (Ethicon, Somerville, NJ) fulfills the requirements at present, but in the near future another braided suture certainly will be available with similar characteristics that will completely absorb in about 1 year. When this new suture becomes available, it should be the suture of choice for all rotator cuff repair situations.

Inserting suture anchors into prepared bone trough requires four very precise steps: 1) the pilot holes are

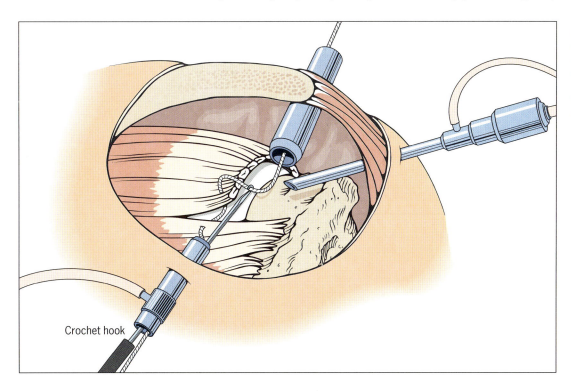

Crochet hook

Figure 10-6. A crochet hook catches the other limb of the suture and pulls it out through the primary cannula.

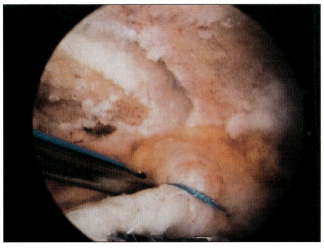

Figure 10-7. The two limbs of the suture are tied together with a loop-handled knot pusher closing the tear.

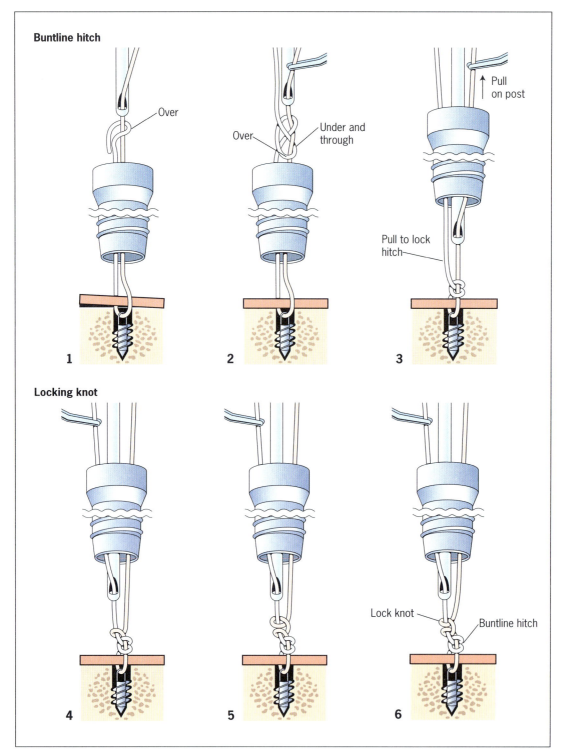

Buntline hitch

1 — Over

2 — Over — Under and through

3 — Pull on post — Pull to lock hitch

Locking knot

4

5

6 — Lock knot — Buntline hitch

Figure 10-8. The "Tennessee slider" is a slip knot that is a combination of a Buntline hitch on the first post and two half-hitches thrown in alternate directions on the opposite post.

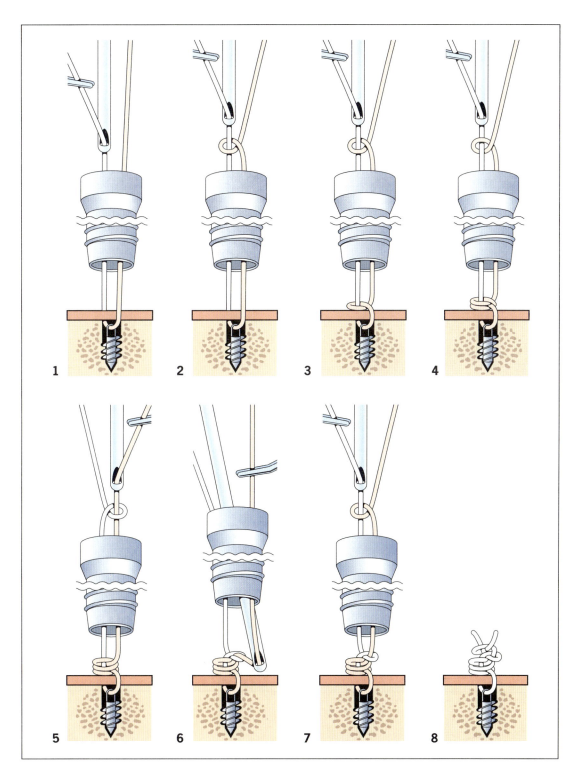

1

2

3

4

5

6

7

8

created; 2) the anchors are implanted; 3) the sutures are passed through the cuff; and 4) the knots are tied. To determine the precise position and angle at which to insert the suture anchors, it is helpful to use a spinal needle as a planning aide while viewing from the lateral portal. The needle is inserted 1 cm lateral to the edge of the acromion in a position that will allow it to approach the prepared trough near the center point. The angle of approach should be approximately 45° to 60° to the articular surface, so that when the anchors are inserted they pass under the compact subchondral bone like tent pegs, thereby best resisting pull-out when stress is applied to the sutures in line with the cuff. The same skin-entry site should permit insertion of all anchors. This also permits them to be inserted in a pattern that will fan out from the central anchor point, ensuring adequate bone stock between each anchor and further increasing the resistance to pull out.

Many styles and sizes of suture anchors are available, and most have adequate holding strength when used properly. Our preference is threaded (screw-in) type anchors. They can be loaded with any desired suture, inserted percutaneously without fear of becoming snagged in the soft tissues, and easily removed if a problem occurs during knot tying or suture breakage. The Revo 4-mm anchor (Linvatec) was designed specifically for rotator cuff repair with the added engineering benefit that if significant stress is applied to the suture before healing has occurred, the failure will likely be through suture breakage rather than through anchor pull-out from bone.

A 2-mm skin stab is made with a #11 knife blade in the spot chosen by the spinal needle guide. The

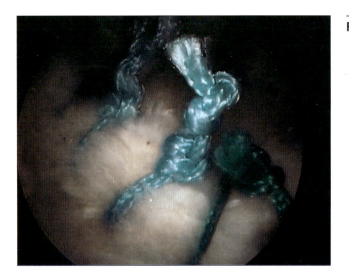

Figure 10-10. The completed side-to-side repair.

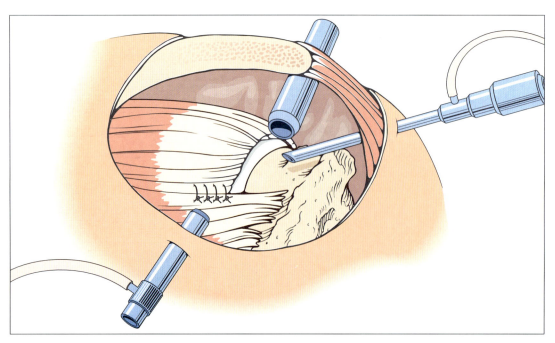

Figure 10-11. After the knots are tied for the side-to-side repair, the free edge of the cuff is approximated much closer to the bony insertion site.

Revo punch (or in the rare case of extremely hard bone, the 2-mm drill) is inserted percutaneously into the bursa and positioned at the posterior end of the bone trough, after making certain that it is angled in a slightly posterior direction. The punch is impacted with an 8-oz mallet until it is completely seated such that the conical portion is completely below the surface (Fig. 10-12). If the punch is not seated deeply enough, difficulty may be encountered in starting the anchor into the pilot hole. The punch is removed from the first hole and repositioned at the anterior end of the trough. Another hole is then made, this time angled in an anterior direction. The central hole (or sometimes two holes) is made last by aiming the punch in a more medial direction, thereby creating a fanning array of the pilot holes.

The first anchor is inserted into the posterior pilot while still viewing with the arthroscope in the lateral or sometimes the anterior portal, whichever affords the best view (Fig. 10-13). The anchor is screwed into the bone until the seating mark on the driver passes below the surface of the bone. The suture is released, and the screwdriver is removed. At this time, the sutures must be pulled to be certain that the anchor is firmly seated. A crochet hook or suture retriever is used through the posterior portal to carry both suture limbs out through the cannula. A guide rod or switching stick is inserted into the cannula, and the cannula is removed and then is replaced over the rod, leaving the sutures outside. This step is important in order to keep the sutures from entangling with subsequent sutures that will be pulled out through the same cannula (Fig. 10-14).

The next anchor is loaded onto the screwdriver using a suture of a different color. By convention, the authors use a dark green suture posteriorly, white in the middle anchor, and light green anteriorly. If a fourth anchor is needed, the authors use a blue suture. The center anchor is inserted, and its suture is retrieved posteriorly and placed outside the cannula, using the guide-rod technique. It is often helpful to change the position of the arthroscope to the posterior or lateral portal to improve visualization while additional anchors are implanted. If four anchors are needed, the next in line from posterior is inserted, and the suture is again retrieved out the back. Finally, the anterior anchor is implanted, but this time the sutures are removed through the anterior portal with the crochet hook.

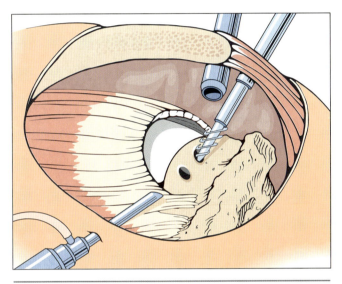

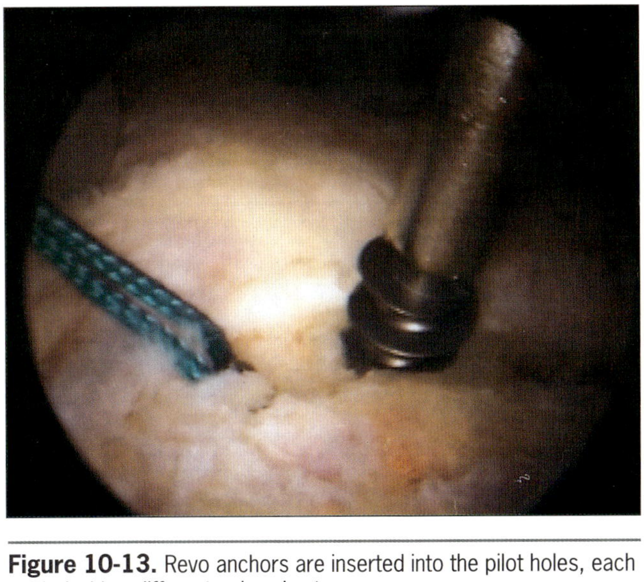

Figure 10-12. A Revo punch (Linvatec) is used to create pilot holes in the prepared trough near the edge of the articular cartilage.

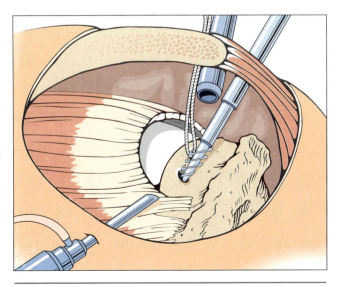

Figure 10-13. Revo anchors are inserted into the pilot holes, each loaded with a different colored suture.

Figure 10-14. An additional anchor is inserted while viewed from an anterior portal.

Passing the sutures through the cuff is the next step. Two standard approaches are available, one through an 8.4-mm lateral operating cannula using the modified Caspari suture punch (Linvatec) or the other using a suture hook through the anterior or posterior portal, either with or without a cannula. The type of stitching technique used can be varied according to the status of the cuff and the number of anchors. A single-pass simple stitch is adequate if the edge of the cuff is relatively strong and multiple anchors are planned. This method tends to roll the edge of the tendon into the bone trough, thus leaving a smooth margin. If the edge of the tendon is thin or if the surgeon wishes to ensure a more substantial grasp of the edge of the tissue, a double-pass mattress stitch or sometimes an end-over roll stitch is preferred. These techniques place more tissue within the stitch pattern, distribute the stress over a wider area, and promote more tendon-to-bone contact at the implantation site. The edge of the suture line is not as flat with this suture method as with the simple sutures, and often the authors use a combination of stitch types for a cuff repair.

If the suture punch is used, an 8.4-mm screw-in type cannula must be inserted into the lateral subacromial portal. It should be placed over a guide rod in the same lateral portal location used for the decompression. A clear cannula is preferred because it improves visualization during knot tying. The anterior suture is addressed first. One limb of the (light green) anterior suture is retrieved through the lateral cannula with a crochet hook (Fig. 10-15). If a mattress stitch is planned, the most anterior of the limbs is passed first. The suture ends are always held with a hemostat clamp if they are hanging free in order to prevent accidental removal during manipulation. The suture punch is loaded with a suture Shuttle Relay and inserted into the 8.4-mm cannula. The bottom jaw of the punch is passed under the cuff and worked into position so that when the needle is sent through the cuff from bottom to top, it will be located a few millimeters anterior to the anterior-most anchor and about 1 cm medial to the cuff edge. The jaws of the punch are closed, and the Shuttle Relay is sent through the needle a few centimeters into the bursa by turning the suture driving wheel on the handle (Fig. 10-16). A miniature grasping clamp holds the end of the Shuttle when it exits the needle tip and guides it out of the anterior cannula while the drive wheel is rolled. Once about half the length of the Shuttle is passed, the jaws of the punch are released and it is removed from the bursa. Because the punch has been modified by cutting a 1-mm slot in the end of the upper jaw, it is possible to close the jaw, thus leaving the Shuttle outside while removing the punch through the cannula. This cannot be done if the punch has not been modified.

The eyelet of the Shuttle is pulled to the outside of the lateral cannula, and 3 cm of the suture is loaded and locked in it. The anterior limb of the Shuttle is pulled carefully, carrying the suture in the eyelet down the lateral cannula, through the cuff from bottom to top and out through the anterior cannula (Fig. 10-17).

The crochet hook is used to grasp the second limb of the anterior suture and carry it out through the lateral cannula. The suture punch is passed again, this time entering the cuff a few millimeters anterior to the anchor position. The Shuttle is pulled out through the anterior portal as before and loaded laterally. By pulling the anterior end of the Shuttle, the second limb of the suture is carried through the cuff to complete the mattress stitch (Fig. 10-18). Both suture

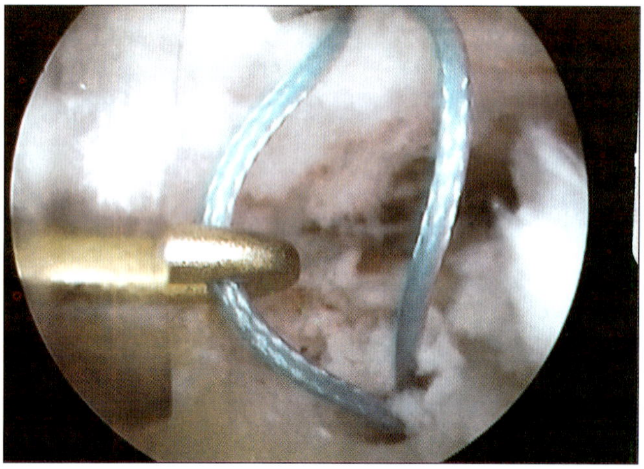

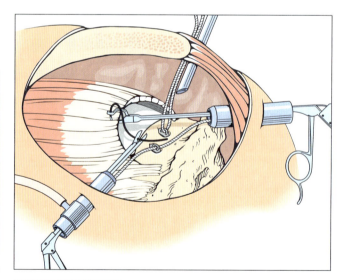

Figure 10-16. The suture punch is inserted down the 8.4-mm lateral cannula and passed through the cuff from bottom to top; one end of the suture is loaded in the eyelet of the Shuttle Relay outside the lateral cannula.

Figure 10-15. A crochet hook pulls one limb of the posterior suture out through the lateral cannula in preparation for passing.

limbs are placed outside the anterior cannula using the guide rod.

In some procedures, it may be easier to pass the Shuttle through the cuff using a suture hook entering either the anterior or posterior portal than to use a suture punch through the lateral portal. Similar to the position used for side-to-side cuff suturing, the arthroscope is positioned in the lateral portal, and two 6-mm operating cannulae are placed in the other two bursal portals. It must be decided which portal affords the better access to the portion of the cuff the surgeon wishes to suture. A probe can be inserted into both the anterior and posterior portals to simulate the path of the suture hook.

After the best access portal has been determined, one limb of the white suture from the middle anchor is retrieved through the other portal. The suture hook may be passed through a cannula if the crescent-shaped hook is chosen, but if a more sharply curved hook seems to provide better access, it may be inserted directly through the portal *without* use of the cannula (Fig. 10-19). The needle is passed through the cuff from top to bottom so that the tip exits near the anchor (Figs. 10-20 and 10-21). The end of the

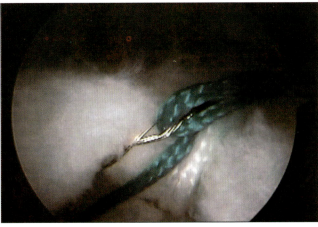

Figure 10-17. The Shuttle is pulled to carry the suture through the cuff from bottom to top.

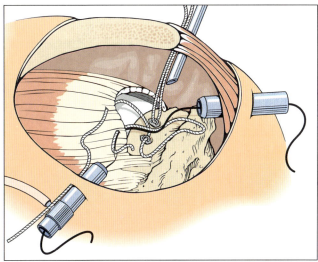

Figure 10-18. The second suture is pulled through the cuff with the Shuttle to complete the mattress suture.

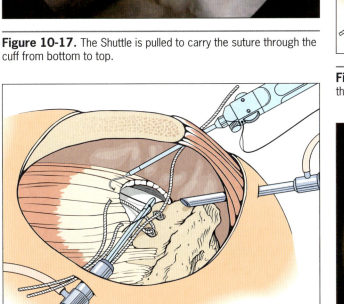

Figure 10-19. An alternative method for passing the Shuttle is using the curved suture hook through either the anterior or posterior portal to pass through the cuff from top to bottom. In this case, it was not necessary to use a cannula, but one limb of the suture must be positioned within the opposite cannula through which the grasper is inserted.

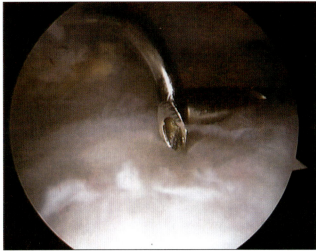

Figure 10-20. Curved suture hook positioned to puncture the cuff from the top while viewing from the lateral portal.

Shuttle is grasped and led out the opposite portal cannula. The suture is loaded into the eyelet and carried back down the cannula, through the cuff from bottom to top, and out the other portal. This forms a simple stitch that, when tied, will roll the end of the tendon into the trough.

The remaining sutures can be passed using either of the above techniques, forming simple or mattress stitches, as desired for the best tendon-edge control. Usually, alternating simple and mattress stitches seems to give the best result (Fig. 10-22).

The final step is to tie the sutures. The arm can usually be maintained in the bursoscopy position of 20° of abduction. The arthroscope is positioned in the posterior portal and the (light green) anterior suture pair is retrieved through the lateral portal. The sutures are tied together using either a "Revo knot" (ie, multiple stacked half-hitches reversing the post after the third and fourth throws) or a sliding knot such as a "Tennessee slider" (buntline hitch followed by two half-hitches on the opposite post) (Fig. 10-23). The knot choice can be made by testing to see if the suture will slide through the tissue and the anchor eyelet easily. If it seems to slide without significant resistance, the sliding knot can be used. If resistance to sliding the suture is present, then the Revo knot is the better choice. The surgeon should be facile and comfortable in tying both knots (Fig. 10-24).

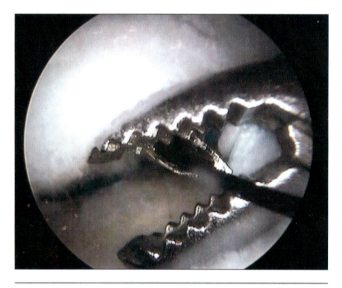

Figure 10-21. A grasping clamp catches the Shuttle as it exits the suture needle on the underside of the cuff.

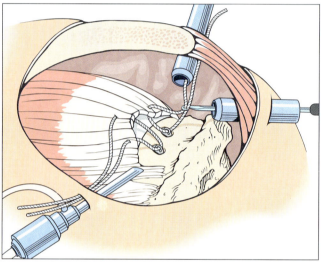

Figure 10-22. The Shuttle pulls the second suture through the cuff, this time directly in line with the anchor to form a simple stitch.

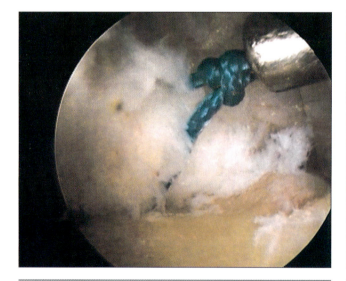

Figure 10-23. Most "simple" stitches can be tied with a Tennessee slider knot, but it is important to test and to be sure the suture will slide easily through the tissue and anchor eyelet *before* the knot is tied.

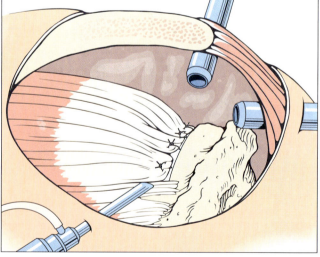

Figure 10-24. The completed repair often includes alternating mattress-type and simple sutures.

POSTOPERATIVE CARE

The shoulder is protected in a neutral rotation brace with a small abduction pillow (Fig. 10-25), such as the UltraSling II (Smith & Nephew DonJoy, Inc, Carlsbad, CA). The patient is encouraged to remove the arm from the sling beginning the first postoperative day to perform active elbow, wrist, and hand exercises. Careful attention should be paid to the axillary skin to guard against development of a rash. Several times during the day, the patient is asked to support the arm in a more abducted position using either a large pillow or the abduction pillow option that is available with the UltraSling II. This accentuated abduction position improves circulation to the cuff and helps prevent adhesions.

After the wounds are inspected at 1 week postoperatively, the patient is instructed to begin gentle pendulum exercises and shoulder shrugs. At first, the circles are small but should enlarge over the next 2 to 3 weeks. Depending on the complexity of the repair, the passive and active assisted elevation may begin between the third and fourth weeks. During this period, exercises in a warm water pool are helpful and comforting. Patients are given a Shoulder Therapy exercise kit and instructional videotape (STK; Breg, Inc, Carlsbad, CA) preoperatively and told *not* to start any exercises until instructed by their doctor. The kit contains a pulley, wand, and rubber exercise cords. The three phases of exercises in the booklet and video can be used progressively while the patient is monitored by the surgeon and physical therapist.

At about the sixth postoperative week, most patients are able to begin active elevation and resisted internal and external rotation exercises. These are begun in the supine position and progressively increase to upright lifts with weights, as strength increases. Most office workers can expect to resume their nonlifting desk work by 3 weeks, but manual workers need 3 to 6 months before a return to work.

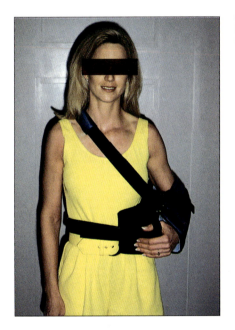

Figure 10-25. The shoulder is protected postoperatively in an UltraSling II (Smith & Nephew DonJoy, Inc, Carlsbad, CA) in slight abduction and neutral rotation.

REFERENCES AND RECOMMENDED READING

Recently published papers of particular interest have been highlighted as:
•• Of outstanding interest

1.•• Snyder SJ: Diagnostic arthroscopy of the shoulder: normal anatomy and variations. *Shoulder Arthroscopy*. Edited by Snyder SJ. New York: McGraw Hill; 1994:23–49.

Excellent review of normal anatomy and systematic point-by-point approach to surgical arthroscopy of the shoulder.

2. Snyder SJ: Evaluation and treatment of the rotator cuff. *Orthop Clin North Am* 1993, 24:173–192.

3. Bigliani LU, Morrison DS, April EW: The morphology of the acromion and its relationship to rotator cuff tears. *Orthop Trans* 1986, 10:216.

4. Snyder SJ, Wuh HCK: A modified classification of the supraspinatus outlet view based on the configuration and the anatomic thickness of the acromion. Paper presented at the American Shoulder and Elbow Surgeons Annual Closed Meeting. Seattle, WA; September 1991.

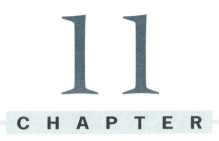

CHAPTER 11

Arthroscopically Assisted Rotator Cuff Repair Using a Mini-Open Incision

Gregory G. Markarian and John W. Uribe

The management of full-thickness rotator cuff tears remains controversial. Rockwood [1,2] advocates conservative management in sedentary patients of advanced age. Other authors [3–7] claim that rotator cuff repair is warranted in full-thickness tears that are symptomatic. These authors' rationale is predicated on the progressive nature of most symptomatic rotator cuff tears. Pain, particularly at night, is the usual presenting complaint. Functional loss occurs most frequently with the massive chronic degenerative tears in the elderly or in patients with acute traumatic conditions. Once humeral head elevation occurs, rotator cuff repair becomes more difficult and less predictable. The end stage of this process is rotator cuff arthropathy. Operative repair provides the best long-term outcome for symptomatic rotator cuff tears.

ARTHROSCOPIC VERSUS OPEN REPAIR: THE ROTATOR CUFF DEBATE

The rationale for an arthroscopically assisted rotator cuff repair with a mini-open incision is quite simply to use the "best of both worlds." Arthroscopy enables the surgeon to visualize intra-articular pathology (loose bodies, glenohumeral chondromalacia, bicipital degeneration, incomplete rotator cuff tears, cleavage tears) that might otherwise be missed, yet that might affect outcome. Arthroscopy also allows for a comprehensive evaluation of the rotator cuff and the subacromial contents. The size, location, and specific tear pattern can be delineated. This is especially true of tears involving the subscapularis tendon, which can be easily overlooked. Most importantly, the surgeon can accurately assess the quality, mobility, and reparability of the cuff tendon. If, during arthroscopic evaluation, the rotator cuff is found to be irreparable, then a simple debridement of the degenerated cuff tissue and inflamed bursa can be performed. Pain is significantly diminished. In these cases, preserving the coracoacromial (CA) arch is critical to prevent possible anterior superior migration of the humeral head. With respect to the actual repair, this is performed through a mini-open deltoid-splitting incision that is an extension of the lateral portal, usually centered over the tear. No difference in morbidity is present; lower cost and quality of fixation are the most compelling reasons for this aspect of the procedure to be followed in an open procedure as opposed to a totally arthroscopic manner.

Bone anchors are expensive, and their strength depends on the quality of bone, which is frequently poor. The mini-open procedure also enables incorporation of a cleavage component into the repair as well as securance of the tendon into a bony trough rather than into a lightly abraded cortical bed. Although the debate continues with respect to completely arthroscopic cuff repair versus open repair, this combined approach incorporates the strong points of both procedures.

PATIENT POSITIONING

General anesthesia is preferred, although interscalene block with sedation can also be performed on patients undergoing rotator cuff repair. Examination under anesthesia is especially important in evaluating any restrictions in preoperative mobility. The patient is then placed in the lateral decubitus position on the beanbag. Axillary roll and kidney rests are used, and all bony prominences are carefully padded. The arm is placed in a traction apparatus with the shoulder at 60° abduction and 15° of frontal flexion (Fig. 11-1). Ten to 12 lbs of traction is normally used to suspend the shoulder.

DIAGNOSTIC GLENOHUMERAL ARTHROSCOPY

A standard posterior portal is established for the arthroscope. After penetrating the subcutaneous tissue, particular attention should be paid so that the trocar is entering through the interval between the infraspinatus and teres minor rather than through the rotator cuff tear itself. Entering through the tear itself limits the ability to evaluate the shoulder accurately. A pump system is routinely used for fluid ingress through the arthroscopic cannula. A standard anterior working portal is then established adjacent to the subscapularis tendon. The glenohumeral joint is evaluated systematically, and each structure is palpated with a blunt probe. Particular consideration is given to the integrity of the biceps tendon and the subscapularis. The biceps tendon is reduced into the joint with the blunt probe, and any fraying is debrided, as are any partial articular surface tears of the rotator cuff. Any cleavage component to the tear is identified and probed. Most rotator cuff tears originate at the rotator interval, progress posteriorly, and are easily visualized through the posterior portal. The posterior extent of large to massive tears, however, is best visualized from the anterior portal.

SUBACROMIAL BURSECTOMY AND DECOMPRESSION

Once the intra-articular pathology has been examined, the arthroscope is removed and the arm is placed in 15° of abduction and 0° of forward elevation while maintaining traction (Fig. 11-2). The same, or in most cases, a new posterior portal is placed, depending on the amount of swelling that has occurred. This portal is approximately 3 cm medial to the posterolateral edge of the acromion

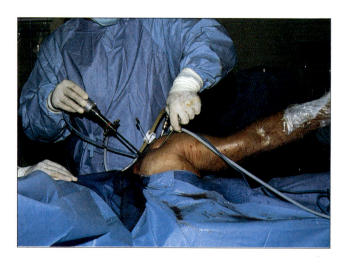

Figure 11-1. Position of the shoulder during glenohumeral arthroscopy. The arm is elevated to 60° of abduction with 15° of forward flexion.

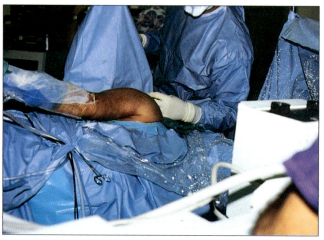

Figure 11-2. Position of the arm before subacromial decompression is performed. The arm is at nearly 10° of abduction, and the horizontal traction is maintained at 12 lbs.

and 1 cm below the acromion. The arthroscopic cannula is introduced into the subacromial space, confirming its position by palpating the undersurface of the acromion. A lateral portal is made 2.5 cm distal to the edge of the acromion and is centered over the observed tear. A working cannula for the arthroscopic instruments is introduced through the lateral portal. To enhance visualization, hypotensive anesthesia and cold saline solution with 1:1000 epinephrine are used. Necessary adequate visualization of the entire cuff can best be done following removal of the subacromial bursa. The bursal side of the rotator cuff is then evaluated by rotating the arm internally and externally. The tear pattern is established, and retracted portions are tested for mobility.

Bursectomy can be performed using a motorized shaver. Gutters around the cuff must also be cleared of inflamed bursa.

Rotator cuff tears may retract posteriorly as well as medially; with chronic tears, substance may be lost (Fig. 11-3). One or two arthroscopic sutures are placed through the retracted edge of the cuff using a suture punch or similar instrument (Figs. 11-4 to 11-6). This is done through the lateral or anterior portal, depending on the direction of retraction. Mobilization may be assisted by cutting the superior and posterior capsules and freeing the tissues with a blunt elevator. Only when reparability has been confirmed should subacromial decompression be performed. Sutures placed into the cuff are left in place to facilitate the open portion of

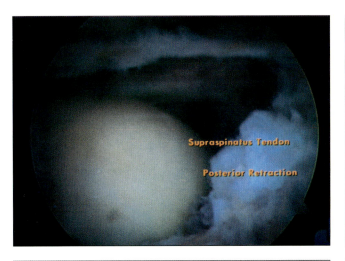

Figure 11-3. Subacromial view of a massive rotator cuff tear. The uncovered humeral head has proximal migration, and the retracted stump of the supraspinatus tendon has some posterior retraction.

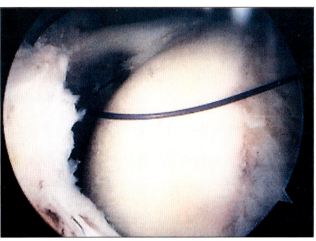

Figure 11-4. The importance of arthroscopy in assessing cuff tear patterns and retraction and the ability to mobilize a rotator cuff tear. A standard 0-PDS suture with a Caspari suture punch is placed in the massive tear.

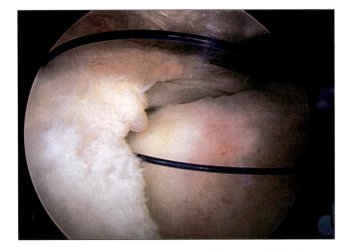

Figure 11-5. Tension is applied to the suture after it has been placed within the massive rotator cuff tear.

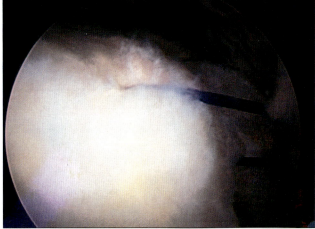

Figure 11-6. A tendon that can be mobilized and pulled back to its insertion along the greater tuberosity. This indicates that the tendon can be repaired and that its insertion can be reestablished through visualization of its tear pattern.

the repair. The authors' preference for ablating the CA ligament complex and exposure of the bony acromion is use of the Arthrocare Electrosurgical device (Arthrocare Co, Sunnyvale, CA). This bipolar multielectrode electrosurgical tool enables rapid tissue ablation with concurrent tissue hemostasis. After exposure of the acromion has been achieved, the acromioplasty is performed with a motorized burr, starting at the anterolateral corner and progressing medially to the acromioclavicular (AC) joint. If AC joint pathology exists concurrently, an arthroscopic resection is performed at that point in the procedure.

A bony subacromial decompression is performed only in patients with type II and type III acromions with evidence of chronic impingement. In patients with adequate subacromial space, the CA arch is preserved, and a simple bursectomy with or without some thinning of the CA ligament is performed. Because of the heterogenicity of rotator cuff tears, it is critical that the surgeon conceptualize the accurate reduction of the tendon before proceeding with the open portion of the repair.

MINI-OPEN REPAIR

The open portion of the repair begins with a simple extension of the lateral portal skin incision to the edge of the acromion. If the subscapularis tendon is involved, a separate anterior incision extending the anterior portal inferiorly is performed. In both cases, the muscle fibers are split bluntly using atraumatic dissection.

Visualization is facilitated by the use of a self-retaining Caspar retractor (Aesculap, Inc, South San Francisco, CA) and by separate retraction under the acromion (Fig. 11-7). The complete extent of the greater tuberosity can be reached with internal and external rotation of the arm. The pattern of the tear determines how the repair should proceed. L-shaped tears should be initially sutured side to side. In U-shaped tears, the repair is more straightforward. Horizontal mattress sutures (or a modification of them) are placed along the edge of the tendon. The authors have found #1 Ethibond suture (Ethicon, Somerville, NJ) on an OS 2 needle to be extremely helpful because of the lower profile of the needle. This is especially useful for suturing the cuff tendon under the acromion. Once all the sutures are in place, the cuff is reduced to its appropriate position along the greater tuberosity. Critical attention to cuff tension is needed. If tension is too great, some medialization of the trough may be required.

Occasionally there is difficulty mobilizing sufficient tissue to cover the humeral head adjacent to the biceps tendon. In these cases, we have found mobilization of the posterior cuff to be much easier than mobilization of the subscapularis. The insertion of the posterior cuff is incised along its attachment on the greater tuberosity. Sutures are placed on the cut edge of the tendon, and the tendon is pulled superiorly. The defect over the posterior humeral head can be closed with absorbable suture or left open.

Trough preparation is performed using a burr to remove the cortical bone cap. A Jensen rongeur is used for removal of cancellous bone (Fig. 11-8). The cancellous bone removed is saved for grafting. The retractor under the acromion is shifted to the inferior aspect of the wound and the soft tissue over the

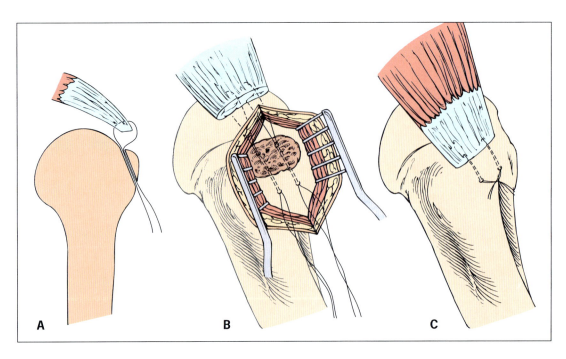

Figure 11-7. The concept and surgical principles involved in deltoid-splitting rotator cuff repair (**A**). By splitting the deltoid anterolaterally through the lateral portal, the entire insertion, from the rotator interval to the posterior aspect of the teres minor, can be visualized through the incision (**B**). **C,** The completed repair.

A   B   C

tuberosity and shaft is elevated. A #5 Ticron needle (Sherwood-Davis & Geck, St. Louis, MO) on a heavy needle driver makes an excellent awl. Holes are placed in the roof of the trough in an eccentric fashion to communicate with the trough. Staggering these holes helps prevent stress risers. The more distally placed the holes are, the better the pull-out strength will be. The number of holes varies with the number of sutures, but need not exceed five or six. Twisted 24-gauge wire is contoured as a suture passer and placed through the holes in the lateral humeral cortex and into the trough. The sutures are placed through the end loop of wire and are pulled through the trough and out to the lateral cortex. Depending on the number of sutures, more than one pair can be brought through each hole. After all the sutures are passed, tension is applied to the sutures, and the tendon is then reduced into the trough (Figs. 11-9 and 11-10). Cancellous bone graft is simultaneously packed over the tendon and into the trough. Beginning with the most anterior sutures, the sutures are tied over the respective bony bridges. To relieve the tension on the knot, the arm can be abducted while the sutures are tied.

After the suture is cut, the free strands are enclosed into a lateral periosteal layer (Fig. 11-11) with 3.0 Vicryl (Ethicon). This is to prevent any irritation from the suture to the subdeltoid fascia. The subdeltoid fascia and deltoid fascia are then closed. Then the remaining layers are closed. Postoperatively, the arms of patients with small and medium tears are placed in a sling; the arms of those with large tears are placed on an abduction pillow. Passive range-of-motion exercise is begun immediately; active assisted range-of-motion exercises are started 5 weeks postoperatively.

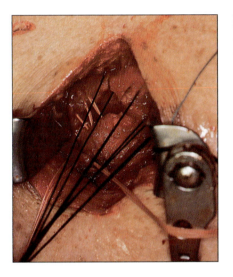

Figure 11-8. A mobilized rotator cuff. The dark sutures will be placed through the bony trough.

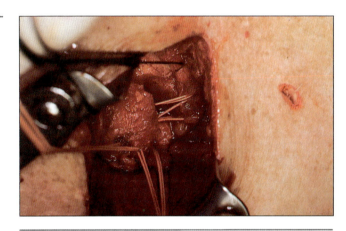

Figure 11-9. The sutures are placed through the bony trough, and the rotator cuff is tensioned into the trough.

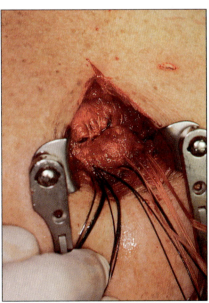

Figure 11-10. The rotator cuff in a reduced position within the trough, with some of the sutures tied.

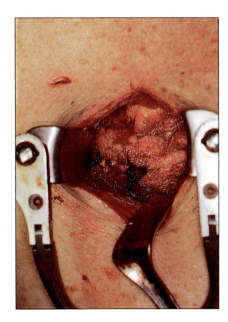

Figure 11-11. Completed repair with the sutures now cut. This provides full visualization of the greater tuberosity.

CONCLUSION

This technique has been performed by the senior author for 12 years. Using the UCLA shoulder scale, this technique was evaluated on a series of 60 consecutive patients with symptomatic full-thickness rotator cuff tears. The average follow-up period for these patients was 73 months. In this series, all cuff tears were repaired, and there was an 86% excellent or good shoulder rating. Arthroscopically assisted rotator cuff repair using a mini-open deltoid-splitting incision exploits the advantage of both arthroscopy and open surgery and is a highly effective technique.

REFERENCES

1. Rockwood CA Jr: Shoulder function following decompression and irreparable cuff lesions. *Orthop Trans* 1984, 8:92.

2. Rockwood CA, Burkhead WZ: Management of patients with massive rotator cuff defects by acromioplasty and rotator cuff debridement. *Orthop Trans* 1988, 12:190–191.

3. Cofield RA: Current concepts review: rotator cuff disease of the shoulder. *J Bone Joint Surg* 1985, 67(suppl A):974–979.

4. Ellman A, Hanker G, Bayer M: Repair of the rotator cuff: end result study of factors influencing reconstruction. *J Bone Joint Surg* 1986, 68(suppl 1):1136–1144.

5. Levy HJ, Uribe JW, Delaney LG: Arthroscopic assisted rotator cuff repair: preliminary results. *Arthroscopy* 1990, 6:55–60.

6. Paulos LE, Rody MA: Arthroscopically enhanced mini-approach to rotator cuff repair. *Arthroscopy* 1991, 7:333.

7. Liu SA, Baker CL: Arthroscopically assisted rotator cuff repair: correlation of functional results with integrity of cuff. *Arthroscopy* 1994, 10:54–60.

12

Avoiding Complications Associated with Arthroscopic Subacromial Decompression, Distal Clavicle Resection, and Rotator Cuff Repair

John S. Rogerson

The technique of arthroscopic subacromial decompression (ASAD) and distal clavicle resection has become an increasingly common procedure for dealing with impingement and acromioclavicular (AC) joint disease. Many surgeons are now routinely combining these arthroscopic decompression techniques with either mini-open or, more recently, completely arthroscopic repair of rotator cuff tears. As with other open operations that have evolved arthroscopically, the learning curve for these procedures is significant and should not be underestimated.

Complications associated with shoulder arthroscopy in general are low. Small, in his 1986 study [1], found a complication rate in subacromial space surgery of 0.76%. However, the complication rate with anterior staple capsulorraphy was 5.3%. The rates excluded clinical failures. In his follow-up study in 1988 [2,3], reporting on complications relating to arthroscopy performed by experienced arthroscopists, the complication rate with shoulder arthroscopy was 0.7% overall, again with the highest rate in anterior capsulorraphy.

Curtis *et al.* [4] reviewed 711 shoulder arthroscopies and found an overall complication rate of 6%. Of the 43 complications, 19 were secondary to postoperative stiffness, six secondary to transient neurologic symptoms, five associated with wound hematomas, and six associated with bruising. One patient each had problems with hardware removal, reflex sympathetic dystrophy, laceration of the cephalic vein, pulmonary embolus, and painful posterior portal, corneal abrasion, and heterotopic bone. The rate increased from 4.5% for arthroscopic procedures to

8.0% for combined arthroscopic and open surgery (*ie*, mini-open cuff repair or stabilization).

Several of the complications associated with shoulder arthroscopy are related to arthroscopic technique in general and are common to other joints that are arthroscopically examined [5]. In a survey sent to arthroscopy association members of the shoulder study group, however, some procedure-specific complications were also identified [6]. This chapter identifies some of the difficulties inherent in these arthroscopic techniques and provides some suggestions for precautions and modifications that may help in their avoidance.

TECHNIQUE-RELATED COMPLICATIONS

Neurologic

For the most part, neurologic complications have been associated with the lateral decubitus position for shoulder arthroscopy (Fig. 12-1). Neuropraxia involving traction injury to the brachial plexus may be secondary to the traction weight, direction of pull, and duration of the surgery. Five to 10 lbs of distal traction is usually adequate for the average patient, and 15 lbs is reserved for larger or well-muscled individuals. Increasing the weight to 20 lbs or more, as was initially done in shoulder arthroscopy, results in changes in the somatosensory-evoked potentials of the musculocutaneous, median, ulnar, and radial nerves, with the musculocutaneous being the most sensitive at all arm positions and traction weights [7].

In a cadaver study, Klein *et al.* [8] demonstrated the greatest brachial plexus strain with the arm at 70° abduction and 30° of forward flexion. The minimum overall strain was noted at 90° of flexion and 0° of abduction, but this resulted in poor visualization.

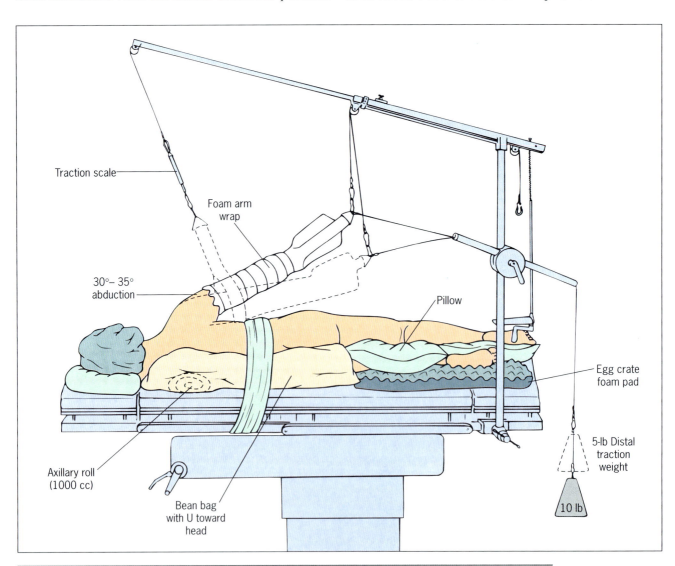

Figure 12-1. The lateral decubitus position (*solid*) with necessary padding and support, and the dual traction technique (*dotted*) with the same padding and 7 to 10 lbs lateral distraction.

They recommended positions of 45° of forward flexion and either 0° or 90° of abduction, depending on the intra-articular region of interest.

Dual traction as described by Gross and Fitzgibbons [9] (see Fig. 12-1) with low distal traction weights on a minimally abducted arm coupled with a laterally directed distraction force appeared to be associated with less compromise to somatosensory-evoked potentials in Pittman et al.'s study [7]. Gross and Fitzgibbons [9] also recommended rolling the patient back about 25° to 30° to orient the glenoid joint surface parallel to the floor. The rollback position coupled with 15° of additional flexion of the arm puts the direction of pull into Klein et al.'s safer zone [8]. No work has been specifically directed at determining the neurologic effects of the laterally directed distraction force in this set-up, but no reported complications have been associated with this type of traction.

For arthroscopic surgery in the subacromial space, minimal abduction (15° to 25°) and 15° of flexion from the rollback position opens up the space and yet does not put excessive strain on the brachial plexus. Excessive forward flexion of the arm brings the tuberosity into contact with the anterior acromial hook, making exposure difficult.

Careful attention needs to be given to the position of the head, which should be as close to exactly neutral as possible. Any sagging of the head down and away from the operative arm increases the strain on the brachial plexus. Overcompensation and excessive propping of the head away from the "down" arm can result in the opposite brachial strain. Careful padding and wrapping of the traction device at the wrist are necessary to avoid compression injury to the sensory branch of the radial nerve with resultant thumb numbness. Moreover, careful padding of the ulnar and peroneal nerves on the downside is necessary [10••]. Time in traction is also a factor, and conversion to an open operation is recommended if the operation is extending past 2 hours or if distention is becoming severe.

The beach-chair position alleviates most of the neurologic concerns already stated [11], but careful positioning and support of the head are still necessary. A case of hypoglossal nerve injury has been reported with this position [12]. Exposure in the subacromial space, however, may be diminished because of loss of distraction. The dual traction technique is not possible with this position.

Anesthetic

General anesthesia provided to the patient in the lateral decubitus position appears safe relative to hypotensive and neurologic problems, so long as proper padding has been established. Interscalene nerve blocks are commonly used for either intraoperative anesthesia or additional postoperative pain relief. A temporary ipsilateral phrenic nerve palsy routinely results from this block but rarely causes pulmonary problems except in patients with preexisting pulmonary insufficiency [13,14].

Esch and Baker [15], however, reported on two patients requiring ventilatory support after interscalene block for ASAD. The anesthesia literature documents various relatively significant complications with interscalene blocks, including bilateral spread affecting both phrenics; complete spinal, bilateral cervical, and thoracic epidural blockade; prolonged Horner's syndrome; auditory disturbance; and cardiac arrest [16–22]. Pneumothorax caused by incorrect needle placement has also been reported [23]. Complications associated with interscalene block appear to be more common when the block is performed after induction of a general anesthetic as opposed to when the patient is awake and a nerve stimulator has been used.

Portal Placement

Direct nerve injury can be associated with incorrect portal placement.

Posterior Portals

The traditional posterior portal as described by Andrews et al. [24] has become the standard position for the initiation of glenohumeral and subacromial arthroscopy. This penetrates the so-called soft spot approximately 1 cm medial and 1 to 2 cm inferior to the posterolateral corner of the acromion. The arthroscope should enter the joint approximately in the interval between the infraspinatus and teres minor muscles. This portal passes through the deltoid, ranging from 2 to 4 cm from the axillary nerve and the posterior humeral circumflex artery, and lies approximately 1 cm lateral to the suprascapular nerve and artery.

Inferior medial migration of this portal as described by Wolf [25] for the central posterior portal or inferior lateral migration for his modified posterior portal [26] places these structures at greater risk. Directing a blunted conical trocar toward the coracoid process provides some increased margin of safety for these posterior portals. Sharp trocars should generally be avoided for shoulder arthroscopy because of the increased risk of neurologic and chondral damage.

Anterior Portals

Several anterior shoulder arthroscopic portals have been described [24,25,27–30]. The anterior superior portals as described by Andrews et al. [24] and Wolf

[25,26] and the superolateral portal described by Laurencin *et al.* [30] are neurologically safe and most useful for subacromial surgery. They are also readily used to provide an anterior viewing portal for glenohumeral work. The central anterior portal in the superior recess above the subscapularis tendon as described by Matthews *et al.* [27] also appears to be safe relative to neurovascular structures. As the surgeon moves inferior to the tip of the coracoid process, the risk to neurovascular structures increases. These portals as described by Wolf (anterior-inferior portal) [25], Resch *et al.* [28], and Davidson and Tibone [29] (anterior-inferior transubscapular) are more useful for arthroscopic instability surgery and are not generally used for subacromial or rotator cuff work (Fig. 12-2).

Superior Portal

The supraclavicular fossa portal was devised by Neviaser [31]; it allowed placement of an additional inflow portal at the posterior superior aspect of the joint, as well as access for superior instrumentation. The suprascapular nerve and artery lie deep and on the inferior surface of the supraspinatus muscle, approximately 2 cm medial to the path of the cannula. Too vertical a passage can injure the suprascapular nerve and artery; too lateral a passage can injure the rotator cuff tendon, particularly if the arm is abducted more than 30° [32]. This portal is no longer routinely needed or used, particularly for subacromial work (Fig. 12-3).

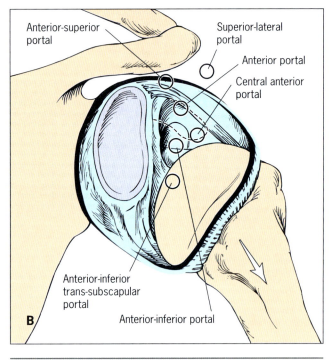

Figure 12-2. External (**A**) and arthroscopic (**B**) views of the anterior portals, including the superolateral [30], anterior-superior [25], anterior [24], central anterior [27], anterior-inferior [25], and anterior-inferior trans-subscapular [28,29] portals.

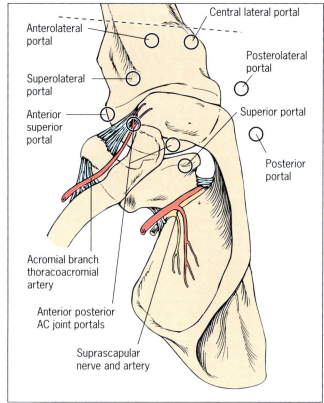

Figure 12-3. Subacromial and superior portals, including the posterior [24], posterolateral [33], central lateral [34,50], anterolateral [33], superolateral [30], anterior-superior [25], anterior and posterior acromioclavicular (AC) [35], and superior [31] portals. *Dotted line* indicates course of axillary nerve 5 cm lateral to the acromial edge.

Subacromial Portals

Multiple subacromial portals have been described for decompression and for AC joint and rotator cuff surgery. These include the traditional posterior portal with angulation of the arthroscope or instrument superiorly into the subacromial bursa, the posterolateral portal [33], the central lateral portal [34], the anterolateral portal, the anterior and posterior AC joint portals [35], and the accessory high portals for anchor placement in rotator cuff surgery (see Fig. 12-3).

The neurologic structure most at risk with the use of these portals is the axillary nerve, which traverses the underside of the deltoid muscle approximately 3 to 5 cm from the acromial margin. If the surgeon keeps the skin incision less than 5 cm from the acromion and directs the trocar toward the subacromial space, as opposed to directly down through the deltoid muscle, axillary nerve problems should be avoided [36]. These portals are best set up after preliminary placement and direct visualization of an 18-gauge needle to ensure the proper orientation for shaving or anchor placement.

Vascular

Problems related to hypotension have been associated with arthroscopy done with the patient in the beach-chair position, especially in elderly or hypertensive patients. Adequate fluid replacement and compression leg stockings may be beneficial to avoid premature termination of the procedure or switching to a lateral decubitus position. Although deep venous thrombosis is rare, it has also been reported with shoulder arthroscopy [37].

Likely, the most common vascular complication with subacromial surgery is bleeding. Because the subacromial area is extensively traversed by veins, frequently inflamed, and not a closed space, bleeding is more troublesome here than at almost any other arthroscopic site. Failure to control bleeding and to maintain visualization and orientation are common sources of complications in subacromial surgery. Use of electrocautery is strongly recommended. Strategies currently used for the control of bleeding include:

- Inject 0.25% bupivacaine with epinephrine into the portals (2 mL) and subacromial space (10 mL) at the beginning of the procedure.
- Incise only the skin to avoid deeper muscle laceration.
- Use a blunted conical trocar for penetration of muscle, joint, and subacromial space.
- Add epinephrine, 10 mL (1:1000) per 3–L bag to only the first irrigation bag.
- Avoid debridement of anterior medial acromion and the undersurface of the AC joint until late in the case.

- Use electrocautery immediately when significant "bleeders" are encountered.
- Increase inflow with large-bore sheath at level of the arthroscope. A pump with independent control of pressure and flow rate is helpful.
- Decrease outflow to maintain pressure. Control suction on shavers and burrs to reduce "red-out." Integrated fluid delivery and shaver systems are helpful for this problem.
- Reduce blood pressure, if the patients' medical condition allows, to maintain systolic pressure of less than 95 to 100 mm Hg.
- Increase pressure on pump or elevate bags to level at which bleeding is well controlled.

Pulmonic

Pneumothorax is a known complication associated with interscalene block anesthesia [23]. There have been rare cases of subcutaneous emphysema, pneumomomediastinum, and potentially life-threatening tension pneumothorax associated with arthroscopic decompression [38].

Soft-Tissue Injury

Skin burns have been reported with shoulder arthroscopy if a noninsulated cautery tip is used with conductive solution. This problem can be avoided if the surgeon uses an insulated tip, or newer bipolar devices for ablation and cautery. These tips can be used safely even in conductive solutions such as normal saline or lactated Ringer's solution.

Sterile water, which was used early on because of its nonconductivity, is injurious to soft tissues. Scattered reports exist of skin and muscle necrosis associated with extremely long procedures using water as an irrigating solution. Glycine (1.5%), used in urologic procedures, and less frequently as an arthroscopic medium, has been associated with transient blindness and is no longer recommended [39].

Extravasation and distention of the soft tissues with saline or lactated Ringer's solution may sometimes produce alarming appearances. Studies have shown, however, that the intramuscular pressures rapidly return to normal at the end of the procedure [40,41]. The effect of soft-tissue distention on the nerves surrounding the shoulder has not been well-documented.

Infection

The infection rate resulting from arthroscopy in general is very low. Johnson et al. [42] reported less than one infection in 2000 new arthroscopies when using 2% glutaraldehyde as a sterilizing agent. Only four infection cases with shoulder arthroscopy have been noted in the literature to date [1,15,43].

Glutaraldehyde solution has been commonly used for instrument sterilization, especially in the outpatient setting. However, instruments must be thoroughly rinsed before use. Even trace amounts (such as may be found in arthroscopic rinse baths) can induce a severe synovial inflammatory reaction [44]. Because of this and because of concerns regarding HIV transmission through the use of glutaraldehyde, sterilization is increasingly being performed by automated sterilization units such as the Steris (peracetic acid; Steris Co, Mentor, OH) [45] or Sterad (gas plasma with hydrogen peroxide; J & J Medical, Arlington, TX) [46].

Equipment Failure

The potential for an equipment failure increases with the complexity of the procedure. Cannulated suture hooks and punches, various suture retrievers, linear punches, and grasping forceps can break off in the joint. Keeping a retrieval instrument, such as the magnetic Golden Retriever suction device (Instrument Makar, Okemos, MI), handy can considerably simplify recapture of metallic peices.

PROCEDURE-RELATED COMPLICATIONS

Arthroscopic Subacromial Decompression

Complications of ASAD include 1) variable bone resection, 2) deltoid detachment, 3) heterotopic bone, and 4) residual coracoacromial ligament (CAL) snapping.

Variable Bone Resection

Variable bone resection is probably the most common complication of ASAD. Both inadequate decompression and excessive resection have been reported. Wolf [47] reviewed 35 patients with failed previous arthro-

scopic surgery of the shoulder. Of these patients, 60% failed because of previous inadequate ASAD; 20 of 21 had complete recovery after further ASAD [47]. Matthews *et al.* [27] and Esch [48] have reported on both acromial and clavicular fractures secondary to excessive resection.

Inaccurate decompression is usually secondary to inadequate preoperative planning with or without poor visualization and orientation during the procedure.

Preoperative Evaluation

Outlet and axillary views are key to evaluating the acromion. The outlet view is used to determine the shape of the acromion (type I, II, or III) and the overall thickness [49,50]. Rockwood and Lyons [51] have described a modified anterior shoulder view that, although helpful in making the diagnosis of impingement, is not beneficial in terms of preoperative planning. On the outlet view, two lines are drawn on the undersurface of the acromion—the first from the front tip of the acromion to the posterior edge, and the second along the posterior half of the undersurface of the acromion extending out anteriorly. The distance between these two lines at the anterior margin approximates the amount of undersurface anterior bone that will be resected (Fig. 12-4).

The axillary view is used to determine the shape of the acromion (cobra-shaped vs square-tipped), as well as to determine whether there is any "anterior acromial protuberance" [52] anterior to the level of the AC joint (Fig. 12-5). This approximates the amount of bone that will be removed anteriorly in addition to the amount of bone that will be taken from the undersurface.

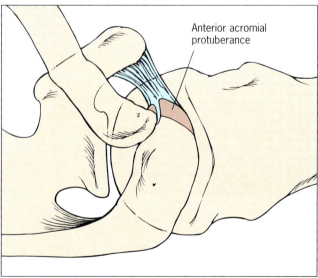

Anterior acromial protuberance

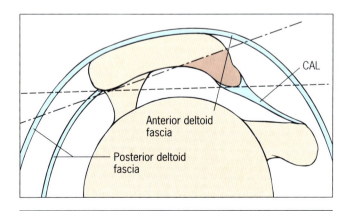

Figure 12-4. Preoperative determination of bone resection shown on an outlet-view radiograph. CAL—coracoacromial ligament. *Shaded area* between *dotted lines* denotes bone resection.

Figure 12-5. Preoperative evaluation (axillary view) of anterior acromial protuberance and the amount of resection needed. *Shaded area* indicates bone resection.

After these measurements have been determined, the two-portal technique of acromioplasty makes it relatively simple to reproduce this resection. It is difficult to obtain a flat acromion when visualizing only from the posterior portal because of the amount of curving away of the acromion from the arthroscope. The acromion may appear flat from medial to lateral and front to back, but may still have a considerable anterior-to-posterior concavity when later viewed from the lateral portal. Placing the arthroscope laterally and then bringing the shaver forward from the posterior portal using the posterior half of the acromion as a "cutting block" [53] helps ensure a straight, flat cut in the sagittal plane. This technique reliably converts a type II or type III acromion to a type I flat surface as demonstrated on postoperative radiographs (Fig. 12-6). The surgeon should be sure to subsequently replace the arthroscope posteriorly and to confirm flatness of the acromion in the medial to lateral plane. The anterior lateral acromial corner is often diffi-cult to visualize from the lateral portal. Good visualization from *both* portals assures a flat, smooth surface.

The surgeon should beware of the thin curved type acromion (type C) [50]. If, on the outlet view, a very thin or curved acromion is found, the cutting block line on the undersurface of the posterior half of the acromion may actually exit from the superior aspect of the acromion, taking off too much anterior bone (Fig. 12-7A). In such cases, the cutting block technique would be inappropriate. In this situation, the original resection technique as described by Ellman [33] is more applicable, that is, removing only a small anterior hook and not producing a type I flat acromion (Fig. 12-7B).

Inadequate Visualization

This finding is usually secondary to excessive bleeding (which can be managed as previously outlined), poor localization of the subdeltoid bursa, or inadequate debridement of the subacromial space. Remembering

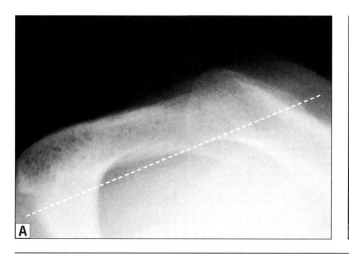
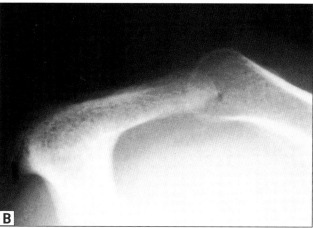

Figure 12-6. A, Preoperative templating for arthroscopic subacromial decompression (ASAD) on outlet-view radiograph. *Dotted line* indicates correct line of bone resection. **B,** Postoperative radiograph of ASAD.

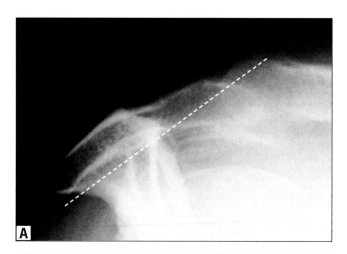
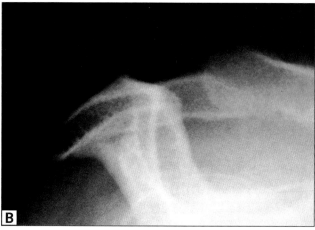

Figure 12-7. Preoperative (**A**) and postoperative (**B**) radiographs of decompression on the thin, curved acromion. *Dotted line* in A indicates excessive bone resection with cutting-block technique. Postoperative radiograph demonstrates more conservative anterior resection with significant increase in anterior acromial humeral distance.

that the bursa is an anterior structure, the surgeon should make every effort when in the subacromial space to direct the arthroscope into what Wuh and Snyder [50] termed the *room with a view*. Time and care should be spent at the beginning of the procedure, debriding the bursitis and the thickened periosteum on the undersurface of the anterior half of the acromion. Some of the posterior bursal curtain may need to be resected to clearly visualize the bony architecture. Debridement can be done with a shaver-burr, or a cautery-ablation system, but the surgeon should be sure to stay on the acromial bone and not deviate into the deltoid fibers. Debridement should be performed from the anterior lateral corner of the acromion toward, but not into, the AC joint, and then posteriorly along the lateral edge of the acromion. Spinal needles are used at the anterior lateral corner and the AC joint to gain better clarification of the bony landmarks.

A burr should next be used to resect 3 to 4 mL of bone, again along the anterior margin of the acromion from the anterior lateral corner to the AC joint, then tapering posteriorly along the lateral edge of the anterior half of the acromion. This improves orientation and visualization when the arthroscope is placed in the lateral portal and the shaver is brought in posteri-

orly. The surgeon should not resect too much anterior bone—only enough to make it easy to delineate the anterior edge of the acromion as seen from the lateral portal. The surgeon should let the shaver from the posterior portal resect most of the bone, coming forward in a smooth, controlled, flat cut (Fig. 12-8). The amount of bone resected is easy to determine by comparing the anterior remaining ledge with the thickness of the burr.

The posterior portal (through the deltoid muscle) must be at the inferior edge of the acromion, and not further below with soft-tissue interposition, so that the shaver does not angulate superiorly in an excessive or artificial manner (Fig. 12-9). Although the same placement of posterior skin incision is used for both glenohumeral and subacromial arthroscopy, the burr needs to puncture the soft tissues right at the inferior edge of the acromion for successful two-portal cutting-block technique.

Deltoid Detachment

Deltoid detachment results from overly aggressive resection at the anterior aspect of the acromion. If no significant anterior acromial protuberance is seen on the axillary radiograph, then simply flattening the

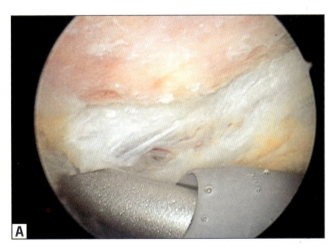

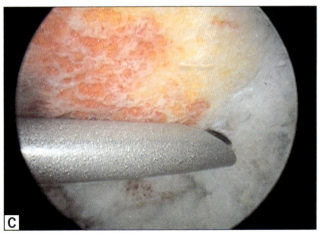

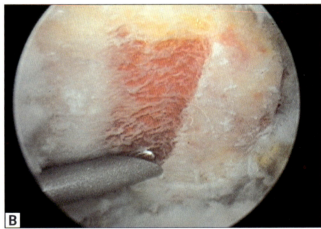

Figure 12-8. Serial intraoperative views of arthroscopic subacromial decompression of the right shoulder. **A,** Conservative anterior resection from the lateral portal with the shaver tip on the cora-coacromial ligament. **B,** Lateral view of the burr starting forward during cutting block resection. **C,** Completed resection with flat acromial undersurface from posterior to anterior and intact deltoid fascia.

undersurface of the acromion will adequately decompress it.

When a protuberance does exist, it usually is an extension of calcification inferiorly into the CAL. Resecting the ligament and the contained bone with subsequent flattening of the acromion will usually eliminate the anterior overhang. Routinely resecting 8 to 10 mm of full-thickness anterior bone (as described for open procedures [51]) from the lateral portal puts the deltoid attachment at significant risk. This damage cannot subsequently be repaired unless the shoulder is then opened. The surgeon should take a small amount of anterior bone from the lateral portal and the bulk of the bone from the posterior portal using the cutting-block technique, thus teasing the bone off anteriorly from the fascia. Deltoid detachment, either open or closed, is arguably the most devastating complication of shoulder surgery and should be avoided [54].

Heterotopic Bone
This finding has been reported to be associated with both acromioplasty and AC resection [55,56]. In the 10 cases reported by Berg *et al.* [55], eight developed recurrent impingement symptoms, with an apparent strong correlation with active spondylitic arthropathy or a profile of hypertrophic pulmonary osteoarthropathy— male, obese, smoker with chronic pulmonary disease. They recommended prophylactic measures (indomethacin or radiotherapy) with these two types of patient groups. The surgeon should also unplug clogged shavers and burrs (or use an accessory gravity drainage portal) to avoid debris ("clouds of snow").

Coracoacromial Ligament
Continued snapping with abduction and rotation maneuvers from an inadequate resection and a rescarring of the CAL do occur occasionally. After bony decompression has been completed, another 5 to 10 mm of ligament can be resected using a shaver, basket punches, or an ablation device. This is especially appropriate if snapping of the biceps tendon or bursal fold on the CAL is an identifiable preoperative complaint. Partial release of the anterolateral band alone may be curative in some athletes engaged in overhead throwing maneuvers [57]. Care should be taken to avoid excessive release of the lateral extension of the ligament along the lateral edge of the acromion. The ligament and deltoid fascia are intimately connected at this location, and release risks the deltoid attachment [58•].

Resection should not be done in the presence of significant degenerative arthritis of the glenohumeral joint or cuff arthropathy with a massive cuff tear, or if future arthroplasty is contemplated [59].

Arthroscopic Distal Clavicle Resection
Thorough clinical and radiologic evaluation of the AC joint should be performed prior to decompression. Significant inferior osteophytes should be noted on the anteroposterior view, and narrowing and sclerosis (degenerative joint disease) or widening and cystic changes (osteolysis) should be noted on the anteroposterior and axillary views. Differential injection into the AC joint instead of into the subacromial bursa may be necessary to confirm AC involvement.

Depending on the findings listed above, a decision must be made preoperatively (if possible) regarding the AC joint and distal clavicle. The surgeon must decide whether to 1) leave the AC joint untouched, 2) bevel the distal clavicle, or 3) perform an arthroscopic distal clavicle resection.

Most early descriptions of ASAD recommended routine beveling of the distal clavicle [33,60].

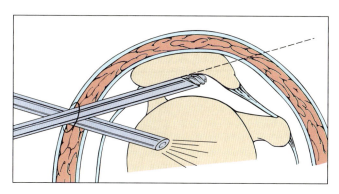

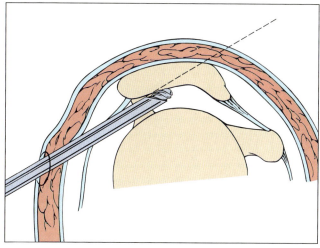

Figure 12-9. A, Although the same skin incision is utilized for both the glenohumeral and subacromial examinations, the trocar penetrates the deeper soft tissues at different levels, so the shaver can be closely applied to the undersurface of the acromion. **B,** If portal or soft-tissue penetration is too inferior, the burr will angulate too far superiorly, and excess resection will occur.

However, this practice destabilizes the AC joint to a certain extent by resecting the weaker inferior ligaments. The author has seen two patients in his own practice (and anecdotal reports from others) who, after decompression and beveling, developed AC joint pain necessitating later distal clavicle resection. Prior to surgery, these patients appeared clinically and radiographically to have normal AC joints.

If there are significant inferior osteophytes off the clavicle, then there is likely already compromise of the inferior AC ligaments and enough direct irritation of the underlying cuff to warrant beveling the tip. As the beveling is performed, downward pressure on the clavicle will bring some of the articular surface into view. If it appears significantly arthritic, then a complete resection of 1.0 to 1.5 cm of clavicle should be performed.

However, in patients with AC joints appearing normal on preoperative clinical and radiographic examinations, the author no longer routinely bevels the clavicle; instead, the medial acromial bone is teased off the capsule and cartilage, much as is done with the deltoid fascia during decompression.

Other complications associated with distal clavicle excision relate to 1) heterotopic bone formation, 2) inadequate resection, 3) underlying muscle injury, and 4) excessive bleeding. Incomplete resection of the superior cortical bone during distal clavicle resection is not uncommon. Clear visualization of this area using either a 30° or 70° arthroscope is necessary to remove all the superior bone (Fig. 12-10). If a cortical eggshell of bone is left behind, elevation or cross-chest maneuvers by the patient will remain painful. The bone will also serve as a nidus of heterotopic bone formation (Fig. 12-11).

The optimal amount of bone to be removed arthroscopically from the tip of the clavicle remains unresolved. If the superior and posterior AC ligaments are well maintained with the resection, the length of clavicle to be removed can be reduced [61]. If the superior and posterior ligaments are violated, however, then the remaining tip of the clavicle becomes more unstable, and further resection is needed [62,63•]. Studies suggest that 1 to 1.5 cm of bone resection would be adequate with use of the arthroscopic technique (Fig. 12-12); 1.5 cm of bone should be resected if the posterior-superior ligaments have been compromised.

Care should be taken to measure the distance between the clavicle and the acromion with two 18-gauge spinal needles placed parallel through the skin

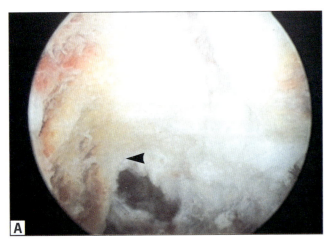

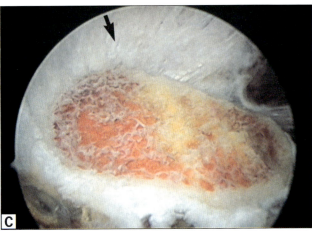

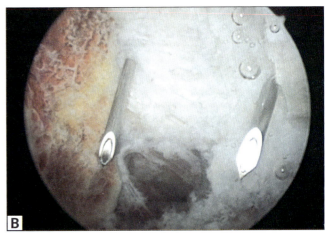

Figure 12-10. A, View from the posterior portal looking up at the acromioclavicular (AC) joint (*arrowhead*) with the inferior half of the distal clavicle already resected from the right shoulder. **B,** Posterior view of the AC space with the distal clavicle resected and two spinal needles placed externally to measure the distance between the clavicle tip and the medial edge of the acromion (*right*). **C,** Lateral view of the clavicle resection with the posterior and superior ligaments intact (*arrow*).

from above. This should be performed at both the anterior and posterior aspects of the clavicle (*see* Fig. 12-10*B*). It is easy to obtain an uneven gap in resection with more bone removed anteriorly than posteriorly, which should be avoided.

Caution should be taken when using unhooded burrs to resect the tip of the clavicle because it is very simple to wrap up the soft underlying cuff musculature in the instrument. The author prefers to use a well-hooded burr with the open side always either facing up or in, toward the cancellous middle of the clavicle. Suction should be low, just sufficient to clear debris.

Vascularity around the tip of the clavicle and AC joint is plentiful. Cauterization of the fat pad beneath the AC joint *before* debridement is helpful. It is also beneficial to outline the tip of the clavicle frequently with the cautery device when it is being resected medially because periosteal vessels are numerous.

Arthroscopic Rotator Cuff Repair

The rotator cuff should be thoroughly evaluated arthroscopically both from the articular and bursal sides. Partial tears are usually well-managed with limited debridement and ASAD. Excessive debridement of partial tears can lead to complete rotator cuff tears if caution is not exercised. Evaluation is aided by placement of "suture markers"—an 18-gauge needle placed from a superior position through the cuff and into the joint with a #1 monofilament suture grasped in the joint and brought out through the anterior portal as the needle is removed. This allows the investigator to closely examine the exact area on the bursal surface of the cuff that corresponds to the torn area on the articular side. Nearly complete tears that will not heal with adequate strength should be completed and repaired [64]. Several clinical studies have demonstrated that repair of rotator cuff tears in

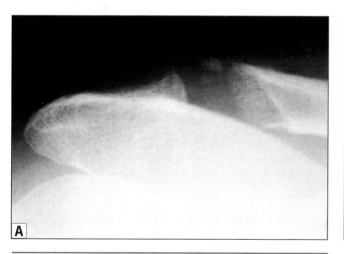
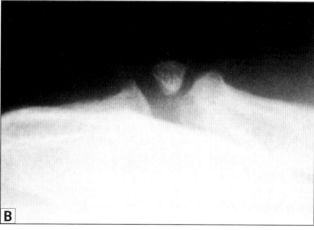

Figure 12-11. Heterotopic bone formation after distal clavicle resection (right shoulder). **A,** Six-month follow-up radiograph showing early heterotopic nidus. **B,** Two-year postoperative radiograph demonstrating mature bone in the A-C interval.

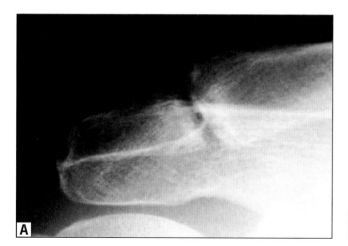
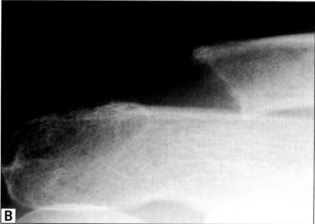

Figure 12-12. Preoperative (**A**) and postoperative (**B**) radiographs of the acromioclavicular resection (right shoulder).

conjunction with ASAD fares better in the long run when compared with simple debridement and decompression [52,64,65].

Failure of fixation of rotator cuff repair is a common problem with both open and arthroscopic repair. This may be due to *mechanical* factors, *biological* factors, or both.

Mechanical Considerations

Several factors related to technique can affect the mechanical strength of rotator cuff repair and increase the likelihood of success. Anchor fixation into bone can be improved by roughening the area of the tuberosity widely to increase the surface area for cuff repair, while decorticating lightly. Creation of deep troughs in the soft cancellous bone lead to anchor pull-out (or tunnel breakage during open techniques). St. Pierre *et al.* [66•] demonstrated good healing in animal studies without the need of a deep trough.

Inserting the anchor at about a 45° angle to the direction of pull (Burkhart's "deadman's angle") [67] results in increased resistance to pull-out and puts the anchor under the stronger subchondral bone medially (*see* Chapter 8, Fig. 8-5). Recent studies also suggest that simple suture may be stronger than mattress sutures in the fixation of tendon to bone in the rotator cuff area [68].

With the 45° "deadman's angle" approach to the bone, the suture is pulled at an acute angle, with repetitive tension over the medial lip of the anchor hole. If the edge is too sharp, fraying and breaking of the suture may ensue. If the initial drill has a slight bevel at the stop point or if the hole is subsequently chamfered, the results of this problem may be diminished.

Biologic Considerations

The vascular involvements of rotator cuff repairs in older patients are always in question. Factors that may affect the blood supply to the repair should be kept in mind. Debriding the edges of a rotator cuff back to bleeding tissue stimulates an acute healing response.

Reducing tension on the rotator cuff repair in its early healing phase improves circulation and healing potential. This reduction can be accomplished by fixing small tears where they appear (*ie*, more medially than the normal tuberosity attachment). Burkhart has described the principle of "margin convergence" [69•] in the reduction of tension on rotator cuff tissue and repairs. By repairing the larger tears with side-to-side sutures medially and then working laterally to fix the remaining Y-shaped or L-shaped tissue to bone using anchors, tension on the repair and susceptibility to anchor pull-out are reduced. This appears to be a valid principle in the author's practice.

The larger the tear, the more beneficial an abduction pillow may be to improve blood flow to the "critical zone" and again reduce tension on sutures. Careful monitoring of postoperative rehabilitation is essential. The goal is to protect the repair and to avoid development of excessive scar tissue formation in the subdeltoid space—a "captured shoulder," as described by Mormino *et al.* [70]. Passive motion is less stressful on the repair in the early phases. Debate exists as to when to allow active abduction; this decision should be influenced by the size, pattern, and vascularity of the tear, as well as the stability of fixation.

Incorrect Diagnosis

Symptoms that persist despite adequate decompression or distal clavicle excision may be secondary to incorrect diagnosis. Decompression in a patient with secondary impingement from underlying anterior instability may often be unsuccessful until the underlying instability has been addressed. Posterior superior impingement is not likely to respond to anterior decompression. Underlying glenohumeral arthritis in weightlifters may negate the beneficial effects of distal clavicle excision for osteolysis. Suprascapular nerve syndrome must be diagnosed using specific neurologic modifications of standard electromyographic technique. A high index of suspicion for this entity must be maintained. Radicular cervical disease, metastatic carcinoma of the scapular neck, Pancost's tumors of the lung, and referred pain to the shoulder from visceral structures are also part of the differential diagnosis. Postoperative pain associated with a cracking sensation is most likely secondary to a fracture of the acromion.

Norwood and Fowler [71] reported on four cases of recurrent symptoms after technically well-performed shoulder arthroscopy, secondary to persistent cuff tears. These appeared to be related to inadequate healing on the articular side of the tendinous portion of the cuff at the posterior portal site. Because larger cannulae are now being used routinely, this problem may become increasingly noted, both anteriorly and posteriorly. If persistent or recurrent pain and weakness occur after arthroscopy, repetition of the arthrogram may be worthwhile. If results are positive, an open repair is likely to be beneficial.

Inadequate Surgical Preparation

Surgical preparation entails not only physician training, preoperative planning, and equipment requirements, but also patient education. Many patients have unrealistic expectations as to the results that arthroscopic surgery can accomplish relative to the shoulder. Education about soft-tissue healing times and scar tissue maturation should help temper unwarranted enthusiasm and activity. Because pain associated with arthroscopic procedures is often reduced, careful monitoring of postoperative activity, especially with rotator cuff repair, is necessary.

Physician preparation is mandatory for successful surgical results. Training at meetings and cadaver laboratories, such as the Orthopedic Learning Center (Chicago, IL), is prudent before attempting new techniques in one's practice. These procedures are equipment intensive, and a step-wise progression from open to mini-open to arthroscopic technique is recommended.

CONCLUSION

Arthroscopic subacromial decompression, distal clavicle excision, and rotator cuff repair are demanding operative procedures. It is hoped that diligent preoperative planning and intraoperative attention to the possible complications presented will increase the potential for successful surgical outcomes.

REFERENCES AND RECOMMENDED READING

Recently published papers of particular interest have been highlighted as:
- Of interest
- • Of outstanding interest

1. Small NC, Committee on Complications of the Arthroscopy Association of North America: Complications in arthroscopy: the knee and other joints. *Arthroscopy* 1986, 2:253–258.

2. Small NC: Complications in arthroscopic surgery performed by experienced arthroscopists. *Arthroscopy* 1988, 4:215–221.

3. Small NC: Complications in arthroscopic surgery of the knee and shoulder. *Orthopedics* 1993, 16:985–988.

4. Curtis AS, Delpezio W, Ferkle RD, *et al.*: Complications of shoulder arthroscopy. Paper presented at the 59th Annual Meeting of the American Academy of Orthopedic Surgeons. Washington, DC; February, 1992.

5. Bigliani LU, Flatow EL, Deliz DD: Complications of shoulder arthroscopy. *Orthop Rev* 1991, 20:743–751.

6. Rogerson JS: Avoiding complications in subacromial surgery. Presented at the AANA Specialty Day at the 61th Annual Meeting of the American Academy of Orthopedic Surgeons. New Orleans, LA; 1994.

7. Pitman MI, Nainzadeh N, Ergas E, *et al.*: The use of somatosensory evoked potentials for detection of neuropraxia during shoulder arthroscopy. *Arthroscopy* 1988, 4:250–255.

8. Klein AH, Franc JC, Mutschlen TA, *et al.*: Measurement of brachial plexus strain in arthroscopy of the shoulder. *Arthroscopy* 1987, 3:45–52.

9. Gross RM, Fitzgibbons TC: Shoulder arthroscopy: a modified approach. *Arthroscopy* 1985, 1:156–159.

10.•• Stanish WD, Peterson DC: Shoulder arthroscopy and nerve injury: pitfalls and prevention. *Arthroscopy* 1995, 11:458–466.

Excellent analysis of all the different etiologies of nerve injuries, including portal placement, traction set-ups, and anesthesia techniques.

11. Skyhar MJ, Altchek DW, Warren RF, *et al.*: Shoulder arthroscopy with the patient in the beach-chair position. *Arthroscopy* 1988, 4:256–259.

12. Mullins RC, Drez D, Cooper J: Hypoglossal nerve palsy after arthroscopy of the shoulder and open operation with the patient in the beach-chair position: a case report. *J Bone Joint Surg Am*, 1992, 74:137–139.

13. Urmey WF, Talts KH, Sharrock NE: One hundred percent incidence of hemi-diaphragmatic paresis associated with interscalene brachial plexus anesthesia as diagnosed by ultrasonography. *Anesth Analg* 1991, 72:498–503.

14. Urmey WF, McDonald M: Hemidiaphragmatic paresis during interscalene brachial plexus block: effects on pulmonary function and chest wall mechanics. *Anesth Analg* 1992, 74:352–357.

15. Esch JC, Baker CL: Complications and pitfalls. In *Arthroscopic Surgery—the Shoulder and Elbow*. Edited by Whipple TL. Philadelphia: JB Lippincott; 1993:221.

16. Dutton RP, Eckhardt WF, Sunder N: Total spinal anesthesia after interscalene blockade of the brachial plexus. *Anesthesiology* 1994, 80:939–941.

17. Gologorsky E, Leanza RF: Contralateral anesthesia following interscalene block. *Anesth Analg* 1992, 75:311–312.

18. Tuominen MK, Pere P, Rosenberg PH: Unintentional arterial catheterization and bupivacaine toxicity associated with continuous interscalene brachial plexus block. *Anesthesiology* 1991, 75:356–358.

19. Cook LB: Unsuspected extradural catheterization in an interscalene block. *Br J Anaesth* 1991, 67:473–475.

20. Edde RR, Deutsch S: Cardiac arrest after interscalene brachial plexus block. *Anesth Analg* 1997, 56:446–447.

21. Sukhani R, Barclay J, Aasen M: Prolonged Horner's syndrome after interscalene block: a management dilemma. *Anesth Analg* 1994, 79:601–603.

22. Rosenberg PH, Lamberg TS, Tarkkila P: Auditory disturbance associated with interscalene brachial plexus block. *Br J Anaesth* 1995, 74:89–91.

23. Abrams SE, Hogan QH: Complications of nerve blocks. In *Anesthesia and Perioperative Complications*. Edited by Benumof JL, Saidman LJ. St. Louis: Mosby; 1992:69–70.

24. Andrews JR, Carson WG, Ortega K: Arthroscopy of the shoulder: technique and normal anatomy. *Am J Sports Med* 1984, 12:1–7.

25. Wolf EM: Anterior portals in shoulder arthroscopy. *Arthroscopy* 1989, 5:201–208.

26. Wolf EM: Arthroscopic shoulder stabilization using suture anchors: technique and results. Presented at the 15th Annual Meeting of the Arthroscopy Association of North America. Washington, DC; 1996.

27. Matthews LS, Zarrens B, Micheal RH, *et al.*: Anterior portal selection for shoulder arthroscopy. *Arthroscopy* 1985, 1:33–39.

28. Resch H, Wykypiel HF, Maurer H, *et al.*: The antero-inferior (transmuscular) approach for arthroscopic repair of the Bankart lesion: an anatomic and clinical study. *Arthroscopy* 1996, 12:309–322.

29. Davidson PA, Tibone JE: Anterior-inferior (5 o'clock) portal for shoulder arthroscopy. *Arthroscopy* 1995, 5:519–525.

30. Laurencin CT, Deutsch A, O'Brien SJ, *et al.*: The superolateral portal for arthroscopy of the shoulder. *Arthroscopy* 1994, 10:255–258.

31. Neviaser TJ: Arthroscopy of the shoulder. *Orthop Clin North Am* 1987, 18:361–367.

32. Souryal TO, Baker CL: Anatomy of the supraclavicular fossa portal in shoulder arthroscopy. *Arthroscopy* 1990, 6:297–300.

33. Ellman H: Arthroscopic subacromial decompression. *Arthroscopy* 1987, 3:173–181.

34. Paulos LE, Harner CD, Parker RD: Arthroscopic subacromial decompression for impingement syndrome of the shoulder. *Tech Orthop* 1988, 3:33–39.

35. Flatow EL, Cordasco FA, McCluskey GM, *et al.*: Arthroscopic resection of the distal clavicle via a superior portal: a critical, quantitative radiographic assessment of bone removal. *Arthroscopy* 1990 6:153–154.

36. Brian WJ, Schauder KK, Tullos HS: The axillary nerve in the relationship to common sports medicine shoulder procedures. *Am J Sports Med* 1986, 14:113–116.

37. Burkhart SS: Deep venous thrombosis after shoulder arthroscopy. *Arthroscopy* 1990, 6:61–63.

38. Lee HC, Dewan N, Crosby L: Subcutaneous emphysema, pneumomediastinum and potentially life threatening tension pneumothorax: pulmonary complications from arthroscopic decompression. *Chest* 1992, 101:1265–1267.

39. Burkhart SS, Barnett CR, Snyder SJ: Transient postoperative blindness as a possible effect of glycine toxicity. *Arthroscopy* 1990, 6:112–114.

40. Lee YF, Cohen L, Tooke SM: Intramuscular deltoid pressure during shoulder arthroscopy. *Arthroscopy* 1989, 5:209–212.

41. Ogilvie-Harris DJ, Boynton E: Arthroscopic acromioplasty: extravasation of fluid into the deltoid muscle. *Arthroscopy* 1990, 6:52–54.

42. Johnson LL, Schneider DA, Austin MD, *et al.*: Two-percent glutaraldehyde: a disinfectant in arthroscopy and arthroscopic surgery. *J Bone Joint Surg* 1982, 64(suppl B)237–239.

43. Ticker JB, Lippe RJ, Barkin DE, *et al.*: Case report: infected suture anchors in the shoulder. *Arthroscopy* 1996, 12:613–615.

44. Harner CD, Mason GC, Few HF, *et al.*: Cidex induced synovitis. *Am J Sports Med* 1989, 17:96–102.

45. Seballos RJ, Walsh AL, Mehta AC: Clinical evaluation of a liquid chemical sterilization system for the flexible bronchoscope. *J Bronchology* 1995, 2:192–199.

46. Caputo RA, Fisher J, Jurzynski V, *et al.*: Validation testing of a gas plasma sterilization system. *Med Dev Diagn Ind* 1993, 15:132–138.

47. Wolf EM: Causes of failed shoulder arthroscopy: a review of 35 revision cases. Presented at the 16th annual meeting of the Arthroscopy Association of North America. San Diego, CA; 1997.

48. Esch JC: Arthroscopic subacromial decompression and post-operative management. *Orthop Clin North Am* 1993, 24:161–171.

49. Bigliani LU, Morrison DS, April EW: The morphology of the acromion and its relationship to rotator cuff tears. *Orthop Trans* 1986, 10:216–228.

50. Wuh HCK, Snyder SJ: Modified classification of the supraspinatus outlet view based on the configuration and the anatomical thickness of the acromion. Paper presented at the 59th Annual Meeting of the American Academy of Orthopedic Surgeons. Washington, DC; February 1992.

51. Rockwood CA Jr, Lyons FR: Shoulder impingement syndrome: diagnosis, radiographic evaluation, and treatment with a modified Neer acromioplasty. *J Bone Joint Surg Am* 1993, 75(suppl A):409–424.

52. Gartsman GM: Arthroscopic acromioplasty for lesions of the rotator cuff. *J Bone Joint Surg Am* 1990, 72:169–180.

53. Sampson TG, Nisbet JK, Glick JM: Precision acromioplasty in arthroscopic subacromial decompression. *Arthroscopy* 1991, 7:301–307.

54. Groh GI, Simoni M, Rolla P, *et al.*: Loss of the deltoid after shoulder operations: an operative disaster. *J Shoulder Elbow Surg* 1994, 3:243–254.

55. Berg EE, Ciullo JV, Oglesby JW: Failure of arthroscopic decompression by subacromial heterotopic ossification causing recurrent impingement. *Arthroscopy* 1994, 10:158–161.

56. Snyder SJ, Banas MP, Karzel RP: The arthroscopic Mumford procedure: an analysis of results. *Arthroscopy* 1995, 11:157–164.

57. Arroyo JS, Rodosky MW, Pollack RG, *et al.*: Arthroscopic resection of the antero-lateral band of the coracoacromial ligament for impingement in the overhead athlete. Presented at 16th Annual Meeting of the Arthroscopy Association of North America. San Diego, CA; 1997.

58.• Edelson JG, Luchs J: Aspects of coracoacromial ligament anatomy of interest to the arthroscopic surgeon. *Arthroscopy* 1995, 6:715–719.

Discusses the anatomic differences between the anterior and the lateral insertion of the coracoacromial ligament and the deltoid fascia and their pertinence to decompression technique.

59. Arntz CT, Jackins S, Matsen FA: Prosthetic replacement of the shoulder for the treatment of defects in the rotator cuff and the surface of the gleno-humeral joint. *J Bone Joint Surg Am* 1993, 75(suppl A):485–491.

60. Esch JE, Ozerkis LR, Helgager JA, *et al*.: Arthroscopic subacromial decompression: results according to the degree of rotator cuff tear. *Arthroscopy* 1988, 4:241–249.

61. Flatow EL, Bigliani LU: Arthroscopic acromioclavicular joint debridement and distal clavicle resection: *Oper Tech Orthop* 1991, 1:240–247.

62. Fukuda K, Craig EV, An K, *et al*.: Biomechanical study of the ligamentous system of the acromioclavicular joint. *J Bone Joint Surg Am* 1986, 68:434–440.

63.• Klimkiewicz J, Sher J, *et al*.: Biomechanical function of the acromioclavicular ligaments in limiting anterior posterior translation of the acromioclavicular joint. Presented at the Open Meeting of the American Shoulder and Elbow Surgeons. San Francisco, CA; 1997.

Demonstrates the importance of the posterior and superior acromioclavicular ligaments for stability.

64. Weber SC: Arthroscopic versus open treatment of significant partial thickness rotator cuff tears. Presented at the Thirteenth Annual Meeting of the Arthroscopy Association of North America. Orlando, FL: 1994.

65. Ryu RK: Arthroscopic subacromial decompression: a clinical review. *Arthroscopy* 1992, 8:141–147.

66.• St. Pierre P, Olson FJ, Elliott JJ, *et al*.: Tendon healing to cortical bone versus a cancellous trough: a biomechanical and histological model in the goat. Presented at the 14th Annual Meeting of the Arthroscopy Association of North America. San Francisco, CA; 1995.

Comparative study of tendon-to-bone biologic healing techniques.

67. Burkhart SS: The deadman theory of suture anchors: observations along a south Texas fence line. *Arthroscopy* 1995, 11:119–123.

68. Burkhart SS, Fisher SP, Nottage WN, *et al*.: Tissue fixation security in transosseous rotator cuff repairs: a mechanical comparison of simple versus mattress sutures. *Arthroscopy* 1996, 12:704–708.

69.• Burkhart SS, Athanasiou KA, Wirth MA: Margin convergence: a method of reducing strain in massive rotator cuff tears. *Arthroscopy* 1996, 12:335–338.

Biomechanical analysis of an important rotator cuff repair concept.

70. Mormino MA, Gross M, McCarthy JA: Captured shoulder: a complication of rotator cuff surgery. *Arthroscopy* 1996, 12:457–461.

71. Norwood LA, Fowler HL: Rotator cuff tears: a shoulder arthroscopy complication. *Am J Sports Med* 1989, 17:837–841.

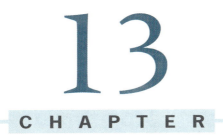

13
CHAPTER

Advances in Elbow Arthroscopy

FELIX H. SAVOIE III, MARK FIELD, AND LARRY D. FIELD

T he elbow is one of the most complex bony articulations in the body. Bone structure and ligamentous connections provide stability and allow motion in two planes: flexion-extension and supination-pronation. Arthroscopically, the bony structures can be readily visualized. The radiocapitellar joint, annular ligament, and anterior aspect of the proximal radioulnar articulation are easily visualized through the medial portals. The coronoid fossa, anterior ulnohumeral joint, and coronoid processes can be seen through the lateral portal (Figs. 13-1 and 13-2).

The posterior capitellar joint, posterior aspect of the proximal radioulnar joint, and the lateral aspect of the ulnohumeral joint are seen through the softspot portal or posterior lateral. The olecranon, olecranon fossa, and medial ulnohumeral joint are best visualized through the posterior central portal and the posterior lateral portals.

The elbow is a tightly constrained joint surrounded closely by important neurovascular structures. Elbow arthroscopy is a procedure that requires careful attention and thorough knowledge of the pertinent anatomy. Elbow arthroscopy was originally introduced in the supine position, but in response to occasional technical difficulties, the techniques for the application of arthroscopy in the prone position were successfully developed. This position avoids the need for special traction or suspension devices. The prone position simplifies orientation for the surgeon by maintaining the humerus proximally and the radius and ulna distally in the arthroscopic fields. For these reasons, this is the position of choice at the authors' institution.

PORTAL ANATOMY

There are numerous access sites around the elbow. Portal sites are determined according to the neurovascular and musculotendinous anatomy to allow safe access to the elbow without significant risk of damage to the surrounding neurovascular structures.

Proximal Anterior Medial Portal

The proximal anterior medial portal, which was first described by Poehling *et al.* [1], lies 2 cm proximal to the medial epicondyle anterior to the intramuscular septum and allows visualization of the anterior aspect of the elbow joint. The ulnar nerve is isolated approximately 3 to 4 mm from this portal site [2] and is the primary structure at risk.

Proximal Anterior Lateral Portal

The newly described proximal anterior lateral portal, which is used routinely at the authors' institution, is positioned 2 cm proximal and 1 cm anterior to the lateral epicondyle. A recent cadaveric study performed by Field *et al.* [3] on 10 specimens showed that this portal remains significantly farther from the radial nerve than do other anterior lateral portal sites. This portal allows for an excellent view of the anterior radiohumeral joint, ulnohumeral joint, and anterior elbow capsular margin.

Posterior Lateral Portal I

The posterior lateral portal is multi-purpose. It is located 3 cm proximal to the olecranon and lateral to the triceps tendon along the lateral border of the humerus. The primary structure at risk is the lateral triceps tendon, which can be avoided by blunt dissection and by remaining close to the posterior humeral cortex when establishing the portal.

Posterior Lateral Portal II

The posterior lateral side of the elbow is accessible by two portal placements anywhere from the soft-spot portal to the standard posterior lateral portal. The

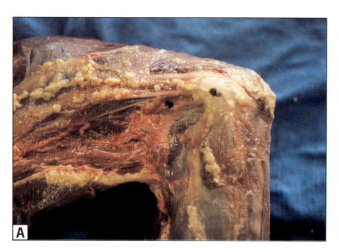

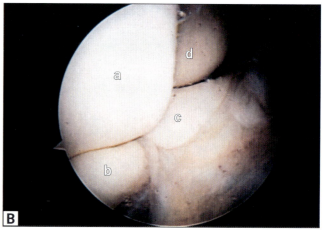

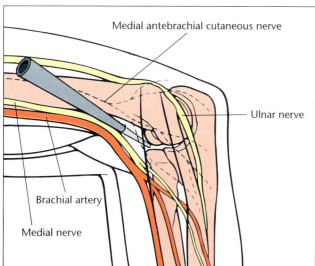

Figure 13-1. Anterosuperior medial portal (proximal anteromedial portal). **A,** Gross anatomic dissection, medial view, of the elbow in the prone position. **B,** Arthroscopic view from the anterosuperior portal showing the trochlea (*a*), coronoid process (*b*), radial head (*c*), and capitellum (*d*). **C,** Gross anatomy of the elbow.

primary structures at risk are the lateral aspect of the triceps tendon and the cartilage of the ulnohumeral joint.

Posterocentral Portal

The posterocentral portal is located 3 cm proximal to the tip of the olecranon in the midline posteriorly. It traverses the most distal part of the triceps muscle and avoids the triceps tendon. The primary structure at risk is the triceps tendon if the portal is established too distally.

Soft-Spot Portal

The entire posterior lateral aspect of the elbow can be used as a portal site for visualization and some rotation of the lateral gutter and posterior radiocapitellar joint. The primary structures at risk are the radiocapitellar joint and the lateral ulnohumeral joint.

ELBOW INSTABILITY

The bony configuration of the joints provides for stability of the elbow to varus and valgus stress, especially at angles less than 20° and greater than 120° of flexion [4]. Between these extremes, stability is provided to a greater degree by the rnedial and lateral ligaments of the elbow as well as by the musculotendinous complexes that cross the joint [5].

The medial ulnar collateral ligament of the elbow is composed of three parts: an anterior oblique ligament, a fan-shaped posterior oblique ligament, and a transverse ligament that is relatively nonfunctional in terms of stability [4–6]. Both the anterior and posterior ligaments originate on the anterior aspect of the medial humeral epicondyle, with the anterior ligament extending distally to insert on the medial aspect of the coronoid process. The anterior ligament is further subdivided into two functionally distinct bands [7]. Under valgus load, the anterior

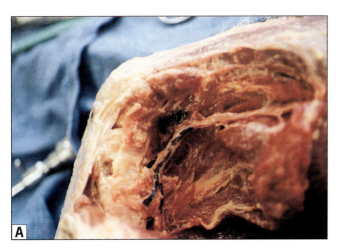
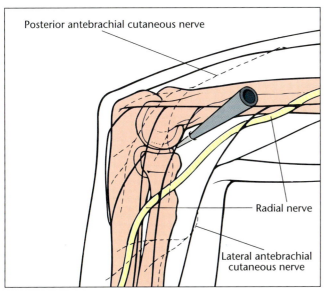
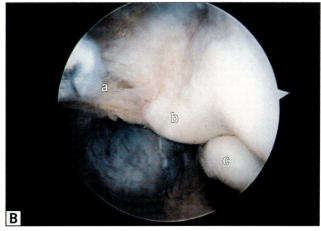

Figure 13-2. Anterosuperior lateral portal (proximal anterolateral portal). **A,** Gross anatomic dissection, lateral view, of the elbow in the prone position. **B,** Arthroscopic view from the anterosuperior (proximal anterolateral portal), showing the coronoid fossa (*a*), trochlea (*b*), and coronoid process (*c*). **C,** Gross anatomy of the elbow.

band is under tension from 0° to 85°, whereas the posterior band is under tension from 55° throughout the rest of flexion. The posterior oblique ligament inserts into the posteromedial aspect of the olecranon and is tight in flexion of more than 60° [8]. The results of sectioning studies indicate that the anterior oblique ligament is the primary stabilizer of the elbow to valgus stress [9–11]. However, in a recently completed biomechanical study performed by Field et al. [3] using 18 cadaveric elbows, complete sectioning of the anterior bundle allowed an average maximum increase in valgus rotation of only 3° over the intact specimens, illustrating the difficulty in sometimes clinically diagnosing ulnar collateral ligament injuries.

The lateral collateral complex shows greater variability than does the medial ulnar collateral ligament but is composed of four structures. The radial collateral ligament originates at the lateral epicondyle and extends distally to insert into the annular ligament of the radioulnar articulation. Its primary function is in providing stability under varus stress. The lateral ulnar collateral ligament also arises from the lateral epicondyle just distal to the radial collateral ligament and extends distally to cover the annular ligament and insert on the lateral side of the ulna and coronoid process. This ligament also functions to stabilize the elbow against varus stress, and rupture of this ligament has been determined by O'Driscoll et al. [12] to be the primary lesion in posterolateral rotatory instability of the elbow. The other two portions of the lateral collateral complex are the annular ligament and the accessory collateral ligament.

Injuries to the medial ulnar collateral ligament are usually caused by chronic overuse of the elbow. Athletes who engage in repeated overhand throwing regularly subject the elbow to valgus forces that may equal or exceed the tensile strength of the medial supporting structures. The anterior oblique ligament is the primary medial stabilizer of the elbow, and forces concentrated in this ligament, along with repeated microtraumatic insult, can lead to attenuation and eventual rupture of this ligament. Undersurface tears of the ulnar collateral ligament, with the external portion of the ligament remaining intact, have recently been reported [6].

In contrast to throwing injuries, repetitive varus stress at the elbow rarely occurs. Thus, lateral collateral ligament injury from an isolated varus stress is uncommon. Incompetency of the lateral collateral ligament complex most commonly occurs following a posterior dislocation of the elbow. Instability may also develop iatrogenically as a result of common extensor tendon release for lateral epicondylitis or radial head excision.

The diagnosis of medial ulnar collateral ligament instability is based on a history of medial elbow pain associated with the acceleration phase of throwing. Ulnar neuropathy is often associated with chronic medial instability [7]. Excessive tightness of the shoulder results in increased stress across the elbow by altering the normal throwing motion. These altered biomechanics can place increased valgus stress around the elbow, causing symptoms over the medial elbow. Thus, if a throwing athlete has medial elbow pain, the shoulder as well should always be examined carefully.

Valgus stress testing of the elbow is performed by taking the patient's hand and placing it underneath the examiner's arm against the side of the examiner's body. The elbow is held at 30° of flexion to relax the bony constraints of the elbow. While one of the examiner's hands applies valgus stress to the elbow, the other hand palpates the medial side of the elbow. Even with complete medial ulnar collateral ligament disruptions, joint opening is often difficult to detect, and the inability of the examiner to appreciate a distinct endpoint in association with pain and local tenderness characterize ligament insufficiency.

O'Driscoll et al. [12] have described a posterolateral rotatory instability test that is useful in diagnosing posterolateral instability. The examination is performed with the patient supine and the shoulder flexed 90°. The wrist is supinated, and then a valgus movement, combined with an axial compressive force, is applied to the elbow as it is fully extended. This maneuver, called a pivot-shift test, may reproduce an apprehensive response in the symptomatic patient.

There are two primary goals of conservative treatment of the symptomatic elbow in throwing athletes. The first objective should be the relief of pain and inflammation. The second objective is to increase the functional strength of the elbow, paying specific attention to the forearm musculature. Operative treatment for medial ulnar collateral injury should be reserved for those patients who fail conservative treatment measures.

Arthroscopy can be used as an aid in diagnosis of valgus instability. Whereas the medial ulnar collateral ligament cannot usually be visualized directly with the arthroscope [13], valgus stress testing can provide indirect evidence of medial ulnar collateral ligament insufficiency through arthroscopic visualization of the most medial aspect of the ulnohumeral articulation from the anterolateral portal with the elbow in 60° to 70° of flexion. In a cadaveric study, Field and Altchek [14] noted that an opening of the ulnohumeral space as small as 1 mm represents a significant injury to the ulnar collateral ligament and may be an indication for reconstruction in symptomatic patients [15]. However, in the authors' experience, many patients with this degree of medial joint opening can be successfully treated with rehabilitation or less extensive procedures.

Arthroscopy is also useful in the diagnosis of lateral collateral ligament insufficiency. Posterolateral rotatory subluxation of the radial head can be easily seen when lateral pivot-shift testing is done while the radiocapitellar joint is viewed from the proximal medial portal.

Reconstruction of the collateral ligaments is an effective way to restore stability to the elbow. Reconstruction of both the medial and lateral ligaments has been described by using autologous graft from ipsilateral palmaris longus, fascia lata, or by a lesser toe extensor. Both of the ligaments are reconstructed by figure-eight placement of the graft using drill holes, and capsular plication, when necessary, is done [10,16].

In cases in which the ligament is traumatically avulsed from humeral origin, it can be repaired using a #2 nonabsorbable suture placed in a Bunnell fashion through the ligament and then repaired to the respective humeral epicondyle through drill holes.

It should be emphasized that Jobe *et al.* [17] and Conway *et al.* [7] performed medial reconstructive procedures in athletes who wished to remain at a highly competitive level of participation. The indications for reconstructive procedures in athletes participating at lower levels of competition is less clear. Valgus instability of the elbow appears to cause little disability in activities of daily living [18,19], and good functional results have been reported after nonoperative treatment of medial ulnar collateral ligament ruptures associated with elbow dislocation [20].

In the authors' practice, most athletes have been successfully treated nonoperatively with the use of global strengthening of the upper extremity and of plyometrics in the selective strengthening of the flexor-pronator musculature.

ELBOW TRAUMA

Management of trauma to the elbow is not generally considered an indication for arthroscopic treatment modalities. However, owing to technical advances in arthroscopy and instrumentation, there are a limited number of indications in which arthroscopic examination and treatment of acute elbow trauma may be beneficial to the patient.

Penetration of the elbow joint by sharp objects or low-velocity missiles needs irrigation and debridement of the joint itself to prevent septic arthritis or to remove intra-articular fragments. In properly selected patients, arthroscopy can alleviate the secondary trauma of a

surgical incision to an already traumatized joint. Absence of or significant distortion of normal landmarks are contraindications to arthroscopy of the elbow. Arthroscopy of an open elbow joint not only provides an excellent means for irrigating the joint, but provides excellent visualization of associated fractures or foreign bodies not visible on radiographs. This provides a significant advantage over arthrotomy. The standard techniques for prone arthroscopy are followed. All aspects of the anterior and posterior compartments of the elbow should be visualized and debrided as necessary. Arthroscopic lavage and debridement does not, however, alleviate the need for open surgical wound debridement and irrigation if indicated.

Arthroscopy can assist in the evaluation and treatment of some intra-articular fractures of the elbow. Fractures of the radial head, coronoid, capitellar, olecranon, and unicondylar humeral can all be considered for arthroscopic or arthroscopically assisted treatment. Arthroscopic evaluation of the elbow allows for excellent assessment of the true extent of injury as well as addressing things such as debridement and removal of traumatic loose bodies associated with elbow fractures (Fig. 13-3). When applicable, the arthroscope can allow fracture reduction and fixation under direct visualization with minimal exposure and dissection.

The authors do not advocate arthroscopically assisted fixation of all articular fractures around the elbow, and the standard of care for treatment of these fractures is still open reduction internal fixation.

Indications for arthroscopy in evaluating and managing acute traumatic injuries to the elbow joint are not well defined. However, with recent advances in instrument technology and the widespread proficiency of arthroscopic skills, there is a place for the

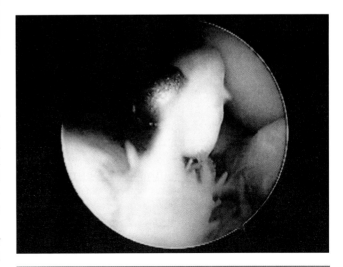

Figure 13-3. View of a large loose body, which was not detected on tomograms, being removed in the anterior compartment, in a patient with a history of a nondisplaced radial head fracture.

arthroscope in enhancing the evaluation and treatment of select intra-articular injuries.

ELBOW ARTHRITIS

The role of arthroscopy in the treatment of arthritic conditions of the elbow continues to evolve. Many diagnostic and therapeutic benefits have been realized in recent years as the techniques for performing elbow arthroscopy have improved.

General techniques such as lavage, debridement, spur excision, and synovectomy employed in the arthroscopic treatment of arthritic conditions of other joints can also be utilized in the elbow. Arthroscopic procedures have been used for conditions unique to the elbow, such as an anterior capsular contracture, valgus and extension overload syndrome, and thickening of the bone bridge between the olecranon fossa and coronoid fossa.

The disadvantages of elbow arthroscopy are largely related to its demanding technical requirements. This is particularly true for arthroscopy of arthritic joints, in which bony landmarks may be distorted or obscured. Elbow arthroscopy is contraindicated when previous surgical procedures have altered the neurovascular anatomy around the elbow, as in anterior transposition of the ulnar nerve. As in other joints, the therapeutic benefits of arthroscopic treatment of arthritic conditions of the elbow may only be temporary. Proper patient selection and attention to technical detail allow arthroscopic techniques to produce quite valuable results in the management of arthritic conditions of the elbow.

When conservative measures fail, the most successful surgical treatment for the painful elbow in rheumatoid arthritis is frequently a synovectomy [21,22]. In general, synovectomy should be reserved for the symptomatic joint with advanced chronic synovial changes and little or no cartilage or bone destruction in which medical management has not been successful. The role of radial head excision with synovectomy remains controversial [21–25].

Arthroscopy allows a complete synovectomy without the need for the large capsular incisions that are required with any open approach (Fig. 13-4). Less postoperative pain allows for early aggressive physical therapy and earlier return of function [26].

The authors have recently reviewed the Mississippi Sports Medicine experience of arthroscopic synovectomy for inflammatory arthritis. Over a 5-year period, 46 elbows were reviewed. All 46 patients had improved motion and decreased pain. One patient developed a synovial fistula that required open excision, two patients required repeat synovectomy, and one patient eventually required total elbow arthroplasty.

Primary osteoarthritis of the elbow is quite rare, accounting for only 1% to 2% of patients presenting with degenerative arthritis [27,28]. Management by nonoperative means is usually successful [29]. Various surgical procedures can be considered when conservative measures fail to provide satisfactory relief of symptoms. Traditional options include prosthetic arthroplasty, interpositional arthroplasty, resection arthroplasty, and arthrodesis of the elbow. Open fenestration of the olecranon fossa and open ulno-humeral arthroplasty have also been described in the treatment of osteoarthritis of the elbow [30,31]. More recently, arthroscopic debridement and spur excision of the olecranon fossa, fenestration, and ulnohumeral arthroplasty have been used.

In the degenerative elbow, landmarks are frequently distorted and safe access more difficult. The prone position allows a more reproducible access and permits easier manipulation of the arm during the arthroscopic procedure. The initial insufflation of the elbow is established through the soft-spot portal. A proximal medial portal is used for initial diagnostic evaluation of the anterior compartment. The changes noted determine the placement of the lateral portal and the need for a transradial capitellar inflow through the posterior soft-spot portal. The lateral portal is used for synovectomy and to debride the radiocapitellar joint, excise the coronoid spurs, and deepen the coronoid fossa. The arthroscope is then switched to the lateral portal, and the proximal medial portal is used to finish the coronoid process and fossa debridement. Trochlea spurs are excised through this portal as well.

The anterior compartment is then evaluated for the need for capsular release or radial head excision. Radial head excision is done by repositioning the

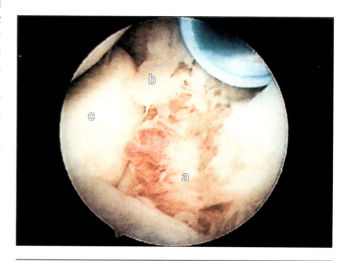

Figure 13-4. Arthroscopy allows a complete synovectomy without large capsular incisions. Synovitis (*a*), the humerus (*b*), and the coronoid process (*c*) are shown in this arthroscopic view.

arthroscope in the proximal superomedial portal, the inflow in the lateral portal, and the instruments through the soft-spot portal. The radial head is then excised from posterior to anterior, using a "cutting-block" technique with medial and lateral sweeps. The resection is continued until full pronation and supination can be easily achieved and no radio-capitellar impingement occurs throughout the normal flexion and extension arc of motion. If full extension cannot be achieved due to capsular contracture, the capsule can be released after olecranon fossa debridement.

The inflow is substituted in the proximal supero-medial portal, and the posterior compartment is evaluated through the posterolateral I or II portal. The olecranon spurs are excised initially with the shaver in the straight posterior portal. The olecranon fossa fenestration, if necessary, is done with the instruments in the same position. Excision of the tip of the olecranon is done using a cutting-block technique similar to that used for the radial head. This is continued until full extension is achieved, with care being taken not to plunge the instrument across the medial aspect of the joint, thereby injuring the ulnar nerve. Olecranon fossa fenestration is best accomplished with the shaver in the posterior central or straight posterior portal. A drill bit may be placed through the cannula for a pilot hole and the fossa enlarged as needed under direct visualization. Care should be taken to not violate the medial or lateral columns of the distal humerus. This is best noted by a change in the texture of the bone when these bony columns are encountered. Fossa resection is continued until full flexion and extension can be achieved.

The senior author has performed arthroscopic debridement and ulnohumeral arthroplasty for degenerative arthritis of the elbow since 1989. The initial 33 patients who underwent this procedure were reviewed at 1 to 5 years follow-up. The average preoperative motion was 30° to 100°. All patients complained of pain with activities of daily living and of popping, catching, and swelling. On follow-up, 31 of the 33 patients (93%) were satisfied with the results of the procedure. In one patient, the arthritis progressed, and total elbow arthroplasty was used to successfully reconstruct the elbow.

MISCELLANEOUS DISORDERS

Lateral Epicondylitis

The patient is first intubated and then positioned prone on the operating table. Two rolled towels are placed longitudinally under the patient's thorax. All bony prominences are well padded. The affected extremity is positioned with the ipsilateral shoulder abducted to 90° and the arm supported in a precut foam holder. The patient's forearm hangs freely over the edge of the operating table, with the elbow flexed to 90°. If needed, an arm tourniquet is then applied proximally.

The affected extremity is then prepared and draped in standard fashion. The following anatomic landmarks are identified and marked: the medial and lateral epicondyles, the radial head, the olecranon, and the ulnar nerve. Potential portal sites are also located and marked.

The surgeon should then distend the joint with approximately 20 to 30 cc of saline through an 18-gauge needle introduced through the direct lateral portal. Maximum distention increases the distance between neurovascular structures and arthroscopic portals, thereby lessening the risk of neurovascular injury. The tubing is removed from the spinal needle, and the backflow of saline is noted in order to confirm adequate intra-articular distention. Extension and supination of the elbow also occurs with intra-articular distention

The superomedial, or proximal medial, portal is established next. It is located approximately 2 cm proximal to the medial epicondyle and 1 cm anterior to the intermuscular septum. All arthroscopic portals are created using a #11 blade to incise the skin, and a blunt hemostat is used to spread the underlying soft tissue. A blunt trocar is inserted into the joint capsule through the proximal portion of the flexor muscle mass near the brachialis muscle. The trocar and sheath are inserted anteriorly to the intermuscular septum, maintaining contact with the anterior aspect of the humerus at all times as the trocar is directed toward the radial head. A 2.7-mm, 30° arthroscope is inserted into the joint, and the diagnostic portion of the procedure is performed.

The authors classified their arthroscopic findings in a consecutive series of 31 patients who were treated surgically for recalcitrant lateral epicondylitis. They found three distinct patterns of pathologic changes in the lateral capsule and at the undersurface of the extensor carpi radialis brevis (ECRB) tendon in these elbows. Type I lesions are those with inflammation and fraying deep to the ECRB without evidence of a frank tear. Type II lesions are linear tears at the undersurface of the ECRB tendon. Type III lesions are retracted, with partial or complete avulsions of the ECRB tendon.

After the pathoanatomy is identified, the supero-lateral portal is established with an 18-gauge spinal needle inserted through the lesion. Using a full-radius resector, the capsule is excised in order to allow identification of the undersurface of the

ECRB tendon. The origin of the ECRB is visualized. Using a curette and motorized shaver, the capsule and the pathologic tendinous attachment of the ECRB are debrided, and the lateral epicondylar ridge is decorticated with an arthroscopic burr, hand-held instruments, or electrocautery device. The limit of epicondylar resection is the lateral collateral ligament posteriorly. Although a 30° arthroscope is adequate for visualization around the corner for most of the procedure, the surgeon may require a 70° arthroscope in rare instances. After release of the ECRB tendon and decortication of the lateral epicondyle, arthroscopic visualization should reveal the overlying muscle belly of the extensor musculature.

Postoperatively, the patient's arm is placed in a sling with the elbow at 90° of flexion, and gentle active and passive range-of-motion exercises are encouraged. The patient progresses to wrist extension strengthening exercises and overall upper extremity rehabilitation exercises.

Olecranon Bursitis

The operating room set-up and instrumentation for arthroscopy of the olecranon bursa are similar to that used in standard elbow arthroscopy, with the patient in the prone position as described earlier in this chapter. Three portals are used for arthroscopic olecranon bursectomy: the lateral, proximal central, and distal central portals. The portals are created using a standard #11 surgical blade followed by a hemostat to spread the soft tissue. Medial portals are not used because of the risk of injury to the ulnar nerve. Excision and adequate resection of the olecranon bursa

can be done using any of the previously mentioned portals for instrumentation and viewing.

Initial examination of the bursal sac usually reveals chronic granulomatous inflammatory tissue. Other deposits, such as rheumatoid tophi or gouty crystals, may be present, depending on concomitant pathologic conditions. Next, a total bursectomy is performed with the surgeon exchanging operative and visualization portals as necessary. Removal of the bursal tissue is complete when an increase in light can be seen through the skin and the triceps tendon and muscle can be visualized. Excision of subcutaneous fat should be minimal. If present, spurs on the olecranon tip should be removed with an arthroscopic burr.

Arthroscopic portals are closed with 3-0 nylon sutures. Postoperative anesthetic injections are rarely used because of the need for an immediate neurological evaluation. A compression dressing is applied for 7 to 10 days. Mobilization of the extremity should be started immediately.

Three basic portals are used in arthroscopic bursal excision: proximal central, distal central, and lateral. The medial aspect is avoided to prevent injury to the ulnar nerve.

The initial view is usually that of chronic inflammation (Fig. 13-5). Often, pieces of granulomatous material, rheumatoid tophi, or gout crystals may be visualized (Fig. 13-6). The arthroscopic shaver can then be inserted into the bursal sac, and inflamed tissue can be excised. The excision should be continued until the entire bursa has been excised. The changing nature of the tissue and the visualization of the light through the skin indicate that the more superficial layer has been excised. Visualization of the

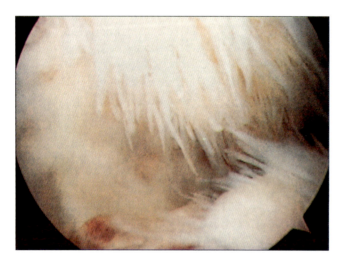

Figure 13-5. Arthroscopic view of the olecranon bursa showing the subcutaneous tissue above the bursal covering of the triceps tendon below.

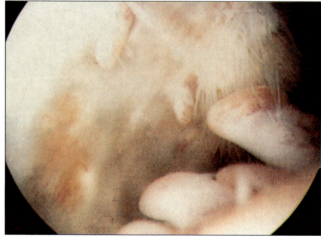

Figure 13-6. Gouty tophi contained within the olecranon bursa.

triceps tendon and fascia indicate excision of the deeper layer of the bursa.

After the excision is completed, a small spur may be noted on the tip of the olecranon. If the triceps is adequately visualized and can be protected, the spur may be excised, using an arthroscopic burr (Fig. 13-7). The authors have limited experience with this procedure. During the past 5 years, only six patients have failed nonoperative management and therefore selected this form of treatment. No patient sustained a recurrence of the bursitis after the procedure was completed. One patient developed a chronic bursal draining fistula from the lateral portal that resolved with packing over a 3-week period. There were no other complications in any other patients.

ELBOW ARTHROFIBROSIS

As the role of arthroscopy has expanded in the treatment of elbow joint pathology, so have the indications. One of these expanded indications for elbow arthroscopy is in the management of elbow arthrofibrosis. Arthrofibrosis of the elbow and the resulting elbow joint contracture may have many etiologies. Although all elbow flexion contractures are not amenable to arthroscopic treatment, contractures with intra-articular etiologies may be well suited to arthroscopic management.

Arthroscopic treatment of elbow flexion contracture allows the surgeon to address the intrinsic or intra-articular causes and manifestations of contracture as well as those extrinsic causes that may be safely reached by this technique, including capsular and collateral ligament contracture and problems with the extensor musculature. However, intrinsic and extrinsic causes of contracture that cannot be safely reached from within the joint are not amenable to arthroscopic management. Flexion contractures secondary to muscle spasticity, cerebral palsy, head injury, skin contracture, or heterotopic ossification may require open surgical procedures.

The primary indication for arthroscopic release of flexion contractures is a painful contracture of 30° or more refractory to conservative management, which results in functional limitation. Contraindications include previous surgical procedures that have altered the neurovascular anatomy around the elbow joint (anterior transposition of the ulnar nerve) and extra-articular deformity (heterotopic bone, displaced anterior fracture of the radial head) that may impinge or entrap the neurovascular structures. A relative contraindication is limited experience with elbow arthroscopy.

The arthroscopic set-up for surgical release of elbow flexion contractures is that of the standard elbow arthroscopy. Insufflation of the elbow is attempted using a standard soft-spot portal. A proximal medial portal is established approximately 2 cm proximal to the medial epicondyle and anterior to the medial intermuscular septum. As with all portal placement, care is taken to avoid injury to the cutaneous nerves by pulling the skin against the scalpel blade during this incision. A blunt trocar is used to palpate the intermuscular septum and is then directed anterior to this structure, penetrating the muscle layers to the capsule of the elbow joint. Joint entrance is then attempted using the blunt trocar. Occasionally, a sharp trocar is needed to penetrate the capsule and allow adequate entrance into the elbow joint. The arthroscope is then introduced through this cannula, and the anterior compartment of the elbow is evaluated.

A proximal lateral portal is then established using an inside-out technique with the Wissenger rod or by direct lateral insertion. Protection of the posterior interosseous nerve is paramount during lateral portal placement. The portal should be just superior to the capitellum, through the capsule and muscular layers. A shaver is used in this area to remove inflamed soft tissues and adhesions from the radial head and coronoid process.

Anterior capsulectomy is initiated after debridement and definition of the anterior intra-articular pathology have been done. The arthroscope is kept in the proximal medial portal, and the shaver is kept in the proximal lateral portal. The capsule is released from the humerus beginning approximately at or near the coronoid fossa and continuing laterally until a complete release of the capsule from the midportion

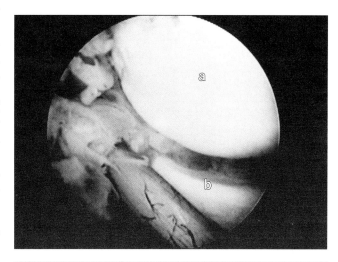

Figure 13-7. View of the anterolateral capsule from the proximal medial portal showing the early stages of debridement of the anterior radiocapitellar joint. The capitellum (a) and the radial head (b) are shown.

of the humerus to the lateral intermuscular septum has been done (Fig. 13-8). The proximal 1 to 2 cm of the capsule should be completely excised to prevent simple elevation of the capsule from the humerus. The arthroscope is then switched to the proximal lateral portal, and the shaver is inserted through the proximal medial portal. The capsular excision is continued medially from the area of release until the intermuscular septum or medial humerus is reached. Care must be taken not to extend the capsular excision past this point and thus risk injury to the ulnar nerve. The proximal half of the capsule is then excised until brachialis fibers are visible from medial to lateral.

To avoid potential neurovascular complications, it is important to confirm that both the arthroscope and shaver are in the joint as well to maintain proximity of the shaver blade to the anterior aspect of the humerus at all times.

After maximum extension through anterior capsular release has been achieved, the instruments are removed from the anterior portals, and a posterolateral and a posterocentral portal are established. The arthroscope is inserted through the posterolateral portal, and the shaver is inserted through the posterocentral portal. Scar tissue and adhesions are removed from the olecranon fossa

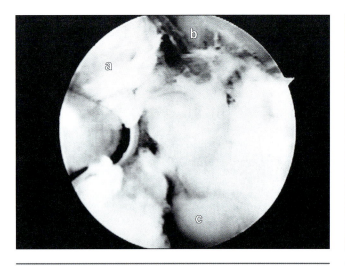

Figure 13-8. The initial phase of the lateral capsular excision as viewed from the proximal superomedial portal. The scar on the capsule (*a*), the humeral cortex (*b*), and the proximal aspect of the capitellum (*c*) are shown.

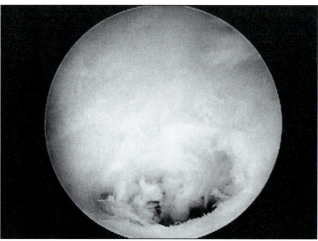

Figure 13-9. Deepening of the olecranon fossa may result in connection of the olecranon fossa to the coronoid fossa and complete excision of this area, increasing both flexion and extension. This represents an arthroscopic variation of the Outerbridge-Kashiwagi procedure, or the ulnohumeral arthroplasty described by Morrey [31].

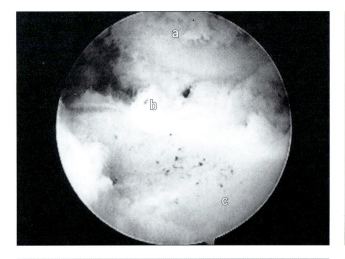

Figure 13-10. In patients with extensive damage to the tip of the olecranon (*c*), excision of the olecranon allows improved extension. The humeral cortex (*a*) and the proximal end of the excised olecranon (*b*) are also shown.

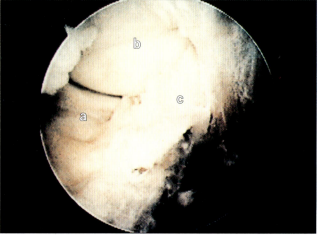

Figure 13-11. Scarring and fibrosis in the posterolateral gutter required debridement, as seen in this view from the posterolateral portal. The olecranon (*a*), radial head (*b*), and a large band of scar tissue (*c*) are shown.

using a full-radius soft tissue shaver blade. A notch-plasty blade or burr may then be used to deepen the olecranon fossa or completely resect it if ulno-humeral arthroplasty is necessary (Fig. 13-9). The olecranon and humerus are then debrided of osteo-phytes, again using a burr or notchplasty-type blade (Fig. 13-10). Olecranon excision is continued until full extension can be obtained.

To increase the point of maximum flexion, all posterior capsular adhesions are debrided from the posterosuperior portion of the elbow joint. Removal of adhesions between the triceps tendon and the posterior humerus should allow increased flexion of the elbow.

The final portion of the release is done by releasing the medial and lateral gutters of scar tissue and adhe-sions. The arthroscope is placed in the posterocentral portal, and the shaver is placed in the posterolateral portal. Excision of adhesions in the lateral gutter is initiated proximally and continues distally. A straight lateral or soft portal may be necessary to adequately debride the posterior radiocapitellar joint, posterior radioulnar joint, and posterolateral plica (Fig. 13-11). The arthroscope is kept in the posterolateral portal, and the shaver is switched to the posterocentral portal for debridement of the medial gutter. A fully hooded side-cutting shaver without suction should be used along the medial gutter to prevent inadvertent injury to the ulnar nerve.

In 1993, Jones and Savoie [32] reported a series of 12 patients who underwent arthroscopic capsular release for elbow flexion contracture. The average preoperative flexion contracture was 38°. The point of maximum flexion increased from 106° to 137°, and pronation and supination were also increased. Furthermore, all patients reported a significant decrease in pain postoperatively.

FUTURE TRENDS

The arthroscope has already been applied to advance techniques in the management of arthritis, trauma, and contractures and as an aid in diagnosing insta-bility around the elbow. These techniques are also still in the evolutionary stage and need to be further refined before their application can become wide-spread. As these changes do occur, one would expect arthroscopic management of these conditions to become a mainstay of treatment but certainly not the only one used. It will simply represent one more approach in the armamentarium of the surgeon in combating these disorders.

REFERENCES

1. Poehling GG, Whipple TL, Sisco L, Goldman B: Elbow arthroscopy: a new technique. *Arthroscopy* 1989, 5:222–224.

2. Adolfsson L: Arthroscopy of the elbow joint: a cadaveric study of portal placement. *J Shoulder Elbow Surg* 1994, 3:53.

3. Field LD, Altchek DW, Warren RF *et al.*: Arthroscopic anatomy of the lateral elbow: a comparison of three portals. *Arthroscopy,* 1994, 10:602–607.

4. Tullos HS, Schwab G, Bennet JB, Wood GW: Factors influencing elbow instability. *Instr Course Lect* 1981, 30:185–199.

5. Schwab GH, Bennett JB, Woods GW, Tullos HS: Biome-chanics of elbow instability; the role of the medial collat-eral ligament. *Clin Orthop* 1980, 146:42–52.

6. Sojbjerg JO, Ovensen J, Nielsen S: Experimental elbow instability after transection of the medial collateral liga-ment. *Clin Orthop* 1987, 218:186–190.

7. Conway JE, Jobe FW, Glousman RE, Pink M: Medial instability of the elbow in throwing athletes: treatment by repair or reconstruction of the ulnar collateral ligament. *J Bone Joint Surg Am* 1992, 74:67–83.

8. Stroyan M, Wilk KE: The functional anatomy of the elbow complex. *J Ortho Sports Phys Ther* 1993, 17:269–288.

9. Callaway GH, Field L, O'Brien S *et al.*: The contribution of medial collateral ligaments to valgus stability of the elbow. Paper presented at the Annual Meeting of the American Academy of Orthopedic Surgeons. Orlando, FL; February 16–21, 1995.

10. Morrey BF, An KN: Articular and ligamentous contribu-tions to the stability of the elbow joint. *Am J Sports Med* 1983, 11:315–319.

11. Morrey BF, Tanaka S, An K: Valgus stability of the elbow. *Clin Orthop* 1991, 265:187–195.

12. O'Driscoll SW, Bell DF, Morray BF: Posterolateral rotator instability of the elbow. *J Bone Joint Surg Am* 1991, 73:440–446.

13. Field LD, Callaway GH, O'Brien SJ, Altchek DW: Arthro-scopic assessment of the medial collateral ligament complex of the elbow. *Am J Sports Med* 1995, 23:396–400.

14. Field LD, Altchek DW: Evaluation of the arthroscopic valgus instability test of the elbow. *Am J Sports Med* 1994, 24:177–181.

15. Timmerman LA, Andrews JR: Undersurface tear of the ulnar collateral ligament in baseball players. *Am J Sports Med* 1994, 22:33–36.

16. Hang YS, Lippert FG III, Spolek GA, *et al.*: Biomechanical study of the pitching elbow. *Int Orthop* 1979, 3:217–223.

17. Jobe FW, Stark H, Lombardo SJ: Reconstruction of the ulnar collateral ligament in athletes. *J Bone Joint Surg Am* 1986, 68:1158–1163.

18. Jobe FW, Nuber G: Throwing injuries of the elbow. *Clin Sports Med* 1986, 5:621–636.

19. Kuroda S, Sakamaki K: Ulnar collateral ligament tears of the elbow joint. *Clin Orthop* 1986, 208:266–271.

20. Josefsson PO, Gentz CF, Johnell O, Wendeberg B: Surgical versus non-surgical treatment of ligamentous injuries following dislocation of the elbow joint: a prospective randomized study. *J Bone Joint Surg Am* 1987, 69:605–608.

21. Inge GAL: Eighty-six cases of chronic synovitis of knee joint treated by synovectomy. *JAMA* 1938, 111:2451.

22. Swett PP: A review of synovectomy. *J Bone Joint Surg* 1938, 20:68.

23. Copeland SA, Taylor JO: Synovectomy of the elbow in rheumatoid arthritis: the place of excision of the head of the radius. *J Bone Joint Surg Br* 1979, 61:69–73.

24. Mackay I, Fitzgerald B, Miller JH: Silastic radial head prosthesis in rheumatoid arthritis. *Act Orthop Scand* 1982, 53:63–66.

25. Rymaszewski L, Mackey I, Amis AA, Miller JH: Long term effects of excision of the radial head in rheumatoid arthritis. *J Bone Joint Surg Br* 1984, 66:109–113.

26. Saito T, Koshino T, Okamoto R: Arthroscopic findings and synovectomy of the rheumatoid elbow. *Techniques Orthop* 1991, 6:7.

27. Collins DH: *The Pathology of Articular and Spinal Diseases.* London: Edward Arnold Co; 1949.

28. Huskisson EC, Dieppe PA, Tucker AK, Cannell LB: Another look at osteoarthritis. *Ann Rheum Dis* 1979, 38:423–428.

29. Doherty M, Preston B: Primary osteoarthritis of the elbow. *Ann Rheum Dis* 1989, 48:743–747.

30. Kashiwagi D: Intraarticular changes of the osteoarthritic elbow, especially about the fossa olecrani. *J Jap Orthop Assoc* 1978, 52:1367.

31. Morrey BF: Primary degenerative arthritis of the elbow: treatment by ulnohumeral arthroplasty. *J Bone Joint Surg Br* 1992, 74:409–413.

32. Jones GS, Savoie FH: Arthroscopic capsular release of flexion contractures (arthrofibrosis) of the elbow. *Arthroscopy* 1993, 9:277–283.

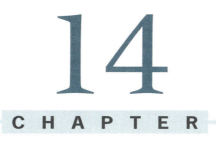

CHAPTER 14

Role of Arthroscopy in the Management of Triangular Fibrocartilage Complex Injuries and Wrist Fractures

GREGORY J. HANKER AND KELLY B. HANKER

During the past decade, arthroscopy of the wrist has become an invaluable surgical procedure that allows detailed examination of intra-articular wrist disorders. The development of new technology and the advancement of minimally invasive surgical techniques have greatly increased the ability of surgeons who specialize in upper extremity operations to provide much more effective treatment for their patients.

Injuries to the wrist joint are extremely common and occur among all age groups. A large portion of these injuries are intra-articular, primarily involving the distal radius, wrist ligaments and fibrocartilage, and carpal bones. Management of fractures of the distal radius has received extensive attention in the orthopedic literature. Intra-articular fractures can be extremely problematic. By their very nature, they disrupt the articulating bony surfaces, and thus markedly impair the smooth gliding motion at both the radiocarpal joint (RCJ) and the distal radioulnar joint (DRUJ). The fracture leads to bleeding within the joint, which incites an inflammatory synovial reaction, eventually resulting in formation of intra-articular scar tissue. Intra-articular fracture debris is commonly found within the joint, further exacerbating development of fibrous adhesions of the wrist joint.

Arthroscopic treatment provides a new dimension of care. Not only can wrist arthroscopy assist with the critical fracture reduction of the intra-articular segments and lavage the joint of hematoma and fracture debris, but it also can discover and treat coincidental injuries to the triangular fibrocartilage complex (TFCC), cartilage, capsule, and intercarpal ligaments. The relatively new technique of arthroscopic-assisted reduction and internal fixation (ARIF) of the displaced distal radius fracture, scaphoid fracture, and other carpal bone injuries is discussed in this chapter in detail.

ACUTE DISTAL RADIUS FRACTURES

In adults with closed distal radius fracture, the physical examination and the posteroanterior and lateral radiographs of the wrist are usually sufficient to determine a treatment plan. If any doubt remains about the complexity of the fracture and the displacement of the fragments, a computed tomographic (CT) scan, magnetic resonance image (MRI), or plane tomograms may be obtained. The intra-articular fracture pattern can be described by any of the many available classification systems that help to accurately depict the type and severity of the fracture and further serve as a basis for treatment and evaluation of outcome [1•]. The extent of the displacement and comminution of the medial fracture complex and the presence of a "die-punch" component continue to present a challenge to fracture reduction and stabilization.

Extra-articular, undisplaced fractures and displaced, stable, reducible fractures are usually managed with cast immobilization and early therapy. Displaced, unstable fractures are best treated with closed reduction under anesthesia and percutaneous K-wire fixation. It is the intra-articular fracture that presents the greatest challenge to the attending physician. Even nondisplaced, stable, intra-articular fractures can be associated with serious ligamentous, capsule, cartilage, or TFCC injuries [2]. Certainly, the displaced, comminuted, and unstable intra-articular fractures require some type of surgical treatment. Closed reduction under anesthesia with percutaneous pinning, external fixation, limited open reduction, open reduction and internal fixation (ORIF), supplemental bone grafting, and ARIF are all viable treatment options [1•].

Arthroscopic examination of ARIF actually *complements* any of the suitably available techniques of fracture care; it does not substitute for well-established surgical techniques to anatomically reduce and stabilize the wrist fracture. Because the primary goal is to restore articular congruity, the arthroscope affords a direct visual tool to monitor the success of the reduction [2,3•,4]. Arthroscopic visualization of the fracture fragments is far superior to either an open arthrotomy or a fluoroscopic image. With the arthroscope in the RCJ, accessory wrist portals can be used to introduce manually or electrically powered instruments to precisely position the fracture fragments. It is the authors' experience that this added degree of accuracy

provided by the ARIF technique should yield superior healing of the joint surface in an anatomic position without fragment displacement or incongruity. This should markedly lessen the possibility of posttraumatic wrist arthrosis. Removal of fracture hematoma and intra-articular fracture debris with shaver should diminish the inflammatory reaction within the joint, and thus lessen postfracture arthrofibrosis.

Of equal importance to accurate fracture reduction, the thorough arthroscopic visualization of the intra-articular ligaments, TFCC, and cartilage allows for discovery of serious injuries that otherwise elude the surgeon. Such associated wrist problems—carpal instability, carpal bone fractures, TFCC tears, and chondral damage—would otherwise remain completely undetected. If these serious associated wrist injuries do go untreated, they will certainly lead to chronic wrist problems long after the fracture has healed [3•,5].

TECHNIQUE OF ARTHROSCOPIC-ASSISTED REDUCTION AND INTERNAL FIXATION

The operating room is set up as it would be for routine wrist arthroscopy [6•,7•,8]. A great deal of equipment might become necessary to carry out the wrist fracture reduction: powered driver to insert K-wires, open reduction sets to install plates and screws, an external fixation set, a small portable fluoroscope or regular C-arm unit, a suspension boom or traction tower, and a radio-translucent hand table. The authors' standard set up is depicted in Figure 14-1. Note that the patient's arm is positioned on the small radio-translucent hand table and may need to be stabilized loosely to the table with a band around the

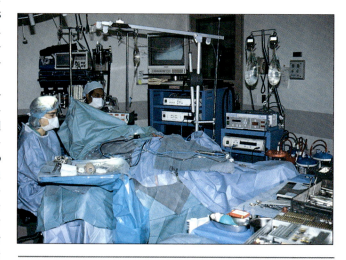

Figure 14-1. Operating room set-up for arthroscopic-assisted reduction and internal fixation. A large operating room is preferred to accommodate the numerous pieces of arthroscopic and surgical equipment.

upper arm. The index, middle, and ring fingers are placed in overhead, longitudinal traction with approximately 10 to 12 lbs of weight. If a boom is used as a suspension device for the injured arm, it must be fastened securely to the opposite side of the operating room table. This will allow adequate space for the fluoroscopic unit to gain 360° access to the wrist. By using a small, portable, self-contained fluoroscopic unit, such as the Xi Scan 1000 (Xi Tec, Inc, Windsor Locks, CT), illustrated in Figure 14-2A, the surgeon has both complete control of the unit and the ease of rapid positioning. The C-arm is positioned parallel to the floor so that it can be moved in, out, and about the vertically oriented wrist. A pneumatic tourniquet is placed proximally on the upper arm; the limb is sterilely prepped, and a drape is placed over the upper extremities.

Initially, the authors perform a closed reduction of the distal radius fracture by direct manual manipulation. Use of the fluoroscope is helpful at this juncture to determine whether anatomic restoration of radial height, inclination, and palmar tilt have been achieved. Some preliminary information about articular congruity can be obtained from the fluoroscopic image, but the surgeon should beware—a significant stepoff in excess of 1 mm can exist despite the image's appearing acceptable. Carpal instability can also be assessed fluoroscopically if there appears to be a widening of the scapholunate joint (SLJ) or lunotriquetral joint (LTJ) on the posteroanterior image.

Using a 10-mL syringe and a 22-gauge hypodermic needle, sterile saline is injected into the RCJ through the dorsoradial (3-4) portal. The Dyonics (Smith & Nephew, Andover, MA) 2.9-mm, short arthroscopic cannula with conical tip obturator is gently placed into the dorsoradial wrist portal. In the vicinity of the dorsoulnar (6-R) portal, a 19-gauge needle is inserted, taking care to avoid injuring the TFCC. The RCJ can now be lavaged with saline solution entering through the 19-gauge needle and exiting thorough the larger cannula. In this way, a good deal of the fracture debris (eg, hematoma, small loose bodies, fibrin clot) can be removed.

The Dyonics 2.7-mm × 30° × 67-mm arthroscope is placed into the cannula at the dorsoradial wrist portal site. Through-and-through fluid irrigation is now initiated, and control is greatly facilitated with the use of a pump, such as the Dyonics Intelijet Fluid Management System (Smith & Nephew). Fluid inflow is through the arthroscope sheath. Systematic examination of the injured wrist joint is performed. Intra-articular visualization is facilitated with the use of a Dyonics EP-1 Shaver System with a Dyonics 2.9-mm full-radius disposable blade (both Smith & Nephew) introduced into the dorsoulnar portal. In most patients, the fracture hematoma is adherent to the articular surface of the distal radius. Complete arthroscopic visualization of the fracture pattern is not possible until all debris has been removed with the shaver. Position of the fracture fragments can now be assessed, but visualization from both the dorsoradial and dorsoulnar wrist portals is necessary. Viewing from the dorsoulnar portal is especially helpful in assessing the reduction of the medial fracture complex or a die-punch type of impaction (Fig. 14-2B).

When all fracture lines can be clearly visualized, the success of the initial reduction can be established. Of equal importance, the surgeon must fully evaluate the integrity of all extrinsic and intrinsic wrist ligaments, the TFCC, capsule, and carpal bone cartilaginous surfaces.

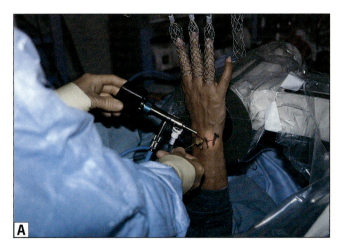

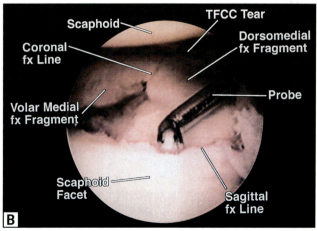

Figure 14-2. A, Instruments can be introduced into the wrist joint to assist with reduction of the displaced fracture fragments while viewing with both the arthroscope and mini C-arm Xi Scan (Xi Tec, Inc, Windsor Locks, CT). **B,** A small joint probe is used to directly manipulate the fracture (fx) fragments. TFCC—triangular fibrocartilage complex.

If articular displacement greater than 1 mm remains, an attempt should be made to manually disimpact the fracture fragments and restore as smooth an articular surface as possible [9]. A dissecting probe can be introduced into the joint to assist with disimpaction and fracture-fragment reduction. Alternatively, a 0.045-in or 0.062-in K-wire can be passed percutaneously into the joint or respective fracture fragments. When placed into the fracture fragment, the K-wire acts as a "joystick" to manipulate the fragment into position. K-wires can also be passed into subchondral areas of the distal radius to assist manipulation. This is especially helpful with reduction of unstable dorsal fracture fragments or a die-punch impacted fragment. The resultant change of position is visualized through the arthroscope, and when a satisfactory reduction is obtained, the wire is drilled across the fracture fragment, securing it in position (Fig. 14-3).

A minidorsal incision can be made over the metaphyseal area of the distal radius, a small Freer elevator (Weck & Pilling Co, Ft. Washington, PA) or 1/4-in osteotome is inserted through the dorsal extensor retinaculum, and an impacted fragment of a die-punch fracture is leveraged upward into an anatomic position. A modification of this technique is to advance the tip of the Freer instrument to the volar cortex of the distal radius fracture, and then leverage distally and volarly to bring the entire distal fracture fragment into anatomic alignment. If a large metaphyseal defect is present after fracture elevation, it is best to install a bone graft, which is most easily obtained from the ipsilateral olecranon.

After reduction of the intra-articular fracture has been confirmed (visually with the arthroscope and radiographically with the fluoroscope), secure fixation

is accomplished. In the authors' experience, this can usually be accomplished with percutaneous K-wires, as depicted in Figure 14-4. If the internal K-wire fixation is secure, a modified "sugar-tong" splint is applied. If, however, concern about stability remains, or if the K-wire purchase is tenuous, it is best to apply a uniplane external fixation device, such as the EBI DFS Distal Radius Fixature/Dyna Fix System (Parsippany, NJ).

Congruity must also be established at the DRUJ. Fracture instability of the medial complex, either dorsomedial or volarmedial, in combination with an avulsion of the TFCC, can lead to DRUJ instability. A congruent reduction of the DRUJ is almost always associated with anatomic restoration of the distal radius fracture. Percutaneous K-wire fixation through the distal ulna, across the DRUJ, and into the distal radius styloid area will not only maintain the congruent alignment of the DRUJ, but also will serve as an additional buttress for an unstable distal radius fracture (see Fig. 14-4).

A displaced ulna styloid fracture through the base of the distal ulna may require percutaneous K-wire fixation. In the authors' experience, ulna styloid fractures are rarely associated with avulsion of the TFCC at its ulnar attachment.

Most importantly, the surgeon should not hesitate to use any combination of surgical techniques that will restore anatomic alignment and secure fixation of these complex fractures.

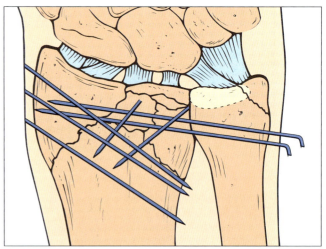

Figure 14-4. Schematic view of K-wire placement. After confirming anatomic reduction of the distal radius fracture both arthroscopically and fluoroscopically, secure fixation is usually obtained by placing two or three 0.045-in K-wires through the radial styloid into the radial shaft. If the dorsomedial fracture complex reduction is difficult to maintain, an additional one or two K-wires should be placed through this fragment. In many patients, the authors also place two additional 0.062-in K-wires through the distal ulna, continuing obliquely into the distal radius to act as an additional buttress for the unstable fracture.

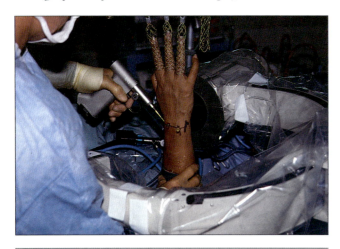

Figure 14-3. K-wires (0.045 in and 0.062 in) are inserted percutaneously through the radial styloid and dorsomedial fracture fragments while they are viewed with both the arthroscope and the mini C-arm Xi Scan.

ASSOCIATED INJURIES

While the arthroscope is being used to examine the wrist fracture pattern, the surgeon should be sure to include a systematic evaluation of all intra-articular soft tissue structures and carpal cartilaginous surfaces. Serious injuries of the intrinsic and extrinsic ligaments, TFCC, capsule, and cartilage surfaces are frequently found. The authors' experience is reviewed in Table 14-1. Subtotal or membranous tear of the intrinsic wrist ligaments should not produce carpal instability but may cause postinjury wrist pain. This type of ligamentous tear is treatable with arthroscopic debridement [10]. Complete intrinsic ligament tear can result in static or dynamic instability. Arthroscopic visualization through the midcarpal portal is especially helpful to ensure that correct alignment is present at the SLJ or LTJ. Treatment options include either open

Table 14-1	Frequency of Associated Intracarpal Soft-Tissue and Cartilage Lesions in Patients with Intra-articular Distal Radius Fractures

Parameter	Frequency, %
Carpal instability	23
Scapholunate instability	15
Lunotriquetral instability	8
DRUJ instability	10
SLL tear	20
LTL tear	10
Radiovolar carpal ligament injury	25
Ulnocarpal ligament injury	55
TFCC tear, acute	65
Class IA	10
Class IB	2
Class IC	13
Class ID	75
Class II, degenerative	15
Perilunate injury pattern	10
Dorsal capsular tear	80
Osteochondral fracture	20
Intra-articular loose bodies	25

DRUJ—distal radioulnar joint; LTL—lunotriquetral ligament; SLL—scapholunate ligament; TFCC—triangular fibrocartilage complex.

repair of the torn ligament or arthroscopically assisted reduction of the carpal dissociation and percutaneous pinning [11].

An extremely common injury, present more often than not, is traumatic tear of the TFCC. TFCC injuries are most easily treated arthroscopically. This will be discussed in detail later in this chapter.

Chondral or osteochondral fractures of the carpal bones are fairly common. Arthroscopy is the only reliable method for diagnosing these cartilage injuries. Arthroscopic treatment consists of debridement of the cartilage flap or a chondroplasty. Loose cartilage fragments should be removed. The surgeon's knowledge of the concomitant existence of these cartilage injuries usually alters prognosis for patients' long-term recovery.

CARPAL BONE FRACTURES

Scaphoid fractures account for approximately 70% of all carpal bone injuries. Because the scaphoid represents an important mechanical link within the carpus, any problem caused by a fracture or ligamentous injury severely alters the kinematics of the wrist joint. The standard of care for a scaphoid fracture is a closed reduction and cast immobilization. ORIF is usually reserved for displaced, irreducible fractures. Wrist arthroscopy can be used in the surgical management of scaphoid fractures. The technique of ARIF is applied to the scaphoid injury. This minimally invasive surgical procedure should lead to a more accurate fracture reduction and decreased surgical morbidity. Of equal importance, associated wrist injuries of the cartilage, intercarpal ligaments, and even the TFCC can be discovered, and appropriate concomitant treatment provided. It is usually necessary to view through both the RCJ and midcarpal joint (MCJ) portals. It is sometimes difficult to fully visualize the waist region through the RCJ portal because of synovitis and capsular connections in this region. The MCJ portal is an excellent viewpoint for seeing the waist and distal pole. After anatomic reduction has been achieved both arthroscopically and fluoroscopically, the authors usually drill three 0.045-in K-wires percutaneously through the distal pole, across the fracture, and into the proximal pole. This stable fixation eliminates motion at the fracture site. The pins are left in place until the fracture is radiographically healed, usually 8 to 12 weeks. An alternative technique using the Herbert-Whipple screw system (Zimmer, Warsaw, IN) has also been quite successful but requires considerably more effort to install the screw [8].

Fractures of the other carpal bones have received less attention than those of the scaphoid, but they present an equal challenge. The authors have treated several patients with dorsal triquetral avulsion fractures whose ulnar-sided wrist pain did not resolve. Dorsal triquetral chip fractures usually heal quickly, within 4 to 8 weeks. When ulnar-sided wrist pain persists for more than 2 months, the treating physician should suspect either a TFCC tear or a lunotriquetral ligament (LTL) injury. At this time, wrist arthroscopy allows for debridement of dorsal capsular scar tissue associated with the chip fracture, thorough evaluation of the ulnar aspect of the wrist for either a central or dorsal TFCC tear, or a partial or complete LTL tear. Both of these associated wrist injuries are quite amenable to arthroscopic treatment.

TRIANGULAR FIBROCARTILAGE COMPLEX INJURIES

Pathology of the TFCC is a common cause of ulnar-sided wrist pain. Patients typically complain of a deep pain, which is worsened with pronation and supination, ulnar deviation, and power grasp. A careful physical examination should make the physician suspicious of a TFCC tear after exclusion of other common causes of ulnar wrist pain, such as extensor or flexor carpi ulnaris tendonitis, extensor carpi ulnaris (ECU) subluxation, ulnocarpal impingement, pisotriquetral or DRUJ problems, intra-articular synovitis caused by inflammatory arthropathy, carpal instability, partial or complete ligament injuries, fractures, and dislocations.

In the authors' experience, the three-compartment wrist arthrogram is currently the best imaging method for diagnosing TFCC tears. However, a high-quality wrist MRI, done by an experienced radiologist, can be equally reliable. Unfortunately, each of these studies has a false-negative rate of between approximately 30% and 40%, and neither study can yield information on the pathophysiologic significance of the lesion [12]. Plane radiographs of the wrist remain quite helpful. Patients with negative ulnar variance are at lower risk for a TFCC tear.

The TFCC injury classification scheme developed by Palmer [13•] is a helpful framework for understanding the nature of these injuries and for deciding appropriate treatment. Class I TFCC lesions result from traumatic injuries, with subclassification based on location of the tear. A class IA lesion represents a tear in the central section of the TFCC. Class IB lesions usually represent an avulsion from the distal ulna, but may also occur at the dorsal peripheral attachment to the wrist capsule. A class IC lesion consists of a disruption of the ulnocarpal ligaments from their volar attachment to the TFCC. A class ID lesion is an avulsion of the TFCC from its radial attachment to the sigmoid notch. These injuries are amenable to arthroscopic treatment. Class II lesions result from progressive degeneration and are staged according to the extent of TFCC wear and tear and deterioration of the surrounding ligamentous and osseous structures.

The focus of this chapter is techniques of wrist arthroscopy that are extremely useful for treatment of traumatic TFCC injuries, concentrating primarily on traumatic tears that occur in association with a distal radius fracture. In the authors' experience, 65% of intra-articular distal radius fractures have an associated TFCC tear. Class ID is the most frequent type (Fig. 14-5A). It is a direct result of the fracture's propagating coronally across the medial fracture complex and into the attachment of the central disk at the sigmoid notch. Class IA is the second most common (Fig. 14-5B). A dorsal peripheral tear, currently

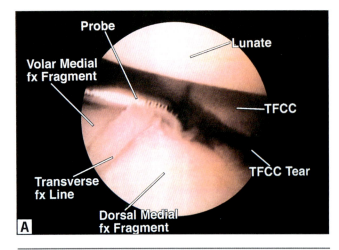

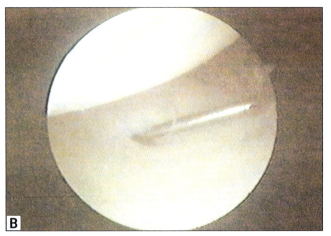

Figure 14-5. A, Arthroscopic appearance of a class ID triangular fibrocartilage complex (TFCC) tear associated with an intra-articular distal radius fracture (fx). Note the coronal fracture line entering directly at the site of tearing of the central disk away from the sigmoid notch. **B,** Arthroscopic appearance of a class IA TFCC tear, which is most often associated with a "sprained" wrist. Note the longitudinally oriented tear is approximately 2 mm ulnar to the sigmoid notch.

considered a variant of a class IB tear, is not uncommon. However, class IB and class IC tears are quite rare.

Arthroscopy of the RCJ is the best way to evaluate the TFCC. On occasion, arthroscopic examination of the DRUJ can lend additional diagnostic information concerning injuries to the undersurface of the TFCC and cartilage of the sigmoid notch and distal ulna. Usually, complete evaluation of the TFCC requires visualization through the dorsoradial, dorsoulnar, and ulnar (6-U) portals. All portions of the TFCC must be inspected and probed because tears can sometimes be quite subtle (*see* Fig. 14-5*B*). The probe acts as an examining finger within the joint and can reveal injuries to the TFCC that were initially overlooked by viewing alone. Thorough evaluation of the TFCC includes the central disk, its origin from the sigmoid notch of the distal radius and its insertion into the base of the ulna; the ulnolunate ligament (ULL) and ulnotriquetral ligament (UTL), with their respective attachments to the volar radioulnar ligament and distally to the lunate and triquetrum; the dorsal attachment to the capsule, dorsal radioulnar ligament, and subsheath of the ECU; the meniscus homologue; and the prestyloid recess.

Not all tears of the TFCC necessarily require surgical treatment. A small, stable class IA linear split in the central disk can sometimes be left untreated. A small, stable volar or dorsal tear can be treated with immobilization of the DRUJ in a modified long arm cast/splint, or "sugar-tong" splint. All other TFCC tears are best treated using wrist arthroscopy. Class IA tears are actually the most common type seen with "sprained" wrists (*see* Fig. 14-5*B*). Arthroscopic appearance of a Class IA tear may vary slightly depending on the thickness of the central disk. This type of tear is vertically oriented from dorsal to palmar and is approximately 2 to 10 mm long. It is located approximately 2 mm ulnar to the sigmoid notch. At this location, the tangentially oriented peripheral fibers meet the randomly oriented central fibers, creating the potential for shear. The goal of treatment is to eliminate any unstable torn tissue through arthroscopic debridement of the avascular, unstable central disk. Biomechanically, this "ectomy" produces no adverse effect on wrist function as long as the peripheral margins of the TFCC remain intact.

Arthroscopic Debridement of Triangular Fibrocartilage Complex Tears

Surgical technique for excision of a class IA or ID TFCC tear (Fig. 14-6) begins when the arthroscope is placed in the dorsoradial portal, because this vantage point usually gives the best view of the entire

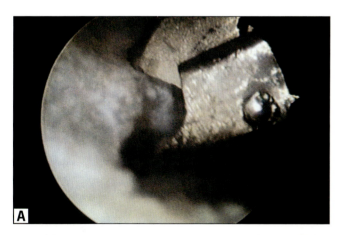

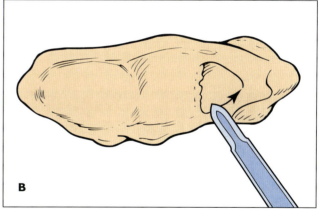

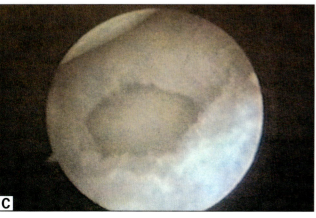

Figure 14-6. A, Arthroscopic view of suction punch debriding torn radiovolar margin of triangular fibrocartilage complex (TFCC). **B,** Either an angled basket rongeur or a curved banana knife can be used to debride the torn dorsal margin of the TFCC. **C,** Arthroscopic view of debrided tear. The unstable central portion of the disk has been excised, and a stable peripheral margin remains.

complex. A Dyonics suction punch is inserted into the dorsoulnar portal, and the radial and volar radial portions of the torn central disk are excised. The arthroscope is then placed into the dorsoulnar portal. The suction punch is placed into the dorsoradial portal, and the ulnar portion of the torn central disk is excised. The dorsal portion of the torn central disk is difficult to excise because of its location. Three options are available to remove this last segment of the TFCC tear. First, an angulated basket rongeur should be used to gain access. If this is not helpful, a 6-U portal should be established. Because the 6-U portal is directly ulnar, instrumentation inserted through this portal has easy access either dorsally, volarly, or at the sigmoid notch attachment. The authors frequently use this 6-U portal to complete the debridement. The final option is to carefully insert a small curved banana knife through the dorsoulnar portal and surgically cut the remaining dorsal margin of torn disk. This last option is cumbersome and somewhat difficult. After the central portion of the disk has been sculpted to a smooth border with the full-radius shaver, the underlying cartilage of the ulna head should be inspected for any pathology. Articulation of the DRUJ is also clearly seen through the central defect.

If the TFCC tear is simply debrided, early motion and occupational therapy are encouraged after 5 to 7 days of postsurgical immobilization in a short arm splint. Patients typically complain of soreness and wrist stiffness for 2 to 4 months. Return of grip strength can easily take 6 months or longer. TFCC debridement alone is not an adequate treatment if the tear is associated with positive ulnar variance or an LTL injury. In a patient with positive ulnar variance, it may be necessary to consider a distal ulnar shortening osteotomy or a distal ulnar recession, such as the "wafer" procedure. LTL tears probably require intercarpal fusion.

Arthroscopic-Assisted Repair of Triangular Fibrocartilage Complex Dorsal Peripheral Tears

The final TFCC injury considered in this chapter is the dorsal peripheral tear, in which the dorsal margin of the TFCC is separated from the dorsal capsule and the subsheath wall of the ECU. This lesion fits neither the classification as a variant of the class IB, or the dorsal equivalent of the class IC. Unique unto itself, it requires its own subclassification. Dorsal peripheral tears are the third most common type of TFCC acute traumatic injury; they are completely amenable to arthroscopically assisted surgical repair and are very similar to peripheral meniscus tears of the knee.

To accomplish reattachment of the torn TFCC, sutures need to be placed through the dorsal capsule and subsheath of the ECU into the dorsal peripheral margin of the TFCC (Fig. 14-7). A 2-cm longitudinal incision is made between the fifth and sixth dorsal wrist extensor tendon compartments. The dorsal sensory branch of the ulnar nerve is protected. The distal third of the extensor retinaculum is incised, and the ECU tendon is retracted ulnarly with the use of a vessel loop. The surgeon now has excellent access to the dorsal capsule and wall of the ECU subsheath. A 1.5-in 20-gauge angiocath is inserted through the capsule, obliquely oriented to also pierce the dorsal peripheral

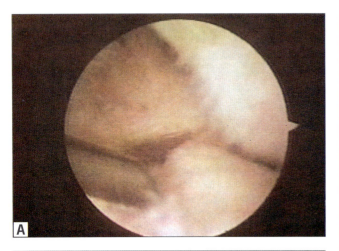

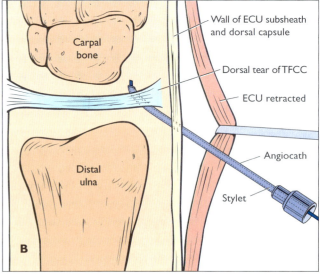

Figure 14-7. A, Arthroscopic view of a dorsal peripheral tear. The torn margins are debrided in preparation for suture repair. **B,** Lateral schematic view. The extensor carpi ulnaris (ECU) tendon is retracted from its compartment, and the angiocath is inserted obliquely through the wall of the ECU subsheath and dorsal capsule. (*continued*)

margin of the detached TFCC and gain a 2-mm purchase. This insertion is monitored arthroscopically with the arthroscope placed in the dorsoradial portal. It is also best to initially freshen the torn margins of the TFCC and capsule with a shaver. With some practice, it becomes fairly easy to place the angiocath properly. As soon as the tip of the angiocath pierces the distal surface of the TFCC, the stylet is removed. A 2-0 Maxon suture (Sherwood-Davis & Geck, St. Louis, MO) is inserted into the angiocath and advanced into the RCJ. While continuing to view arthroscopically, a narrow-tip mosquito clamp is inserted through the

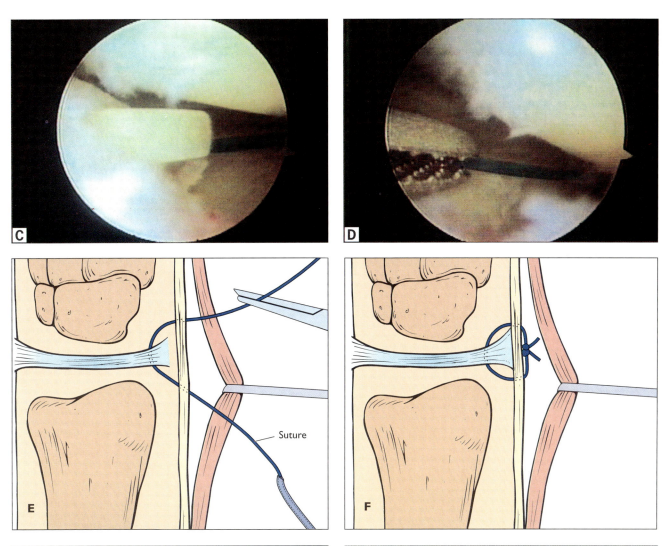

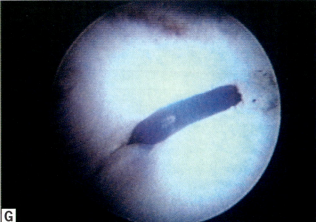

Figure 14-7. (*continued*) **C,** Arthroscopic view of angiocath tip penetrating the dorsal margin of the TFCC. The Maxon 2-0 suture (Sherwood-Davis & Geck, St. Louis, MO) is seen to exit just beyond the catheter tip. **D,** Arthroscopic view of clamp grasping the suture after the catheter has been removed. **E,** The mosquito clamp is withdrawn, and the suture is secured. The angiocath is withdrawn. Both suture ends are now exterior to the joint with a secure purchase on the dorsal peripheral margin of the torn TFCC. This process is repeated in order to place a second suture just ulnar to the first. **F,** With the forearm in neutral rotation, the sutures are tied tightly over the ECU subsheath and the dorsal capsule. **G,** Arthroscopic view of the tied suture. The dorsal peripheral tear has been closed.

dorsal capsule, slightly distally to the location of the angiocath. Under arthroscopic control, the protruding suture is grasped and withdrawn along with the angiocath. A secure ligature is now in place to pull the torn margin of the TFCC against the wall of the dorsal capsule. A second stitch is placed just ulnar to the first. Usually two stitches yield a secure repair of the dorsal peripheral TFCC tear. The stitches should be tied securely, and the ECU should be returned to its compartment. The DRUJ is immobilized in neutral position for 4 weeks, in a modified "sugar-tong" splint, to allow for soft-tissue healing.

Whipple [8] has developed a small joint suturing system (The Intec; Linvatec, Largo, FL). The disposable cannulated needle set is quick and simple to use [14]. Poehling [15] uses a Tuohy needle technique, which is also effective.

Class ID tears can be successfully repaired with a technique that places drill holes coronally across the distal radius. A suture can then be placed through the 6-U portal, into the radial aspect of the torn TFCC, and then into the drilled holes. The suture needles exit at the radial styloid. A cut down is necessary over the radial styloid to safely tie the suture [16]. This technique is moderately difficult to perform, and the authors favor simple excision of the torn central disk.

Class IC tears are rare, and there is very limited experience in their arthroscopic treatment. Partial class IC tears are amenable to arthroscopic debridement. This is usually done with the arthroscope in the dorsoulnar portal and the shaver in the 6-U portal. A complete tear of the ulnocarpal ligaments with instability may require open repair of the ULL and UTL complex. Class IB tears are rare and usually occur in conjunction with bony injury to the ulna styloid. They are amenable to ARIF, in which sutures are placed through the ulnarmost aspect of the TFCC to anchor it back to bone.

Recent experience indicates that arthroscopic debridement and arthroscopically assisted repair of TFCC tears are extremely effective treatments for these painful wrist injuries.

CONCLUSION

Wrist arthroscopy has dramatically increased the ability to evaluate and treat wrist disorders. The technique is especially helpful in the treatment of intra-articular wrist fractures, such as those involving the distal radius and carpals, and in the debridement and assisted repair of acute, traumatic TFCC tears.

REFERENCES AND RECOMMENDED READING

Recently published papers of particular interest have been highlighted as:
•   Of interest

1.•   Fernandez DL, Jupiter JB: *Fractures of the Distal Radius.* New York: Springer Verlag; 1996.

A comprehensive text on the practical approach to management of distal radius fractures.

2.   Hanker GJ: Arthroscopic evaluation of intraarticular distal radius fractures. Presented at the 46th Annual Meeting of the American Society for Surgery of the Hand. Orlando, FL; October, 1991.

3.•   Hanker GJ: Intraarticular fractures of the distal radius. In *Operative Arthroscopy,* edn 2. Edited by McGinty JB. New York: Lippincott-Raven Publishers; 1996:987–997.

The author thoroughly describes the use of wrist arthroscopy as an adjunct technique to assist with intra-articular distal radius fracture reduction.

4.   Cooney WP III, Berger RA: Treatment of complex fractures of the distal radius: combined use of internal and external fixation and arthroscopic reduction. *Hand Clin* 1993, 9:603–612.

5.   Geissler WB, Freeland AE, Savoie FH, *et al.*: Intracarpal soft tissue lesions associated with an intra-articular fracture of the distal end of the radius. *J Hand Surg* 1996, 78(suppl A):357–365.

6.•   Whipple TL, Poehling GG, Roth JH: Surgical technique for wrist arthroscopy. In *Operative Arthroscopy,* edn 2. Edited by McGinty JB. New York: Lippincott-Raven Publishers; 1996:927–935.

The authors present a comprehensive review of the surgical technique for diagnostic and therapeutic wrist arthroscopy, including set-up, portal placement, and technique for viewing the wrist joint.

7.•   Poehling GG, Chabon SJ, Siegel DB: Diagnostic and operative arthroscopy. In *The Wrist.* Edited by Gelberman RH. New York: Raven Press; 1994:21–45.

The authors describe indications, preoperative planning, and multiple diagnostic and surgical techniques available for successfully performing wrist arthroscopy.

8.   Whipple TL: *Arthroscopic surgery—The Wrist.* Philadelphia: JB Lippincott; 1992.

9.   Knirk JL, Jupiter JB: Intra-articular fractures of the distal end of the radius in young adults. *J Bone J Surg* 1986, 68(suppl A):647–659.

10.   Ruch DS, Poehling GG: Arthroscopic management of partial scapholunate and lunotriquetral injuries of the wrist. *J Hand Surg* 1996, 21(suppl A):412–417.

11. Cooney WP, Berger RA: Interosseous ligamentous injuries of the wrist. In *Operative Arthroscopy*, edn 2. Edited by McGinty JB. New York: Lippincott-Raven Publishers; 1996:1023–1032.

12. Hanker GJ, Lynch TP, Flannigan BD, *et al.*: Chronic wrist pain : spin-echo and short tau inversion recovery—MR imaging and conventional and MR arthrography. *Radiology* 1992, 182:205–211.

13.• Palmer AK, Harris PG: Classification and arthroscopic treatment of triangular fibrocartilage complex lesions. In *Operative Arthroscopy*, edn 2. Edited by McGinty JB. New York: Lippincott-Raven Publishers; 1996:1015–1022.

A description of the Palmer classification of triangular fibrocartilage complex lesions and the arthroscopic technique for their surgical treatment.

14. Corso SJ, Savoie FH, Geissler WB, *et al.*: Arthroscopic repair of peripheral avulsions of the triangular fibrocartilage complex of the wrist: a multicenter study. *Arthroscopy* 1997, 13:78–84.

15. deAraujo W, Poehling GG, Kuzma GR: New Tuohy needle technique for triangular fibrocartilage complex repair: preliminary studies. *Arthroscopy* 1996, 12:699–703.

16. Trumble TE, Gilbert M, Vedder N: Arthroscopic repair of the triangular fibrocartilage complex. *Arthroscopy* 1996, 12:588–597.

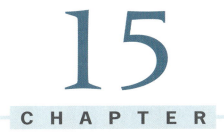

CHAPTER 15

State of the Art
Hip Arthroscopic Techniques

ANDREW H.N. ROBINSON AND RICHARD N. VILLAR

The popularity of hip arthroscopy has lagged behind that shown for operating on many other joints. This may result from the technical difficulty of the procedure or the perceived infrequency of indications for its use. In 1931, Burman [1] stated that "it is manifestly impossible to insert a needle between the head of the femur and the acetabulum." However, during the past 20 years considerable technical advances have been made that allow safe access to the joint with good visualization.

In 1977, Gross [2] reported the use of arthroscopy in the adolescent hip affected with chondrolysis, secondary to a slipped upper femoral epiphysis. Subsequent reports have documented other indications, such as the removal of cement from the acetabulum following total hip arthroplasty [3] and as a means of synovial biopsy [4].

During the past two decades, both the acceptance of hip arthroscopy and the frequency of publications discussing it have increased. Although the indications for it are less common than are those for knee arthroscopy, it is a useful surgical tool. The purpose of this chapter is to detail the surgical techniques, outline the indications, and review the results of hip arthroscopy.

INSTRUMENTATION

Many of the instruments used for hip arthroscopy are identical to those used for knee surgery, and as with knee surgery, the arthroscopy hook is the most useful. Electrical instruments can greatly ease hip arthroscopy (Fig. 15-1). Both manual and electrical instruments are available with curved handles; this makes the insertion of the instrument into the hip joint more difficult but can ease access around the femoral head to more remote parts of the joint.

The most useful blades are the 4.5-mm concave and convex full-radius chondroplasty blades (Smith & Nephew Endoscopy, Oklahoma City, OK). The recommended blades are either convex or concave to avoid scuffing the femoral head. The chondroplasty blade is used for the trimming of chondral or osteochondral flaps. A synovectomy blade is occasionally used for its end-cutting capability, particularly in the acetabular notch.

The instruments (Fig. 15-2) are inserted through a 5.7-mm diameter disposable arthroscopic cannula (Smith and Nephew Endoscopy). The cannula both protects the soft tissues and eases instrument manipulation.

Also useful is an 8- or 10-mm diameter laparoscopy cannula, down which a large bore suction catheter (Techniko-Deltaflo; Niko Surgical, Stonehouse, Gloucestershire, England) can be passed to remove large loose bodies.

Arthroscope

The most commonly used arthroscope for hip arthroscopy is the 70°, 4.5-mm instrument. The 70° viewing direction gives the widest field of view, while maintaining surgical orientation. The hip joint is deep, with relatively fixed soft tissues surrounding it; this makes it difficult to manipulate the arthroscope to change the field of view. Thus, rotation of the arthroscope and a side-viewing direction are of greater importance to obtain a complete view of the joint.

In most patients, a standard-length arthroscope is sufficient. The use of longer arthroscopes (22.5 cm) is desirable in the obese patient. Use of a camera preserves sterility and is preferable. Video recording or still photography are available, depending on the surgeon's preference.

Irrigation System

Good fluid flow is essential. It is possible to use the arthroscope in the hip using saline administered through a standard intravenous fluid administration set. Considerable debris or bleeding can be encountered during instrumentation, and for this reason a pressure bag is helpful. The pressure increases flow and tamponades bleeding. Fluid management systems that provide high fluid flow at controlled pressures are ideal.

A 15-gauge cardiac needle is used for the fluid inflow, and the arthroscope sheath is used as the outflow. Frequent checks should be made to avoid loss of portal position and the consequent extravasation of fluid into the soft tissues.

TECHNIQUE
Operating Room Layout

Hip arthroscopy requires a great deal of equipment in the operating room. The room must accommodate the

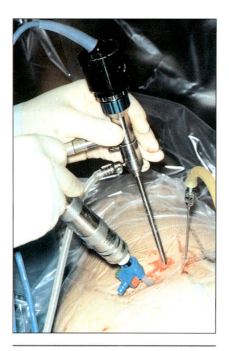

Figure 15-1. Power shaver in use, using three lateral portals. The anterior needle is used as a fluid inflow. The outflow is through the arthroscope sheath. (©Richard N. Villar.)

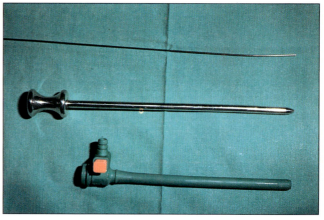

Figure 15-2. The Nitinol guidewire (Smith & Nephew Endoscopy, Oklahoma City, OK) shown with the blunt, cannulated trocar and the 5.7-mm diameter operative portal. (©Andrew H.N. Robinson.)

distraction apparatus, a camera stack, an image intensifier, and the surgical and anesthetic staff. A well-organized layout is necessary. The image intensifier is positioned horizontally, with the surgeon positioned cephalad to it.

Hip Distraction

Dorfman and Boyer [5] noted that the hip is divided into two regions. The peripheral region consists of synovium, femoral neck, peripheral femoral head, and labrum. This can be visualized without traction. The articular surfaces require traction for proper viewing. The latter are most commonly of interest; consequently, distraction systems have been developed. These must be atraumatic and distract the hip in a controlled way without the use of excessive force.

Eriksson *et al.* [6] showed that the force required to distract the hip joint 10 mm could be reduced from 900 N to 300 to 500 N with anesthetic muscular relaxation. The hip joint is further held in the close-packed position by the surface tension of the synovial fluid. When attempting to distract the hip, a vacuum is created in this fluid. By inserting a needle and allowing air into the joint, the pressures are equalized, allowing the joint to open. This release of the vacuum halves the force required to distract the hip.

There are two methods for distracting the hip joint. A standard orthopedic traction table can be used. This position is preferred by Byrd [7], who described good access and visualization in 20 hips using this technique. The patient is positioned supine with the foot in a boot. The hip is extended and abducted 25°. An oversized perineal bollard is inserted. The bollard applies lateral force to the proximal femur, which together with simultaneous longitudinal traction, causes a resultant pull aligned along the femoral neck. In the later cases, a force transducer was incorporated into the footplate. The supine position uses equipment that is available in most surgical departments. It allows easier access to the anterior portal, and in the obese patient the adipose tissue falls away posteriorly, according to Byrd.

Alternatively, a specialized hip distracter, such as the Arthronix hip distracter (Arthronix Co, New City, NY), can be used. With this, the patient is positioned in the lateral decubitus position. This distracter also has a perineal bollard to provide pull along the femoral neck. There is a force transducer.

The authors use the lateral position with a specialized distracter (Fig. 15-3). This provides reproducible distraction, which is easily achieved because greater lateralizing forces can be used with the perineal bollard in this position. Using 25 kg of distraction can distract the joint by 1.5 to 3.0 cm in the absence of muscle relaxation, therefore, muscle relaxation is not routinely used.

The patient is positioned in the lateral position, with the head as near to the top of the table as possible. The foot is firmly secured into the traction boot. The perineal bar is then positioned between the legs as close to the perineum as possible. The traction boot is engaged in the traction frame. The frame is then padded, and the leg is strapped to it. The leg should be abducted about 30° to relax the superolateral capsule and ease distraction. The perineal bollard is only now attached to the table. It is then lifted until the patient is almost, but not fully, lifted off the operating table. This lateralizes the distraction force.

The image intensifier is positioned to take an oblique anteroposterior view. The radiography source is positioned on the same side as the surgeon, and this end of the C-arm is positioned slightly toward the caudal end of the table to provide a slightly oblique anteroposterior view. The arm is tilted toward the feet. These two maneuvers increase the standing room available to the surgeon.

An image of the hip is obtained. The image should ideally be positioned at the top of the screen so that as the hip is distracted, it stays within the radiologic field. This prevents repositioning during the procedure.

At this stage, a trial distraction is performed. The aim is to establish that the hip is distractible. The force required is usually about 25 kg, but forces up to 50 kg may be needed. This distraction is performed under intensification. The surgeon wishes to see the joint space open; often a radiolucent crescent is seen in the joint space as the joint surfaces separate. Full distraction requires the vacuum to be released. After distractibility has been established, the traction is released, and the patient is prepared and draped. This minimizes traction time and is called a "trial of distraction."

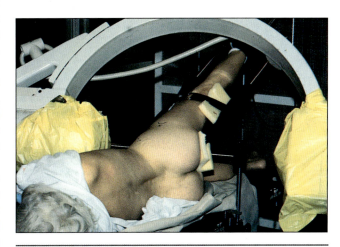

Figure 15-3. The patient in the lateral position. (©Richard N. Villar.)

The skin is prepared across to the symphysis pubis. A sterile, adhesive isolation drape designed for use with the dynamic hip screw (Steridrape 1017; 3M Healthcare, St. Paul, MN) provides a convenient draping system. Square draping is quite acceptable.

Portals

The lateral, anterior, and posterior portals are described here. In the authors' practice, the lateral is the diagnostic and operative workhorse. Hasan and Al-Sabiti [8] described a medial portal, which is presumably based on the medial "Ludloff" approach to the hip.

Types of Portals

Lateral Portal

The lateral portal is positioned approximately 2 cm above the greater trochanter. It is often necessary to use several separate lateral portals to insert instruments, irrigation needles, and the arthroscope into the joint. An area from the posterior border of the greater trochanter forward to the anterior portal can be used.

A portal is established by inserting a 22-gauge spinal needle into the joint under image intensifier control. When the joint is entered, the stylette is removed. Air can then enter the joint, and an air arthrogram can be performed to confirm position within the joint. With pressure equalization and release of the vacuum, the joint opens. The joint is distended with 10 to 30 mL of 0.9% saline solution.

The spinal needle is removed, and a 15-gauge needle is inserted (Fig. 15-4). The image intensifier is used to confirm position. A second 15-gauge needle is inserted into the joint anterior to the first needle (Fig. 15-5A). This functions as the irrigation fluid inflow, and the arthroscope sheath functions as the outflow. Free fluid flow between the needles establishes that both are in the joint.

A Nitinol guidewire (Smith & Nephew Endoscopy) is inserted into the joint through the first needle. This wire ideally passes freely to the cotyloid fossa, without touching the dome of the femoral head. This allows passage of larger instruments into the joint without scuffing the articular cartilage.

A 1-cm incision is made in the skin using a #11 scalpel blade around the guidewire. The arthroscope sheath, with a sharp, cannulated obturator, is next passed over the guidewire and into the joint. The sharp obturator is only used until it is felt to penetrate the joint capsule; this is done by feel under image intensifier control. The sharp obturator is exchanged for a blunt, cannulated obturator, and the sheath is advanced toward the cotyloid fossa (Fig. 15-5B), when both wire and obturator are removed. A standard length, 4.5-mm, 70° arthroscope can then be inserted down the sheath into the joint.

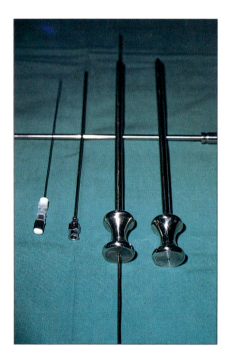

Figure 15-4. The needles and trocars inserted into the joint, in sequence from *left* to *right*. The Nitinol guidewire (Smith & Nephew Endoscopy, Oklahoma City, OK) is shown within the cannulated, sharp trocar. (©Andrew H.N. Robinson.)

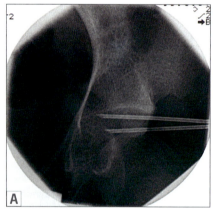 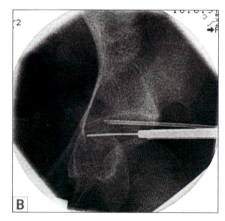

Figure 15-5. Image intensifier films. **A,** Two 15-gauge needles passing into the distracted joint. The dome of the femoral head is avoided, and the needles ideally pass into the cotyloid fossa. **B,** The trocar and blunt obturator being passed over the Nitinol guidewire (Smith & Nephew Endoscopy, Oklahoma City, OK) into the joint. (©Andrew H.N. Robinson.)

Anterior Portal

This portal is easiest to set up with the patient positioned supine on a standard traction table. The hip is abducted 25°. Image intensification and a trial of traction are performed, as previously described.

The anterior portal is situated at the intersection of a vertical line dropped down from the anterior superior iliac spine and a horizontal line across from the tip of the greater trochanter. The femoral artery should always be palpated and marked before the start of surgery.

The technique for opening the portal is the same as that already given. This portal provides good access to the inferior recess of the hip joint, in particular for loose body removal. Access to the posterior joint is poor.

Posterior Portal

The posterior portal has been described by Goldman *et al.* [9]. They described an open technique because of the obvious danger to the sciatic nerve. An open posterior approach to the hip is used, including division of the short rotators. The arthroscope is then inserted under direct visualization through the capsule into the joint. Goldman used this approach for the removal of a bullet embedded in the posterior part of the femoral head.

Establishing Portals

When establishing an operative portal, a 15-gauge needle is inserted into the joint. It is preferable to do this under arthroscopic visualization, because placing the needle close to the site of the pathology makes the procedure much easier. After the portal has been established, little opportunity exists to maneuver the instruments. The 5.7-mm diameter portal (*see* Fig. 15-1) is inserted over the guidewire using a large, sharp-tipped, cannulated trocar. When the tip of the sharp trocar is seen to enter the joint, the blunt obturator is substituted.

After the cannula has been inserted, the arthroscopic hook and other instruments can be inserted through it. The portal can be cut off short at this stage; this is necessary if the instruments are too short, and it allows a greater arc of movement of the instrument within the joint.

Additional Tips

As with any arthroscopic technique, hip arthroscopy is best performed by those with knowledge of the problems and the methods for avoiding them. The major problems of diagnostic arthroscopy can be overcome by using a tried and tested set-up that works. There are a few extra tricks required to perform surgery:

1. The use of a fluid management system is helpful to control bleeding, which cannot be controlled by using a tourniquet, as can be done in knee surgery.
2. For debridement, the use of powered instruments, as outlined previously, is helpful. If curved instruments are available, they can help with access. However, there is no substitute for initial accurate localization of the portal.
3. Loose bodies are best washed or sucked out of the joint. The smaller ones can be removed by positioning the arthroscope close to them, turning off the irrigation, and then removing the arthroscope, allowing the debris to flow out through the sheath. The larger ones are best removed through a wide bore (8- to 10-mm) cannula with either fluid flow or suction. The last resort is to push them below the transverse ligament so they become entrapped in the inferior recess of the hip.
4. The final "trick" is to know that everything cannot be achieved in every hip all the time. Sometimes, an open procedure is preferable to difficult arthroscopy that causes excessive articular and periarticular damage.

ANATOMY OF THE HIP JOINT

The cadaveric extra-articular anatomy of the hip joint is well described in standard anatomic texts. Byrd *et al.* [10••] performed cadaver studies on portal placement. They found that there was a safe zone over the top of the whole breadth of the greater trochanter. The anterior portal does place at risk branches of the lateral cutaneous nerve of the thigh; however, at this level the nerve has divided into three branches. The *in vivo*, intra-articular anatomy was described by Keene and Villar [11••].

Femoral Head

Dvorak *et al.* [12] found that by using fluid distention of the joint alone, 80% of the femoral head could be seen using lateral and anterior portals. The fovea and inferior part of the femoral head are best visualized from the anterior approach, although they can also be seen from the lateral approach when distraction is good.

Acetabulum and Ligamentum Teres

Approximately 90% of the acetabulum can be visualized from the lateral portal. The superolateral rim is difficult to visualize from this portal because of its proximity to the site of the arthroscope's entry through the capsule. Just above and anterior to the cotyloid fossa, there is often an area of thin, rough hyaline cartilage that may be confused with early degenerative change (Fig. 15-6A). This normal finding is known as the *stellate crease*. The crease may be the remnants of the point of fusion of the triradiate cartilage, with the iliopubic groove representing a failure of fusion [13]. A stellate crease may also be seen posteriorly.

The cotyloid fossa is lined with dense fibrous tissue. In the lower two thirds it is covered by adipose tissue (Fig. 15-6B). Toward the end of an arthroscopy procedure, this area can become inflamed and appear as if synovitis is present. This synovitis is surgically induced and is a normal finding. The transverse ligament can be seen inferiorly. Below this ligament is the inferior recess, a common hiding place for loose bodies. It is sometimes necessary to use the anterior portal to better visualize this area. The ligamentum teres arises from the posteroinferior portion of the acetabular fossa, and inserts into the femoral head (Fig. 15-6C).

Acetabular Labrum and Zona Orbicularis

In the majority of cases, the labrum is well visualized; it is thinner anteroinferiorly than posterosuperiorly. The labrum overlies the hyaline cartilage of the acetabulum, except for an area at the margin of the acetabulum, where it is separated by a distinct "labral groove" (Fig. 15-6D). The synovium abuts against the labrum to form the perilabral sulcus. That part of the labrum close to the entry portal may not be visualized; in this case, a second portal is needed. On the other hand, the labrum may not be visualized if it is everted.

The zona orbicularis is an hourglass-shaped condensation of the hip capsule. It is sometimes seen indenting the hip synovium and can be mistaken for the labrum.

INDICATIONS AND RESULTS OF HIP ARTHROSCOPY

From a technique that was "manifestly impossible" in 1931 [1], hip arthroscopy has developed into a widely used technique. By the late 1980s, the technique was recognized as a procedure restricted to use by a few experts [14,15]. The restriction was caused by the technical requirements of the surgery. The technique is now well established, and many of the limitations have been resolved. However, the indications are widely questioned. The frequency of indications for hip arthroscopy in the senior author's practice is shown in Table 15-1. These indications can be divided into two categories, diagnostic and operative.

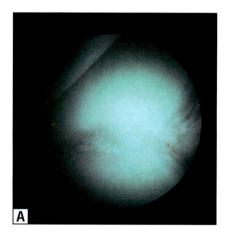
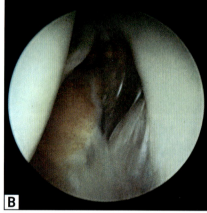
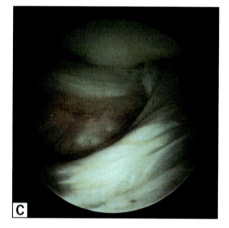
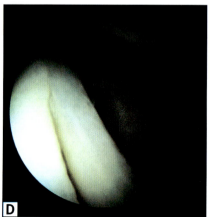

Figure 15-6. A, Left acetabulum, looking anteriorly. Note the pronounced stellate crease. **B,** The cotyloid fossa of the left hip, looking inferiorly. The femoral head is to the *left*. The fossa is lined with dense connective tissue. **C,** The banded appearance of the ligamentum teres is shown. It passes from the cotyloid fossa to insert into the femoral head. **D,** The acetabular labrum overlies the articular cartilage at the acetabular perimeter. The labral groove is clearly shown. The perilabral sulcus is lined with synovium and extends around the labral margin. (©Richard N. Villar.)

Diagnostic Indications

Glick [16] has shown that in 40% of hips that defied diagnosis by clinical or other radiographic means, hip arthroscopy could provide an answer. In the authors' current practice, pathology is seen in 80% of patients with hip pain of unknown cause. This does not mean that the viewed pathology is always the cause of symptoms.

Edwards *et al.* [17•] compared magnetic resonance imaging (MRI) of the hip with arthroscopy in 23 patients with no radiologic evidence of osteoarthritis. Labral tears, osteochondral loose bodies, and chondral defects smaller than 1 cm in diameter were more reliably seen by hip arthroscopy than by MRI. However, with the advent of MR arthrography, radiologic accuracy may be improved [18].

With increasing interest being shown in osteotomies around the hip for the treatment of degenerative disease, the arthroscope provides an attractive way of preoperatively assessing the joint surface.

Operative Indications

Osteoarthritis

The hip arthroscope can be used to remove osteochondral flaps and impinging osteophytes in the degenerate hip. The arthroscope is also a convenient way to wash out the joint (Fig. 15-7*A*).

Arthroscopic debridement of osteoarthritis has unpredictable results. However, up to 60% of unselected patients report symptomatic relief 6 months after arthroscopic debridement [19]. Selection of those

Table 15-1	Indications for Hip Arthroscopy

Indication	Patients, %
Undiagnosed hip pain	35
Osteoarthritis	30
Labral pathology	10
Loose bodies	10
Osteochondral defects	5
Sepsis	
Ligamentum teres	10
Trauma	
Synovitis	

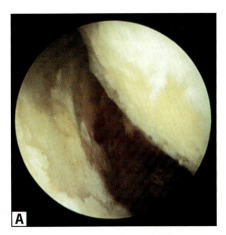
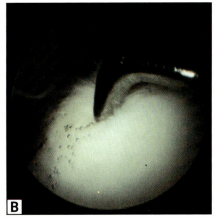
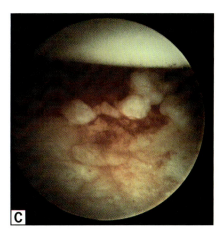
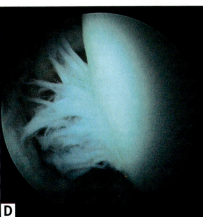

Figure 15-7. A, Gross osteoarthritic destruction of the hip. **B,** A probe demonstrating softening of the femoral head cartilage in chondromalacia coxae. **C,** Multiple loose bodies of synovial osteochondromatosis. **D,** A ligamentum teres tear on the femoral head. This was debrided with power instruments. (©Richard N. Villar.)

patients who are less than 50 years of age with a good range of motion can improve the percentage of patients symptomatically improved to 70% at 2 years.

Articular Cartilage

Osteochondritis dissecans of the hip joint is not widely reported. When present, it usually affects the superior portion of the femoral head. The defect is amenable to debridement, and there is sometimes a loose body that can be removed.

Chondromalacia coxae (Fig. 15-7B), with softening of the femoral head cartilage, has been reported [20]. Hip arthroscopy has led to symptomatic improvement patients without associated dysplasia.

The arthroscope certainly has a role to play in the assessment of osteochondral defects of the hip. The defects can be debrided and drilled arthroscopically, and there is the potential for osteochondral allografting or chondrocyte transplantation in the future.

Removal of Loose Bodies

Loose bodies in the hip have numerous causative pathologies. They can be single or multiple from Perthes' disease, previous trauma, osteochondritis dissecans, or synovial osteochondromatosis.

In synovial osteochondromatosis, multiple loose bodies are present (Fig. 15-7C) that can be removed arthroscopically [21], improving hip function [22]. Keene and Villar [23] reported the removal of intra-articular bony fragments after traumatic hip dislocation. After dislocation, distraction of the hip is easy; however, great care must be taken to minimize the risk of vascular damage to the hip during distraction.

Foreign bodies can also be removed from the normal or prosthetic hip. Goldman et al. [9] used a semi-open technique to remove a bullet from the posterior aspect of the femoral head. In hip arthroplasty, Vakili et al. [3] described cement and trochanteric wires entrapped between the femoral and acetabular components of a total hip arthroplasty. They were unable to remove the debris but managed to displace them from between the bearing surfaces to an area considered safe. Nordt et al. [24] were able to arthroscopically remove both cement and wire from joint replacements.

Ligamentum Teres Rupture

Gray and Villar [25] have recently reported on 20 patients who had a rupture of the ligamentum teres (Figure 15-7D). These patients were identified in 472 consecutive hip arthroscopies. The patients presented with either groin pain, thigh pain, or clicking of the hip. The ruptures are divided into types 1, 2, and 3. Type 1 is a complete rupture after surgery or trauma, type 2 is a partial rupture, and type 3 involves a degenerate ligamentum associated with an osteoarthritic joint. The significance of these pathologies remains unclear at present.

Acetabular Labrum Tears

Acetabular labral tears are a cause of hip pain and clicking. Resection of the tear is associated with relief or cure of symptoms in 89% of affected patients [26]. The tears can be visualized and treated arthroscopically [27•]. The tears can be located anywhere on the labrum, although they are most commonly located anteriorly (62%). The tears can either be classified by etiology into degenerative (49%), traumatic (19%), congenital (5%), and idiopathic (27%), or by configuration into radial flap (57%), radial fibrillated (22%), longitudinal peripheral (16%), and unstable (5%).

Lage et al. [27•] identified two teenage girls with generalized joint laxity who had instability of the labrum, which resulted in subluxation during internal and external rotation performed at the time of arthroscopy. They initially presented with "clicky hips."

Synovitis

Synovectomy for both synovitis [28] and for the treatment of pigmented villonodular synovitis [29] has been described. The results are uncertain, but it has been suggested that the arthroscope may make it possible to make a diagnosis earlier; therefore, arthroscopic synovectomy may be more effective.

Frich et al. [30] reported an intra-articular plica bridging the space between the femoral head and the roof of the acetabulum in two patients. They resected this arthroscopically.

Avascular Necrosis of the Hip

Ide et al. [31] have suggested that arthroscopy of the hip is indicated in the presence of avascular necrosis (AVN). The senior author has personal experience of two patients with AVN whose femoral heads collapsed within 3 months of having arthroscopic surgery. AVN is therefore regarded as a relative contraindication to hip arthroscopy, although it is unclear if it is the arthroscopy itself, traction, or the natural history of the disease that is the problem. Glick [32] also suggested that arthroscopy of the hip in the presence of AVN could add insult to injury.

Hip Sepsis

Numerous reports of septic arthritis of the hip being treated by arthroscopic washout have been published. Chung et al. [33] reported nine cases of septic arthritis in children between 2 and 7 years old who were treated with arthroscopic lavage. He used manual traction and reported good results. No recurrences were reported, and all had a good outcome. Blitzer [34] has reported similarly good results in adults. Bould *et al.* [35] reported arthroscopic clearance of the infective focus as late as 2 months from the onset of symptoms, although considerable damage to the hip joint was present after such a long-delayed diagnosis.

The Immature Hip

In 1977, Gross [2] reported arthroscopy of the child's hip in untreated hip dysplasia. More recently, Hasan and Al-Sabiti [8] have described the arthroscopic findings in children between 1 and 2 years of age with untreated congenital dislocation of the hip. They used a medial portal, just below the adductor origin, to insert the arthroscope. They did not attempt to debride the structures blocking reduction, but this is a potential area of development.

Gross [2] has reported 32 hip arthroscopies in children with a variety of conditions. He concluded that arthroscopy did not improve diagnosis or treatment. Schindler *et al.* [36], on the other hand, found that of 24 arthroscopies performed in adolescents with a mean age of 16 years, eight were diagnostic, and 16 were therapeutic. The diagnosis was altered in 11 patients. The diagnoses were of osteochondral defects; chondromalacia; and synovitis, which was biopsied. The therapeutic procedures performed included shaving of chondromalacia and the removal of loose bodies in Legg-Calvé-Perthes disease. The latter of these procedures was found to be the most worthwhile. Of the patients undergoing therapeutic arthroscopies, nine of 16 improved.

Futami *et al.* [37] reported the results of arthroscopic surgery on five patients with slipped capital femoral epiphyses. All of the patients had synovitis, four had anterosuperior acetabular erosion, and three had posterolateral labral damage. Symptoms improved postoperatively, and there were no complications recorded.

Suzuki *et al.* [38] reported pain relief in Legg-Calvé-Perthes disease from arthroscopic lavage of the hip in those patients who were not willing to rely solely on bed rest for relief. The joint was noted to have reactive synovial proliferation.

COMPLICATIONS

Little definitive data exists on the incidence of complications of hip arthroscopy. Glick [32] reported eight transient nerve palsies and one instance of instrument breakage in a series of 60 patients arthroscoped during a 4-year period. Several patients also had articular cartilage scuffing during the procedure. Thus, with a complication rate of more than 20%, hip arthroscopy is more prone to problems than is knee arthroscopy, in which the rate is lower than 2%. However, as

Funke and Munzinger [39••] reported, complications occur early in the learning curve, and with care and experience the incidence can be reduced.

In addition to Glick's report of four pudendal nerve and four sciatic nerve injuries, Villar [19] has reported a femoral nerve palsy that recovered after 6 hours. Eriksson *et al.* [6] reported dysesthesia from damage to the lateral cutaneous nerve of the thigh from the anterior portal.

Neurapraxias and other soft-tissue injury can also be caused by traction or extravasation of fluid. Funke and Munzinger [39••] reported a case of abdominal pain from retroperitoneal leakage of fluid in a patient under regional anesthesia. The procedure had to be abandoned. Consequently, they no longer use regional anesthesia.

Perineal tears and hematomata can be caused by the perineal bar, both in the supine and lateral positions. This is a particular problem in the posterior commissure of females. There are no reports of sepsis secondary to hip arthroscopy.

Avoidance of Complications

To reduce the complication rate, Villar [40] recommends that careful attention should be paid to patient positioning and padding, and care must be taken with the perineal bar. Excessive flexion or extension of the hip should be avoided. This can stretch the sciatic and femoral nerves, respectively.

Brumback *et al.* [41] showed that traction forces greater than 50 kg are only safe if applied for a short time during femoral nailing. The development of pudendal nerve palsy correlated with the magnitude of the traction force more closely than with traction time. However, the authors keep both traction force and time to an absolute minimum.

Surgeons should preoperatively exclude patients in whom access would be unacceptably traumatic, that is, those with widespread osteophytosis, protrusio acetabuli, and repeated previous surgery. Presentation of a poor range of motion at the preoperative examination implies that access may be difficult.

Lastly, the technique for establishing portals must be well established. The guidewire technique minimizes the trauma of portal creation. The senior author uses the lateral portal routinely; only on rare occasions is the anterior used. Care must be taken to avoid fluid extravasation and cartilage scuffing.

FUTURE DEVELOPMENTS

Hip arthroscopy will undoubtedly change in the future. Indications will alter. In the management of developmental hip dysplasia, it may be possible to debride the soft tissues and reduce the previously irreducible hip. In the dysplastic hip, the arthroscope is already a valuable tool for assessing the hip and determining the best orientation of the osteotomy; in the future, arthroscopy may even be used for intraoperative control of the osteotomy.

Chondrocyte grafting of osteochondral defects in the knee is already performed. Due to the location of the hip joint, open grafting is less attractive; however, arthroscopic techniques could make grafting the hip an attractive proposition.

CONCLUSION

Hip arthroscopy remains technically demanding; however, with training and the availability of the correct equipment, large hip units should have at least one surgeon performing the procedure.

Although hip arthroscopy is unlikely to be as frequently indicated as is knee arthroscopy, it has an important contribution to make both as a diagnostic and an operative tool in the hip surgeon's repertoire. It has already contributed to better understanding of the acetabular labrum and ligamentum teres and the management of the associated pathology. It has unquestionable merit in the treatment of many hip diseases, such as osteoarthritis in the young patient and septic arthritis. With selective usage, it will be an invaluable technique for assessing hips thought suitable for osteotomy, and potentially for guiding chondral repair therapies in the future.

REFERENCES AND RECOMMENDED READING

Recently published papers of particular interest have been highlighted as:
- • Of interest
- •• Of outstanding interest

1. Burman MS: Arthroscopy or the direct visualisation of joints: an experimental cadaver study. *J Bone Joint Surg Br* 1931, 13:669–695.

2. Gross RH: Arthroscopy in hip disorders in children. *Orthop Rev* 1977, 6:43–49.

3. Vakili F, Salvati EA, Warren RF: Entrapped foreign body within the acetabular cup in total hip replacement. *Clin Orthop Rel Res* 1980, 150:159–162.

4. Holgersson S, Brattstrom H, Mogensen B, *et al.*: Arthroscopy of the hip in juvenile chronic arthritis. *J Paediatr Orthop* 1981, 1:273–278.

5. Dorfman H, Boyer T: Letter to the editor. *Arthroscopy* 1996, 12:264–266.

6. Eriksson E, Arvidsson I, Arvidsson H: Diagnostic and operative arthroscopy of the hip. *Orthopedics* 1986, 9:169–176.

7. Byrd JWT: Hip arthroscopy utilizing the supine position. *Arthroscopy* 1994, 10:275–280.

8. Hasan ARH, Al-Sabiti A: Arthroscopy of the hip in congenital dislocation [abstract]. *J Bone Joint Surg Br* 1995, 77(*Orthop Proc* suppl I):3.

9. Goldman A, Minkoff J, Price A, *et al.*: A posterior arthroscopic approach to bullet extraction from the hip. *J Trauma* 1987, 27:1294–1300.

10.•• Byrd JW, Pappas JN, Pedley MJ: Hip arthroscopy: an anatomic study of portal placement and relationship to the extra-articular structures. *Arthroscopy* 1995, 11:418–423.
Classic text describing the anatomy of portal placement and the structures placed at risk by use of such portals.

11.•• Keene GS, Villar RN: Arthroscopic anatomy of the hip: an in vivo study. *Arthroscopy* 1994, 10:392–399.
A description of the intra-articular anatomy of the hip joint seen at arthroscopy.

12. Dvorak M, Duncan CP, Day B: Arthroscopic anatomy of the hip. *Arthroscopy* 1990, 6:264–273.

13. Santori N, Villar RN: The iliopubic groove: failure of triradiate fusion. *J Anatomy*, in press.

14. Glick JM, Sampson TG, Gordon RB, *et al.*: Hip arthroscopy by the lateral approach. *Arthroscopy* 1987, 3:4–12.

15. Dorfmann H, Boyer Th, Henry P, *et al.*: A simple approach to hip arthroscopy [abstract]. *Arthroscopy* 1988, 4:141–142.

16. Glick JM: Hip arthroscopy. In *Operative Arthroscopy.* Edited by McGinty JB. New York: Raven; 1991:663–676.

17.• Edwards DJ, Lomas D, Villar RN: Diagnosis of the painful hip by magnetic resonance imaging and arthroscopy. *J Bone Joint Surg Br* 1995, 77:374–376.
A comparative study of the abnormalities seen during arthroscopic procedures, compared with those seen with use of magnetic resonance imaging.

18. Leunig M, Werlen S, Ungersböck A, *et al.*: Evaluation of the acetabular labrum by MR arthrography. *J Bone Joint Surg Br* 1997, 79:230–234.

19. Villar RN: Arthroscopic debridement of the hip. *J Bone Joint Surg Br* 1991, 73(*Orthop Proc* suppl II):170–171.

20. Norman-Taylor FH, Mannion SJ, Villar RN: Chondromalacia coxae. *Hip International* 1995, 5:121–123.

21. Witwity T, Uhlmann RD, Fischer J: Arthroscopic management of chondromatosis of the hip joint. *Arthroscopy* 1988, 4:55–56.

22. Bull TM, Selzer G, Villar RN: Arthroscopic management of synovial chondromatosis of the hip. *Knee Surg, Sports Traumatol, Arthroscopy*, in press.

23. Keene G, Villar RN: Arthroscopic loose body retrieval following traumatic hip dislocation. *Injury* 1994, 25:507–510.

24. Nordt W, Giangarra CE, Levy IM, *et al.*: Arthroscopic removal of entrapped debris following dislocation of a total hip arthroplasty. *Arthroscopy* 1987, 3:196–198.

25. Gray AJR, Villar RN: Rupture of the ligamentum teres of the hip: an arthroscopic classification. *J Bone Surg Br (Orthop Proc* suppl I) 1997, 79:96.

26. Fitzgerald RH: Acetabular labrum tears: diagnosis and treatment. *Clin Orth Rel Res* 1995, 311:60–68.

27.• Lage LA, Patel JV, Villar RN: The acetabular labral tear: an arthroscopic classification. *Arthroscopy* 1996, 12:269–272.

A description of the etiology and morphology of labral tears seen during arthroscopic procedures.

28. Gondolph-Zink B, Puhl W, Noack W: Semiarthroscopic synovectomy of the hip. *Int Orthop* 1988, 12:31–35.

29. Janssens X, Van Meirhaeghe J, Verdonk R, *et al.*: Diagnostic arthroscopy of the hip joint in pigmented villonodular synovitis. *Arthroscopy* 1987, 3:283–287.

30. Frich LH, Lauritzen J, Juhl M: Arthroscopy in the diagnosis and treatment of hip disorders. *Orthopaedics* 1989, 12:389–392.

31. Ide T, Akamasu N, Nakajima I: Arthroscopic surgery of the hip joint. *Arthroscopy* 1991, 7:204–211.

32. Glick JM: Complications of hip arthroscopy by the lateral approach. In *Current Management of Complications in Orthopedics. Arthroscopic Surgery.* Edited by Sherman OH, Minkoff J. Baltimore: Williams & Wilkins; 1990:193–201.

33. Chung WK, Slater GL, Bates EH: Treatment of septic arthritis of the hip by arthroscopic lavage. *J Pediatr Orthop* 1993, 13:444–446.

34. Blitzer CM: Arthroscopic management of septic arthritis of the hip. *Arthroscopy* 1993, 9:414–416.

35. Bould M, Edwards D, Villar RN: Arthroscopic diagnosis of septic arthritis of the hip joint. *Arthroscopy* 1993, 9:707–708.

36. Schindler A, Lechevalier JJC, Rao NS, *et al.*: Diagnostic and therapeutic arthroscopy of the hip in children and adolescents: evaluation of the results. *J Pediatr Orthop* 1995, 15:317–321.

37. Futami T, Kasahara Y, Suzuki S, *et al.*: Arthroscopy for slipped capital femoral epiphysis. *J Pediatr Orthop* 1992, 12:592–597.

38. Suzuki S, Kasahara Y, Seto Y, *et al.*: Arthroscopy in 19 children with Perthes' disease. *Acta Orthop Scand* 1994, 65:581–584.

39.•• Funke EL, Munzinger U: Complications in hip arthroscopy. *Arthroscopy* 1996, 12:156–159.

Review of the current literature concerning the complications of hip arthroscopy.

40. Villar RN: *Hip Arthroscopy.* Oxford: Butterworth-Heinemann; 1992.

41. Brumback R, Scott-Ellison T, Molligaan H, *et al.*: Pudendal nerve palsy complicating intramedullary nailing of the femur. *J Bone Joint Surg Am* 1992, 74:1450–1455.

16

Arthroscopy of the Posterior Subtalar Joint

J. SERGE PARISIEN

Subtalar arthroscopy was first described by Parisien and Vangsness [1] in 1985. Using six fresh lower-extremity cadaver specimens and two amputation specimens, with two different-sized arthroscopes (2.2 mm and 2.7 mm), they reported a technique for examination of the posterior subtalar joint. Since the original description, more reports dealing with the surgical aspect of the technique have followed [2–6,7••,8•,9,10].

ANATOMY

The subtalar joint is divided into anterior (talocalcaneonavicular) and posterior (talocalcaneal) articulations (Fig. 16-1). These articulations are separated by the tarsal canal and sinus tarsi. Sulci on the undersurface of the talus and superior surface of the os calcis form the tarsal canal. The lateral opening of the tarsal canal is called the *sinus tarsi*. The tarsal canal makes a 45° angle with the lateral border of the calcaneus. Within this canal, the medial root of the inferior extensor retinaculum, the cervical and talocalcaneal interosseous ligaments, fatty tissue, and blood vessels are found. According to Cahill [11], the cervical ligament plays a major role in limiting inversion. Ligamentous support of the subtalar joint has been reviewed by Harper [12]. He described this supporting ligament as consisting of superficial, intermediate, and deep layers. The superficial layer comprised the lateral talocalcaneal ligament, the posterior talocalcaneal ligament, the medial talocalcaneal ligament, the lateral root of the inferior extensor retinaculum, and the calcaneal fibular ligament. The intermediate layer is formed by the intermediate root of the inferior extensor retinaculum and the cervical ligament. The deep layer comprises the medial root of the inferior extensor retinaculum and the interosseous talocalcaneal ligament. The talocalcaneonavicular, or anterior subtalar joint, is composed of the talus, the posterior surface of the tarsal navicular, the anterior surface of the calcaneus, and the plantar calcaneonavicular, or spring ligament. The posterior part of the capsule of this anterior subtalar joint forms the anterior part of the interosseous talocalcaneal ligament. The posterior talocalcaneal, or posterior subtalar joint, is a synovium-lined articulation formed by the posterior convex calcaneal facet of the talus and the posterior concave talar facet of the calcaneus. Its long axis is placed obliquely at 40° to the midline of the foot. The articulation is directed upward with a convex orientation. The joint capsule is reinforced laterally by the lateral talocalcaneal ligament and the calcaneal-fibular ligament. This joint has a posterior capsular pouch with small lateral, medial, and anterior recesses, as well. On a more superficial level, the peroneal tendons, the sural nerve, and the small saphenous vein are located behind the lateral malleolus.

PORTALS

Two main portals are available for arthroscopy of the posterior subtalar joint: the *anterolateral* and *posterolateral* portals (Fig. 16-2). The anterolateral portal is located approximately 2 cm anterior and 1 cm distal to the tip of the lateral malleolus. The posterolateral portal is located either at the level of the tip of the lateral malleolus or 5 mm proximal to the tip. Developing it too proximally places the arthroscope into the posterior aspect of the talocrural joint. This portal is placed close to the Achilles tendon to avoid injury to the sural nerve and short saphenous vein. Two acces-

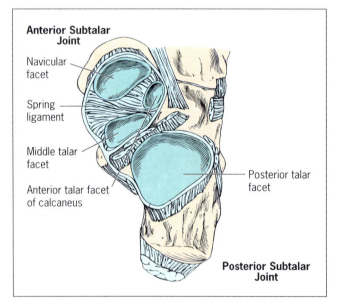

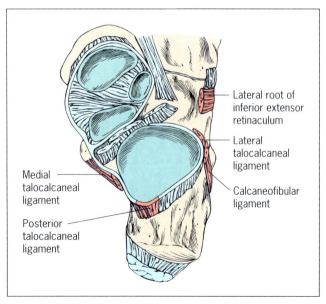

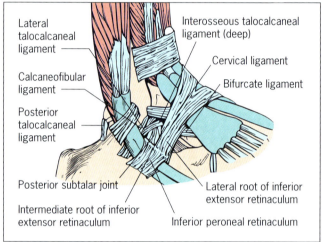

Figure 16-1. A, The subtalar joints. **B**, Lateral view of the right ankle showing the peripheral ligaments. **C**, Axial view of the ankle showing the peripheral ligaments. (*Adapted from* Ferkel [7••]; with permission.)

sory portals can also be established. The accessory anterolateral portal can be placed slightly anterior and proximal to the anterolateral portal. The accessory posterolateral portal can be placed anterior to the posterolateral portal closer to the peroneal tendons. The accessory portals are most useful for the placement of inflow cannula to keep the capsule distended. With the use of the accessory anterolateral portal, branches of the superficial peroneal nerve can be injured. With the use of the accessory posterolateral portal, the sural nerve is at risk [13•].

INSTRUMENTATION

Small short arthroscopes from 1.9 to 2.7 mm in diameter with 30° angulation are used to perform the

procedure. The standard 30°, 5-mm arthroscope can be used in some situations. A 70° arthroscope is very helpful during surgery. A small joint shaver, set with a 1.9-mm or 2.9-mm shaver blade and small abrader, are also needed (Figs. 16-3 and 16-4). Joint distention is obtained using a gravity system instead of the infusion pump. Joint distraction can be performed manually by an assistant, and a mechanical distractor is usually not necessary.

INDICATIONS FOR SUBTALAR JOINT ARTHROSCOPY

At present, many disorders of the subtalar joint can be evaluated successfully by the use of special radiographic projections, contrast arthrography, computed tomography scanning, and magnetic resonance imaging [14–20]. There are, however, some selective situations in which direct visualization is very critical in the management of the disorder.

Subtalar joint arthroscopy can be used for visual assessment of the articular surfaces when persistent pain is present in the subtalar area after a chronic ankle sprain or a fracture of the os calcis. In cases of

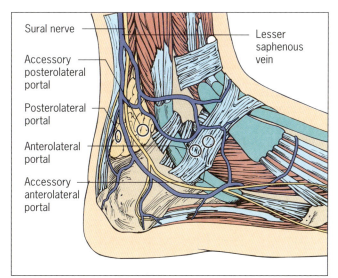

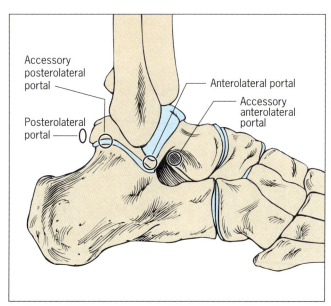

Figure 16-2. The subtalar portals with neurovascular structures (**A**) and with the soft tissues removed (**B**).

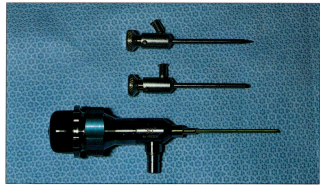

Figure 16-3. A 2.7-mm short 30° video arthroscope (*bottom*) with trocar and cannula (*top*) (Smith & Nephew Dyonics, Andover, MA).

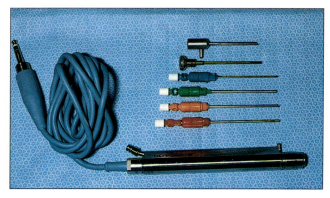

Figure 16-4. Motorized instrumentation system with various surgical blades (top) and motorized shaver (bottom) (Smith & Nephew Dyonics, Andover, MA).

degenerative or inflammatory arthritis, joint assessment can be performed, and lavage or biopsy can be done at the same time. Some surgical procedures, such as debridement of chondromalacic area, removal of loose bodies, excision of adhesions, and debridement of osteochondral lesions, can be performed. Most recent indications have included excision of painful os trigonum, management of sinus tarsi syndrome, arthrodesis of the subtalar joint, and management of the displaced intra-articular fracture of the calcaneus.

SURGICAL TECHNIQUE

The patient is placed in the lateral decubitus or supine position with a sandbag under the buttocks (Fig. 16-5). A tourniquet is applied over the thigh and can be inflated if necessary. If diagnostic arthroscopy of the subtalar joint is indicated at the time an arthroscopic procedure is performed on the ankle, the subtalar joint arthroscopy should be done first to avoid obliteration of the landmarks by fluid extravasation following ankle arthroscopy. A marking pen is used to indicate landmarks. The posterior subtalar joint is distended with an 18-gauge needle placed into the anterolateral portal. The distention is obtained with approximately 5 to 10 mL of normal saline. With the joint distended, the posterolateral portal is developed by placing another spinal needle close to the Achilles tendon at the level of the tip of the lateral malleolus. The anterior needle is removed, and a small incision is made in the area of the needle insertion. The smooth obturator is directed superiorly and posteriorly. Overhead irrigation is used with the inflow placed through the arthroscope. Initially, the posterior needle can be used for outflow. From the anterior portal, the following structures can be visualized: the synovial lining of the posterior aspect of the interosseous talo-calcaneal ligament, the anterolateral corner of the joint, the lateral gutter with the lateral capsule, the articular cartilage of the posterior facet of the talus, and the calcaneus. Moving the arthroscope more posteriorly and into the joint allows visualization of the midportion of the talus and the calcaneus and posterolateral gutter. By switching portals, the arthroscope is placed in the posterior portal and the outflow cannula anteriorly. Visualization of the lateral gutter with the capsular reflections of the lateral talocalcaneal ligament and calcaneofibular ligaments is achieved. Then visualization of the posterolateral recess, the posterior capsular pouch, and the posteromedial recess complete the diagnostic examination of the subtalar joint (Fig. 16-6).

For a diagnostic arthroscopy of the subtalar joint to minimize injury to the sural nerve, a single anterior portal can be used with a 70° arthroscope, and a spinal needle is used posteriorly for outflow. Following diagnostic exploration of the joint, the portals are closed with nylon sutures, and a compression dressing is applied over the ankle. Range of motion exercises can be started the same day, and full weight bearing is allowed as tolerated by the patient.

If surgical arthroscopy of the subtalar joint is contemplated, two portals are necessary, with an accessory anterolateral or posterolateral portal at times. The following procedures can be performed. In selected cases of degenerative joint disease of the posterior subtalar joint, the chondromalacic area can be shaved, followed by excision of osteophyte and partial synovectomy. In arthrofibrosis, a small obturator can be used first to break the adhesions, followed by their excision with a motorized shaver (Fig. 16-7). Excision of loose bodies (Fig. 16-8) preferably should be performed from an anterior portal. However, if the fragment must be removed from the

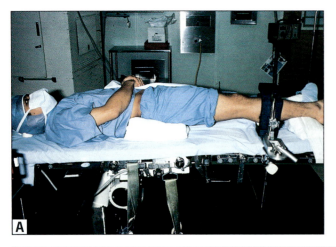
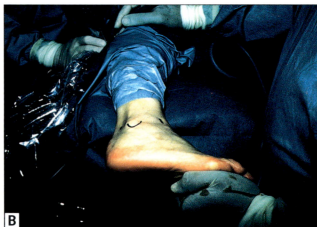

Figure 16-5. A, Patient positioning for ankle and subtalar joint arthroscopy. **B,** Ankle joint after preparation and draping.

posterolateral portal, a vertical incision in the skin should be made, followed by the use of a small hemostat to spread the wound down to the capsule to avoid neurovascular injury.

In patients with sinus tarsi syndrome, debridement of the interosseous ligament and fibro-fatty tissue in the lateral aspect of the sinus can be performed under arthroscopic visualization

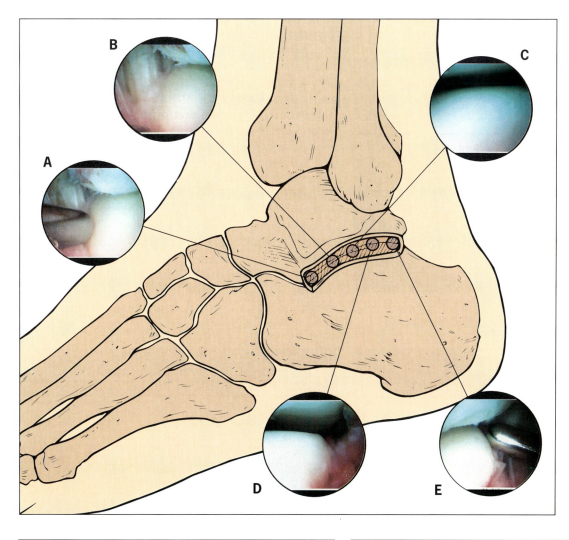

Figure 16-6. Arthroscopic visualization of various areas of the posterior subtalar joint in a patient with subtalar instability. Shown are the interosseous ligament area (**A**), anterior aspect of the joint (**B**), midaspect (**C**), posterior aspect (**D**), and posterior pouch of the subtalar joint (**E**). (*Adaped from* Parisien [5]; with permission.)

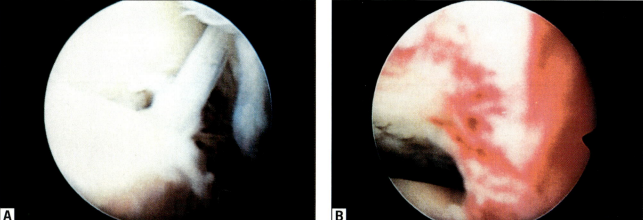

Figure 16-7. Arthrofibrosis of the posterior subtalar joint. **A**, Band of adhesion at the lateral aspect of the subtalar joint. **B**, Wider band of adhesion with reactive synovium.

(Fig. 16-9). In patients with chronic pain resulting from a symptomatic os trigonum, arthroscopic excision of nonunited fragment can be performed. The use of a 70° arthroscope from the anterolateral portal facilitates instrumentation through a posterolateral portal. During excision of an os trigonum, the tip of the instrument should always be visualized to avoid injury to the flexor hallucis longus and posteromedial neurovascular bundle, which are located medially. Osteochondral lesions of the talocalcaneal joint can be managed arthroscopically using two portals (Fig. 16-10). Following excision of the lesion, a small burr is used to abrade the osteochondral defect down to bleeding bone. The patient should not bear weight on the ankle and should keep it immobilized for a few days in a posterior splint to minimize swelling.

In selected cases of osteoarthritis, arthrodesis of the posterior subtalar joint can be performed arthroscopically. This is usually performed in patients with degenerative arthritis confined to the subtalar joint without deformity of the foot. After debridement of the soft tissue and resection of the articular cartilage with a curette or shaver, the subchondral bone is superficially abraded down to bleeding bone. A self-tapping 6.5-mm cannulated capsular screw is used to maintain the reduction. Tasto [9] has advocated the use of a small lamina spreader during the procedure to improve visualization and facilitate the maneuvering of surgical instruments.

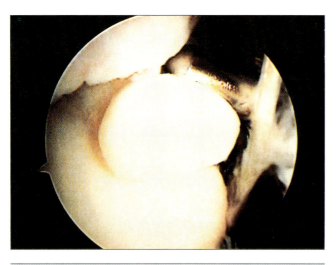

Figure 16-8. Loose body in posterior subtalar joint.

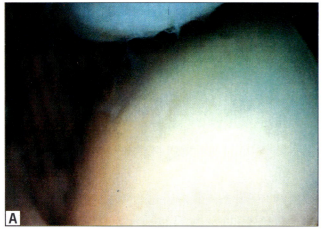

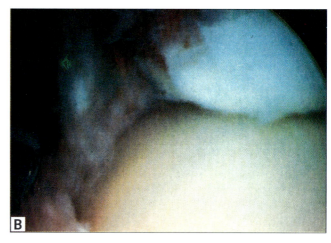

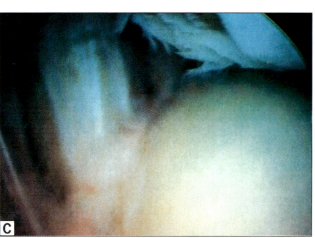

Figure 16-9. Debridement of interosseous ligament in sinus tarsi syndrome. **A**, Reactive synovium and fibro-fatty tissue in front of the interosseous ligament. **B**, Same area during debridement. **C**, Same area post-debridement.

RESULTS

Diagnostic and arthroscopic surgery of the subtalar joint have been used by Williams and Ferkel [6,7••] in 75 patients. They recently reported experience with 50 patients. A total of 21 patients had only diagnostic arthroscopy. In 29 patients, surgical procedures were performed for various pathologies, such as synovitis, degenerative joint disease, sinus tarsi syndrome, chondromalacia, symptomatic os trigonum, arthrofibrosis, loose bodies, and osteochondral lesion of the talus. The overall results were good to excellent in 86%. The author's results have been similar in a smaller group of patients. There were five cases of arthrofibrosis in post-fracture complications, seven cases of chondromalacia in posttraumatic situations, two cases of osteochondral lesions, four cases of synovitis, and one case of sinus tarsi dysfunction. In 14 patients with generalized lateral ankle pain, diagnostic subtalar arthroscopy was performed, as was an ankle arthroscopic procedure. There were no complications (infection, neurologic disturbances) in either group. Tasto [9] reported the results of arthroscopic subtalar arthrodesis in nine patients without complications. With an average follow-up of 7 months, the average time to union in his series was 10 weeks. More recently, Seo and Choi [10] reported their preliminary results of the use of subtalar arthroscopy in the management of displaced intra-articular calcaneal fractures in five patients. They reported satisfactory anatomic reduction in four patients, without major complications.

CONCLUSION

Subtalar joint arthroscopy is, at present, part of the armamentarium of the foot and ankle surgeon for the assessment and management of various disorders of the subtalar joint. Many procedures can be performed in selected situations without morbidity and complications for the patient, if careful attention is paid to the anatomy of the area, the technical details, and proper patient selection.

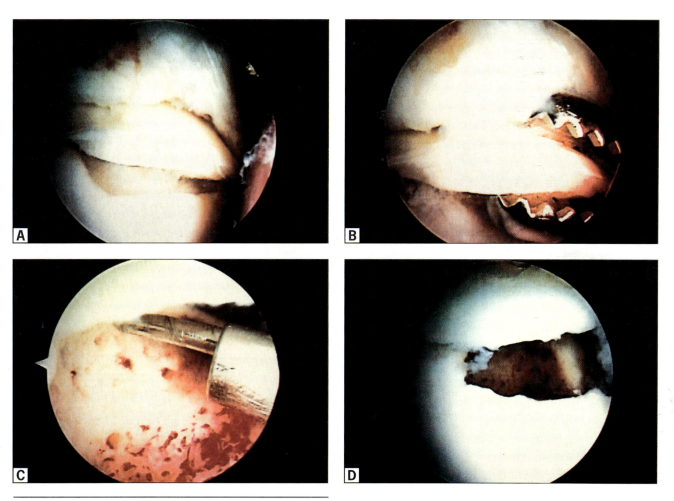

Figure 16-10. Osteochondral lesion of the posterior subtalar joint, calcanear area. Various steps of excision and drilling. **A,** Loose osteochondral fragment in the posterior subtalar joint. **B,** Grasping forceps excising the fragment. **C,** Crater following excision. **D,** Drilling of the crater.

REFERENCES AND RECOMMENDED READING

Recently published papers of particular interest have been highlighted as:

• Of interest

•• Of outstanding interest

1. Parisien JS, Vangsness T: Arthroscopy of the subtalar joint: an experimental approach. *Arthroscopy* 1985, 1:53.

2. Parisien JS: Arthroscopy of the subtalar joint. In *Foot and Ankle Arthroscopy*, edn. 2. Edited by Guhl J. Thorofare, NJ: Slack; 1993:171–176.

3. Parisien JS: Arthroscopy of the ankle and posterior subtalar joints. In *Disorders of the Foot and Ankle*. Edited by Jahss MH. Philadelphia: WB Saunders; 1991:205–235.

4. Parisien JS: Arthroscopy of the posterior subtalar joint: a preliminary report. *Foot Ankle* 1986, 6:219–224.

5. Parisien JS: Arthroscopy of the posterior subtalar joint and great toe. In *Techniques in Therapeutic Arthroscopy*. Edited by Parisien JS. New York: Raven Press; 1993:20:1–10.

6. Williams MM, Ferkel RD: Subtalar arthroscopy; indications, technique, and results. *Arthroscopy* 1994, 10:345.

7.•• Ferkel RD: Subtalar arthroscopy. In *Arthroscopic Surgery: The Foot and Ankle*. Edited by Ferkel R. Philadelphia: Lippincott-Raven Publishers; 1996:231–254.

Excellent chapter on indications and techniques of subtalar joint arthroscopy by a surgeon with vast experience.

8.• Frey C, Gasser S, Feder K: Arthroscopy of the subtalar joint. *Foot Ankle* 1994, 15:425.

Good description of various portals for subtalar joint arthroscopy.

9. Tasto JP: Subtalar arthrodesis. Presented at Arthroscopy Association of North America. Orlando, FL; February, 1995.

10. Seo SS, Choi JS: Arthroscopic management of displaced intraarticular calcaneal fractures. Proceedings of the First Biennial Congress, International Society of Arthroscopy, Knee Surgery and Orthopaedic Sports Medicine. Buenos Aires, Argentina; May 11–16, 1997: 283.

11. Cahill DR: The anatomy and function of the contents of the human tarsal sinus and canal. *Anat Rec* 1965, 153:1–18.

12. Harper MC: The lateral ligamentous support of the subtalar joint. *Foot Ankle* 1991, 12:354–358.

13.• Lawrence SJ, Botte MJ: The sural nerve in the foot and ankle: an anatomic study with clinical and surgical implications. *Foot Ankle* 1994, 15:490–494.

This paper should be read by every foot and ankle surgeon in order to avoid sural nerve injury during foot surgery.

14. Beaudet F, Dixon J: Posterior subtalar joint synoviography and corticoid injection of rheumatoid arthritis. *Ann Rheum Dis* 1981, 40:132–135.

15. Resnick D: Radiology of the talocalcaneal articulations. *Radiology* 1974, 3:581–586.

16. Tailard W, Meyer J, Garcia J, Blanc Y: The sinus tarsi syndrome. *Int Orthop* 1981, 5:117–130.

17. Isherwood I: A radiographical approach to the subtalar joint. *J Bone Joint Surg (Br)* 1961, 43:566–574.

18. Smith RW, Staple TW: Computerized tomography (CT) scanning technique of the hindfoot. *Clin Orthop* 1983, 177:34–38.

19. Beltran J, Munchow AM, Khabiri H, *et al.*: Ligament of the lateral aspect of the ankle and sinus tarsi: an MR Imaging study. *Radiology* 1990, 177:455–458.

20. Goossens M, Destoop N, Claessens H, Van Der Straeten C: Posterior subtalar joint arthrography. *Clin Orthop* 1988, 249:248–255.

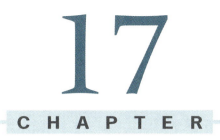

CHAPTER 17

Translaminar Epidural Endoscopic Technique

Daniel Julio De Antoni and María Laura Claro

The translaminar epidural endoscopic technique was originally developed in 1985 and was used for the first time in 1986 as a means for treating all types and sizes of herniated lumbar discs situated from L_2 to S_1 or elsewhere with minimum invasiveness and total visualization. Conventional instruments for arthroscopic surgery, as well as specific instruments adapted for triangulation, were used. The operational space was created through the smallest possible incision and through tissue irrigation.

HISTORY

In 1955, Ottolenghi [1] published a paper on his radiographically guided procedure for biopsy aspiration of the vertebral bodies and discs. In 1975, Hijikata and Yamagishi [2] developed the percutaneous nucleotomy, using a posterolateral approach to puncture the disc to extract the nucleus pulposus. In the United States, Kambin [3,4] popularized approaches to the lumbar disc through a posterolateral percutaneous procedure, under radiographic guidance. Schreiber and Suezawa [5,6] in Switzerland had earlier developed a similar technique.

ANATOMY

Normal arthroscopic anatomy must be clearly understood to allow better comprehension of pathologic conditions that are considered appropriate for this technique [7,8•].

The following anatomic parameters should be recalled: proximal and distal laminal edges, ligamentum flavum, articular capsules of the articular facet, and the intersection of the superior facet with the lamina. Moreover, beyond the ligamentum flavum and inside the vertebral canal, the epidural fat, and dural tissue, the shoulder and the axilla of the nerve root, the posterior longitudinal ligament and its lateral expansion, the intervertebral disc, the lateral recess, and the foramen must all be recognized (Fig. 17-1).

These parameters should be used as a base to understand the localization of the surgical approach. Extreme care must be taken to enter the vertebral canal in close proximity to the superior edge of the root. This point is placed in the angle created by the intersection of the proximal lamina with the articular apophysis (Fig. 17-2).

INDICATIONS

A precise diagnosis is essential in order to apply this technique. Improvisation should be avoided, and the technique should not be used as a diagnostic method because very important structures, such as the nerve roots, are at risk [7,8•]. Using noninvasive diagnostic methods such as computed tomography (CT), radiography, and magnetic resonance imaging (MRI), it is possible to isolate the cause of pain and the exact localization of the pathology.

The procedure is indicated in patients with single-level, unilateral, intraforaminal, and extradural pathology. It is also indicated in disc herniation of any size because it makes therapy possible even in patients experiencing total invasion of the vertebral canal (Fig. 17-3). In some patients, the pathology is present in more than one area. These multiple sites may be treated simultaneously by the same method, whether they are one space below, one space above, or unilateral. This method makes it possible to operate on three spaces more or less simultaneously. It could also be used for radicular compressions caused by facet hypertrophy with or without concomitant disc herniation.

CONTRAINDICATIONS

The translaminar epidural endoscopic technique is not indicated for use in other spinal pathologies, such as tumors, scoliosis, narrow canal with multiple osteophytosis, pathologies associated with segmentary stability, spondylolisthesis, degenerative spondylolisthesis, and general or localized infections, and never in patients with previous surgery. It is also relatively contraindicated or of only limited use in multilevel pathology, multiple osteophytes of the posterior vertebral body, and severe bilateral hypertrophy of articular facets of one or more segments.

PATIENT SELECTION

Patients are selected according to the basic principles of conventional surgery. The symptoms and findings on physical examination must correlate with the level to be operated on. The following should be present before endoscopic microdiscectomy is chosen: long evolution of lumbar pain, evident radiculopathy, sensory and motor deficit, reflex abnormalities, positive tension signs, positive MRI findings, and unilateral symptomatology. These patients should not have had previous surgery [7,8•].

SURGICAL PROCEDURE
Set-up

The operating room should be equipped with basic arthroscopic surgery instruments, that is, high-resolu-

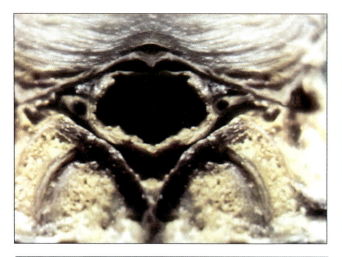

Figure 17-1. In this anatomic dissection, the relationships between the disc, annulus, posterior longitudinal ligaments (and their lateral expansion), dural sac, origin of the nerve roots, lateral recess, articular facets, and ligamentum flavum are illustrated.

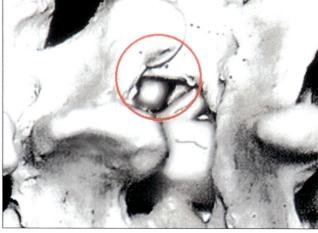

Figure 17-2. Working zone (*circled*) in the joint between the proximal lamina border and the superior articular facet, allowing access to the root and disc.

tion camera and monitor, light source, shaver, and pump irrigation system. To visualize the space and explore it until the endoscopic system is connected, it is necessary to use an image intensifier (C-arm). This is placed perpendicularly to the patient, level with the lumbar spine. The anesthesia apparatus is placed at the patient's head.

The instrumentation table should include 30° and 70° arthroscopes with wide angles, a variable-pressure pump irrigation system with a 6-mm access cannula, a shaver with a full-radius blade, an abrader, an acromionizer, and a special protective cannula.

Additional equipment needed includes a probe; a laminar dissector (to separate the muscular planes and create a virtual cavity); a dissector to open the ligamentum flavum; baskets of several sizes and different angles; and a work cannula open in its dorsal part. In cases of adherence, the root can be gently manipulated with a blunt spatula. An operative scalpel, 30 cm long with a lateral cutting edge; and the basket forceps, 23 cm long, 2, 3, and 4 mm upbiting; and two types of angulation are used to evacuate the disc material. The shaver should be used *before* opening the ligamentum flavum and then followed by kerrison rongeurs if lateral bony resection is required.

Anesthesia

General anesthesia is used because it allows greater certainty to both surgeon and patient. Peridural anesthesia is not recommended for use because of the use of an irrigation pump.

Patient Positioning

The patient, who has previously undergone general anesthesia, is positioned in the lateral decubitus posi-tion with the affected side superior and the knees flexed to keep the interlaminar space open as wide as possible. This position is achieved with a bolster placed under the down side of the patient. Also with this lateral position, intra-abdominal pressure is reduced, thereby decreasing epidural venous pressure. It allows free flow out of the saline solution and facili-tates the procedure. The surgeon and the assistant face the patient's spine, with a nurse positioned at the patient's feet.

Surgical Technique

The proper space to be operated on is localized with an image intensifier. A 2-cm long paraspinal incision is introduced approximately 1 cm laterally to the midline for instrumentation and outflow of the saline-solution irrigation. An open space on the proximal lamina is created by dissecting the muscular plane insertions until they reach the articular apophysis (Fig. 17-4). Using a portal 2 cm from the anterior approach, an arthroscope with 25° to 30° wide-angle view is introduced (Fig. 17-5). Depending on which side the hernia is located, the arthroscope is directed accordingly: from distal to proximal if the hernia is on the left, and from proximal to distal if it is on the right. Thus, we are prepared to triangulate. The arthroscope is now placed in close proximity to the articular facets. Once the irrigation pump is connected, it is imperative that the liquid flows freely through the working portal. At this point, shaving of the lamina and ligamentum flavum is performed under direct visualization.

The location of the proximal lamina's border, artic-ular facets, and ligamentum flavum must be identi-fied. The sublaminar portion of this ligament is detached. Depending on preoperative strategy, if a

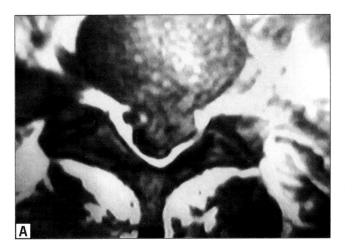
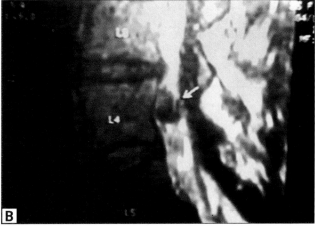

Figure 17-3. A, Disc herniation filling the larger part of the vertebral canal and compressing most of the root and dural sac. **B,** Hernia (*arrow*) that has migrated into the vertebral canal.

small lamina's border or articular facet's resection was planned, it should be undertaken *before* opening the ligamentum flavum, which serves as a shield (Fig. 17-6). The opening of this ligament in its lateral portion near the articular apophysis is made next, with a blunt dissector designed for this purpose. The endoscope is introduced through the gap to visualize the working space, fatty deposits, and epidural vessels. The lateral ligamentum flavum is resected using an appropriately sized basket, so that the opening is widened by the ventral facet of articular apophysis and the sublaminar portion of the ligamentum flavum (Fig. 17-7). Inside the canal, the following structures must be recognized, in this order: epidural fat and dural tissue, shoulder and axilla of nerve root (Fig. 17-8), posterior longitudinal ligament, intervertebral disc, lateral recess, and foramen.

After exploring these structures, the root retractor, which can function as a working cannula, is introduced (Fig. 17-9). In this manner, the shoulder of the root is free of adherences typically found as a result of the local inflammatory process. The root is retracted toward the medial line, and the herniated disc is observed. The strategy to follow next depends on the characteristics of the disc.

In cases of protruded discs, the posterior longitudinal ligament, its lateral expansion, and the annular fibers of the intervertebral disc will normally not be damaged. A scalpel with a single cutting edge is now introduced through the cannula into the most protruded area, at which point it should be directed distally and laterally (Fig. 17-10). After this maneuver is accomplished, the forceps is introduced through the cannula to extract the degenerated nucleus pulposus material.

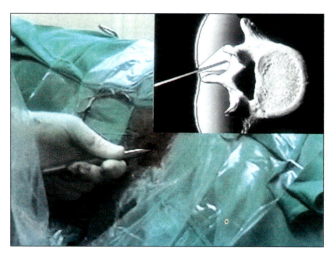

Figure 17-4. Virtual space up to the articular apophysis is created by the path of periostotome through muscular layers. A graphic illustration of the path created by the instrument is shown in the *inset*.

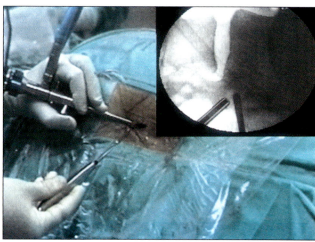

Figure 17-5. Arthroscope and periostotome in position within the working area. The radiographic view is shown in the *inset*.

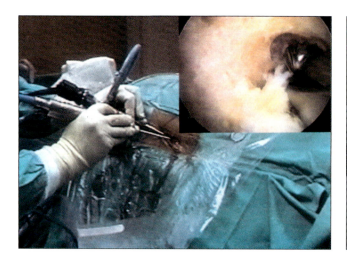

Figure 17-6. Drilling of articular facets. The arthroscopic view is shown in the *inset*.

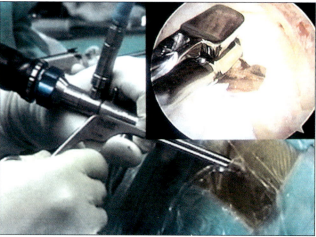

Figure 17-7. A window is made with basket for access into the vertebral canal. The arthroscopic view is shown in the *inset*.

The inside of the disc is now evaluated. When an extruded herniated disc is treated, the herniated material is usually found without retention of annular fibers, and the posterior longitudinal ligament is usually lacerated. For these reasons, to retract the nerve root and free it from adhesions, it is generally necessary to extract the material using 4-mm forceps, taking extreme care to avoid lacerations of the dural sac (Fig. 17-11).

If the patient's condition suggests pathologic migration, an exploration of the vertebral canal is made with the help of the 70° wide-angle lens. This exploration is performed using a probing hook that must remain under arthroscopic visualization in a field of almost 360°. This maneuver allows localization of migrated tissue without enlargement by further bony resection. The migrated material must be placed in the approach window before it can be extracted.

In cases of foraminal hernias, those that can be approached by the inside of the vertebral canal are appropriate for this procedure. In these cases, before opening the ligamentum flavum, the ventral facet of articular apophysis should be drilled. The lateral part of the ligamentum flavum is also resected to open a lateral breach and extract the herniated disc.

These varying mechanisms to treat herniated discs are determined by location, that is, by using the patient's description of the site of the affected segment, its peripheral manifestations, and by using the indispensable assistance of MRIs and radiographs.

During the entire procedure, an irrigation pump is set at high flow and low pressure, which creates improved visualization through the liquid medium. This procedure also makes electrocoagulation generally unnecessary. Pressure at 20 mm Hg is maintained

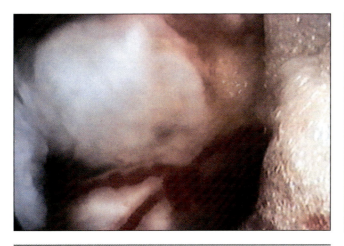

Figure 17-8. Axillary zone. The nerve root is at the *top*, and the epidural sac is at the *bottom*. Through the axilla, an extruded hernia can be seen.

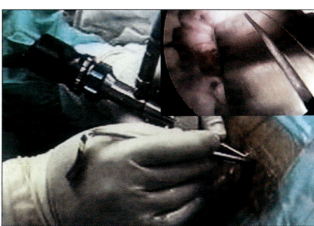

Figure 17-9. The working cannula is inserted to retract the nerve root. The arthroscopic view is shown in the *inset*.

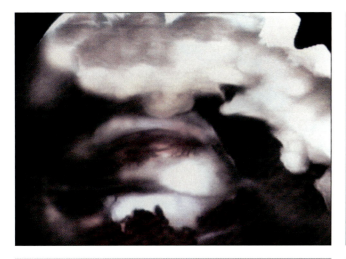

Figure 17-10. Nerve root with its vascularization is seen in the 1° plane; the prominent protrusion of the herniated disc is shown in the 2° plane. To the *right* and at the *top*, the articular facet and ligamentum flavum are shown.

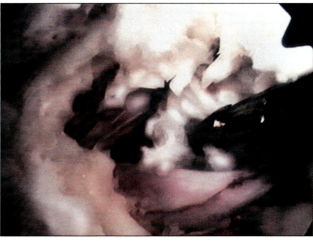

Figure 17-11. Extraction of the extruded hernia.

throughout surgery, higher only intermittently if bleeding requires it.

The saline-solution outflow by the working portal must be constantly controlled to avoid creation of high pressure within the vertebral canal; the pump is used to irrigate and wash away blood. After the herniated disc has been extracted and the operated space re-explored, the nerve root must be examined to ensure that it is free. Instrumentation is then removed, and the skin is sutured with nylon, after which a small dressing and a brace are applied to the area.

POSTOPERATIVE REHABILITATION

The patient must remain positioned during the first 12 to 24 postoperative hours in the decubitus position, and oral antibiotics and analgesics must be given. The patient is permitted to walk 7 days after discharge from the hospital. Long-term physical therapy is indicated after ambulation is resumed.

RESULTS

Results of translaminar epidural endoscopy were presented at the 15th Annual Fall Course of the Arthroscopy Association of North America (Palm Desert, 1996) and the First Biennial Congress of ISAKOS (Buenos Aires, 1997). In a selection of 190 patients who had been operated on between 1986 and 1995 for herniations of the lumbar disc, 100 (52.63%) of the hernias were located in the fourth disc, and 90 (47.36%) were located in the fifth disc. Protrusions were found in 40 patients (21.05%), extrusions in 120 (63.15%), and migrated herniation in 30 (15.78%). Good results were obtained in 92.89%, fair results in 6.03%, and poor results in only 1.08%.

COMPLICATIONS

There was a single intraoperative accident, a dural sac rupture of 3 to 4 mm. Sutures were not required, and the recovery was fast and favorable. No other complications (*eg*, cauda equina syndrome, recurrences, infections, thromboembolisms, reactions to anesthetics, mortality) were present.

CONCLUSION

Translaminar lumbar epidural endoscopy is a minimally invasive surgical technique that brings a new element to arthroscopic surgery. Minimum invasiveness has been kept in all the cases (100%), even though there were variable difficulties because of technical impediments that were not solved by currently available instrumentation. Even so, no patients required reoperation.

In all patients, maximum visualization and instrumental accuracy were achieved. It was possible to extract all types of hernia and to free compromised roots through dynamic exploration of the vertebral canal and use of various optical lenses without requiring bony resection.

Because this technique requires permanent irrigation of the tissues, bleeding is constantly controlled so that hemostasis by electrocoagulation is unnecessary. This form of irrigation, already common in arthroscopic surgery, also works against infection. This technique improves the exactitude of extraction of the affected tissue, and because it avoids the overload segmentary instability caused by surgery, it also helps to reduce possible complications. Use of this technique also results in greater comfort in the postoperative period, a faster recovery, and earlier resumption of work.

REFERENCES AND RECOMMENDED READING

Recently published papers of particular interest have been highlighted as:
•   Of interest

1. Ottolenghi C: Diagnosis of orthopaedic lesions by aspiration biopsy: results of 1061 punctures. *J Bone J Surg Am* 1955, 37:443–464.

2. Hijikata S, Yamagishi H: Percutaneous discectomy: a new treatment method for lumbar disk herniation. *J Toden Hosp* 1975, 5:13.

3. Kambin P, Gellman A: Percutaneous lateral diskectomy of the spine. *Clin Orthop* 1983, 174:127–132.

4. Kambin P: Arthroscopy microdiscectomy. *J Arthroscopy* 1992, 8:287–295.

5. Schreiber A, Suezawa Y: Transdiscoscopic percutaneous nucleotomy in disk herniation. *Orthop Rev* 1986, 15:35–38.

6. Schreiber A, Suezawa Y: Does percutaneous nucleotomy with discoscopy replace conventional discectomy? Eight years of experience and results in treatment of herniated lumbar disk. *Clin Orthop* 1989, 238:35–42.

7. De Antoni D, Claro ML: Cirugía artroscopica del disco lumbar. *Rev Arg Artr* 1994, 1:81–85.

8.• De Antoni D, Claro ML, Poehling G, *et al.*: Translaminar lumbar epidural endoscopy: anatomy, technique and indications. *J Arthroscopy* 1996, 12:330–334.

The original surgery technique is described, and comparison with other surgery techniques is made.

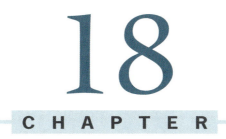

18
CHAPTER

Arthroscopic Evaluation and Treatment of the Problematic Total Knee Arthroplasty

JESS H. LONNER AND J. SERGE PARISIEN

otal knee arthroplasty has proven to be effective for the treatment of advanced arthrosis and inflammatory arthritis, with survivorship, pain relief, and improved mobility reported to be in excess of 90% at 10 to 15 years after implantation [1–3]. Despite these impressive results, pain, instability, dysfunction, stiffness, or septic and aseptic failures inevitably occur in a small number of patients. Although the majority of these problems may be diagnosed by a combination of clinical evaluation and imaging or laboratory studies, there are times when the painful or dysfunctional total knee arthroplasty has no clear etiology. In these circumstances, arthroscopic evaluation may play a valuable role. Additionally, several entities, including patellar subluxation, acute infection, arthrofibrosis, impinging pseudomeniscus, popliteus tendon impingement, or loose body, may be effectively treated by arthroscopy, obviating the need for arthrotomy [4•,5–9, 10•,11,12•,13–20].

CONDITIONS AMENABLE TO ARTHROSCOPY AFTER TOTAL KNEE ARTHROPLASTY
Infection

Pain after total knee arthroplasty should be considered to be caused by infection until proven otherwise. Although most cases of sepsis are easily diagnosed with careful history, physical examination, standing radiographs, serologic studies, and joint aspiration (with cell count and culture), occasionally these problems are occult and the studies are nondiagnostic; thus, arthroscopic evaluation is warranted. In the absence of identifiable mechanical or anatomic reasons for symptoms, or when infection is suspected, synovial fluid and tissue should be cultured and sent for a cell count. Interface tissue for frozen and permanent section histoanalysis can be diagnostic of occult infection, even in the absence of bacterial growth [21••].

Implant retention in the setting of deep infection has met with limited success. However, it remains a viable option for acute infections diagnosed within 3 weeks of implantation, provided the components are not loose, the host is immunocompetent, and the bacteria are sensitive to appropriate antibiotics. In such situations, thorough debridement of scar, synovium, and devitalized tissue is essential. This may be performed by arthrotomy or arthroscopy [5]. When arthroscopic debridement is chosen, multiple portals may be necessary in order to adequately address dense scar and ensure meticulous debridement, particularly in the medial and lateral gutters and posterior capsular recess.

Pseudomeniscus

New onset of pain may also represent an impinging pseudomeniscus, which usually localizes to the posteromedial or posterolateral joint line [6,12•] (Fig.18-1). Meniscal regeneration following total knee arthroplasty is a recognized phenomenon, postulated to be a metaplastic event, with compressed mesenchymal-derived cells differentiating into fibrocartilaginous tissue [12•]. As an isolated pathologic entity, clinical findings are nonspecific, and diagnostic studies are usually normal; however, a lidocaine injection test may eliminate the posterior pain that characteristically occurs in flexion. Frequently the diagnosis is unclear until arthroscopic visualization. Excision of the offending tissue should effect prompt relief.

Polyethylene Wear

Polyethylene wear remains a prominent undefeated nemesis in total knee arthroplasty and a common cause of late aseptic implant loosening. Early polyethylene wear may present with asymptomatic swelling; effusion; progressive deformity; clicking; or rarely, pain. It is at this stage that traditional studies, particularly radiographs, may fail to establish a diagnosis [11,16,20,22]. Arthroscopic findings typically include extensive synovitis with polyethylene debris embedded in the synovium and polyethylene wear of the tibial and patellar components (Fig. 18-2).

Polyethylene wear may range from pitting, cracking, and abrasion to severe delamination. In advanced cases, in which diagnosis can generally be made radiographically, exposed metal tibial or patellar base plates and femoral component burnishing may be seen arthroscopically as well. Arthroscopic synovectomy may provide short-term symptomatic relief; however, the authors recommend polyethylene exchange prior to the initiation of osteolysis and implant loosening, or revision arthroplasty if required.

Arthrofibrosis

Arthrofibrosis, secondary to the formation of dense intra-articular adhesions, is a source of stiffness after total knee arthroplasty [6,7,9,10•,13,15]. The problem may range in severity from isolated infrapatellar adhesions to more diffuse scarring of the suprapatellar pouch, medial and lateral gutters, and posterior capsule (Fig. 18-3). A constellation of presenting symptoms commonly includes stiffness, pain, clunking or clicking, and diminished patellar excursion.

Manipulation becomes more difficult, and the risk of supracondylar femur fracture or patellar tendon rupture increases as the scar matures; therefore, it may be advisable to refrain from manipulation unless it is performed within the first 6 to 12 weeks after arthroplasty.

Even with isolated peripatellar fibrosis, multiple ancillary arthroscopic portals may be necessary to adequately debride the scar and adhesions [6,15]. Lateral retinacular release may facilitate patellar excursion and subsequent flexion. After comprehensive scar debridement, manipulation is advisable to

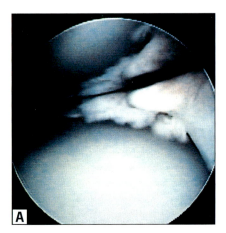 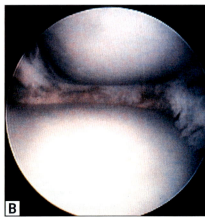

Figure 18-1. Symptomatic pseudomeniscus in the lateral compartment of the left knee before (**A**) and after (**B**) excision.

lyse further periarticular fibrosis or quadriceps adhesion to the anterior femur. Indwelling epidural analgesia and aggressive postoperative physiotherapy may help maintain motion after adhesiolysis.

Patellar Dysfunction

Patellar subluxation or dislocation after total knee arthroplasty may result from component malposition, oversizing, soft tissue imbalance, or acute dehiscence of the medial arthrotomy repair. When patellar maltracking is attributable to soft-tissue imbalance, it may be addressed with lateral retinacular release [6,9]. Clinical examination is diagnostic in most cases, identifying tightness of the lateral retinaculum, patellar apprehension, or a characteristic "J-sign." Skyline-view radiographs also contribute to the diagnosis. Arthroscopic evaluation should include assessment of patellar tracking and overhang through a controlled arc of motion, using a combination of inferolateral, superolateral, or medial parapatellar portals. In general, symptomatic relief and improved patellar

tracking are noted promptly, unless the etiology is more complex than soft-tissue imbalance.

The so-called "patellar clunk syndrome" is a noted complication in posterior stabilized arthroplasties. In this entity, a retropatellar fibrous nodule becomes entrapped in the intercondylar housing of the femoral component. As the knee continues into extension, the nodule snaps free, causing a characteristic clunk. Arthroscopic excision of the nodule can effectively relieve symptoms and improve function [6,14].

Miscellaneous Disorders

Arthroscopy may also be effective at diagnosing and removing loose bodies within the joint, including cement fragments, modular screws, or bone debris. Occult polyethylene disassociation from its tibial or patellar metal backing has also been reported to be a source of dysfunction after arthroplasty, with an uncertain diagnosis until arthroscopic identification is made (Figs. 18-4 to 18-8). The popliteus tendon may rub over a lateral femoral condylar osteophyte or an

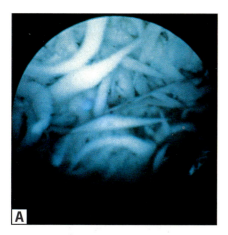
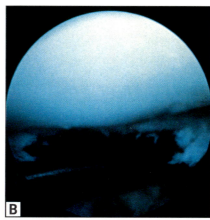

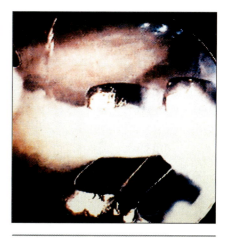

Figure 18-2. Polyethylene wear causing extensive synovitis. **A,** Synovitis in the suprapatellar pouch. **B,** Visualization of the retropatellar area.

Figure 18-3. Excision of fibrous band in arthrofibrosis.

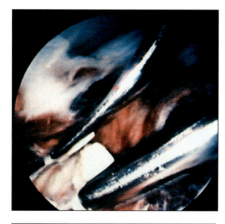
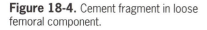

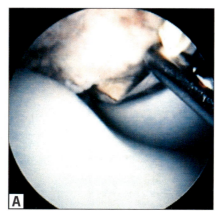

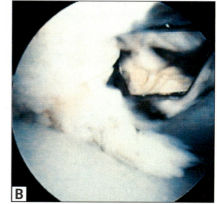

Figure 18-4. Cement fragment in loose femoral component.

Figure 18-5. Loose prosthesis with probe on femoral component (**A**) showing instability between the cement and bone interface (**B**).

oversized femoral prosthesis, resulting in a characteristically painful snapping. Arthroscopic release of the tendon may successfully relieve symptoms [4•]. Finally, posterior cruciate ligament (PCL) retention in total knee arthroplasty may limit flexion if the ligament is too tight. In cases in which initial balancing of the PCL was insufficient, arthroscopic release may improve motion arc and eliminate associated pain [7]. It is important, however, to recognize that PCL release should not be used to address flexion contractures, as this may increase flexion laxity and have no or minimal effect on extension.

GENERAL PRINCIPLES OF ARTHROSCOPIC TECHNIQUE IN TOTAL KNEE ARTHROPLASTY

Arthroscopic surgery of the knee is performed under general, regional, or local anesthesia. A tourniquet may be used if necessary. Although no prospective studies have addressed the use of antibiotics prior to arthroscopy after total knee arthroplasty, the authors prefer to administer an appropriate dose of a parenteral first-generation cephalosporin (*eg*, cefazolin) 5 minutes

prior to surgery, if the patient is not allergic to it. Standard arthroscopy portals and instruments are used. Additional ancillary portals should be considered to facilitate visualization and intervention. The basic tenets of arthroscopic technique are followed; however, the procedure may be more difficult because of intra-articular adhesions, an altered level of the joint line, and glare off the metal femoral component. Scratching the metal or polyethylene components may jeopardize component longevity and obviously should be avoided [4•,5–9,10•,11,12•,13–20].

Although postoperative infection has not been reported in most series, a retrospective study by Sisto and Cook [23] reported a 4% incidence of infection after arthroscopy in 96 knee-replacement patients who underwent 142 subsequent arthroscopic surgeries of the affected knee. The average time between joint replacement and arthroscopic intervention was 49 months. Many of the patients had only patellofemoral joint replacement or unicompartmental replacement, and infection prior to arthroscopy may not have been adequately ruled out [23]. Nonetheless, safeguards should be taken to minimize the risk of infection,

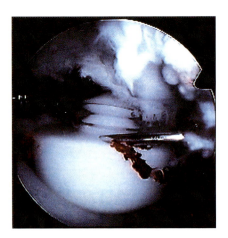

Figure 18-6. Loose patella prosthesis in a patient with painful clunk of the left knee after injury.

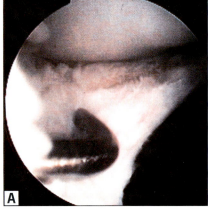

Figure 18-7. Hypertrophic band causing retropatellar symptoms before (**A**) and after (**B**) excision.

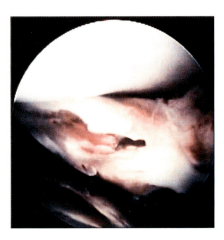

Figure 18-8. Symptomatic hypertrophic band retropatellar area.

including careful patient selection, the use of perioperative antibiotics, adherence to aseptic technique, and copious knee irrigation.

RESULTS

Fourteen patients with symptomatic total knee arthroplasties were arthroscopically evaluated and treated, on average, 23.5 months after implantation. A preliminary report was presented at the Annual Meeting of the North American Arthroscopy Association in 1996 [19]. Presenting symptoms included pain [14], swelling [6], stiffness [3], locking [2], and "clunking" [1]. Preoperative evaluation failed to establish a diagnosis in nine patients. Arthroscopic examination yielded or confirmed a diagnosis in each case, including arthrofibrosis [3], impinging posterolateral pseudomeniscus [5], fibrous retropatellar and suprapatellar band [2], tight lateral capsule and patellar subluxation [2], patellar component dissociation, and aseptic femoral component loosening with loose cement fragments [2]. No patients had infections. Pain relief, improved patellar tracking, or

increased knee motion were noted in each patient treated arthroscopically. Two patients underwent revision arthroplasty to address the loose components. There were no postoperative complications.

CONCLUSION

Arthroscopy can play a limited but valuable role after total knee arthroplasty. It is a safe and effective mechanism for diagnosing a variety of occult processes after total knee arthroplasty and has been proven effective for the treatment of several conditions. Basic principles of arthroscopic technique should be followed, recognizing that it may be difficult because of intra-articular adhesions, an elevated joint line, and glare off the femoral component. The procedure is technically demanding and should be limited to appropriately selected patients and performed by surgeons skilled in arthroscopic techniques to avoid scuffing the prostheses. If appropriately performed, arthroscopy can play an important role in the dysfunctional total knee arthroplasty, avoiding the morbidity of formal arthrotomy, and without compromising future procedures.

REFERENCES AND RECOMMENDED READING

Recently published papers of particular interest have been highlighted as:
* Of interest
** Of outstanding interest

1. Ranawat CS, Flynn WF, Saddler S, *et al.*: Long-term results of the total condylar knee arthroplasty. *Clin Orthop* 1993, 286:94–102.

2. Scott RD, Volatile TB: Twelve years' experience with posterior cruciate-retaining total knee arthroplasty. *Clin Orthop* 1986, 205:100–107.

3. Stern SH, Insall JN: Posterior stabilized prostheses: results after follow-up of nine to twelve years. *J Bone Joint Surg Am* 1992, 74(suppl A):980–986.

4.• Allardyce TJ, Scuderi GR, Insall JN: Arthroscopic treatment of popliteus tendon dysfunction following total knee arthroplasty. *J Arthroplasty* 1997, 12:353–355.
Two patients with popliteus tendon dysfunction were treated with arthroscopic release of the tendon from its femoral insertion.

5. Flood JN, Kolarik DB: Arthroscopic irrigation and debridement of infected total knee arthroplasty: report on two cases. *Arthroscopy* 1988, 4:182–186.

6. Bocell JR, Thorpe CD, Tullos HS: Arthroscopic treatment of symptomatic total knee arthroplasty. *Clin Orthop* 1991, 271:125–134.

7. Campbell ED: Arthroscopy in total knee replacements. *Arthroscopy* 1987, 3:31–35.

8. Davis PF, Bocell JR, Tullos HS: Dissociation of the tibial component in total knee replacements. *Clin Orthop* 1991, 272:199–204.

9. Johnson DR, Friedman RF, McGinty JB, *et al.*: The role of arthroscopy in the problem total knee replacement. *Arthroscopy* 1990, 6:30–32.

10.• Markel DC, Luessenhop CP, Windsor RE, Sculco TA: Arthroscopic treatment of peripatellar fibrosis after total knee arthroplasty. *J Arthroplasty* 1996, 11:293–297.
Arthroscopic management of peripatellar fibrosis, although recommended, was found unpredictable in 48 total knee arthroplasties.

11. Mintz L, Tsao AK, McCrae CR, *et al.*: The arthroscopic evaluation and characteristics of severe polyethylene wear in total knee arthroplasty. *Clin Orthop* 1991, 273:215–221.

12.• Scher DM, Paumier JC, DiCesare PE: Pseudomeniscus following total knee arthroplasty as a cause of persistent knee pain. *J Arthroplasty* 1997, 12:114–118.
Report of successful arthroscopic treatment of pseudomeniscus following total knee arthroplasty.

13. Sprague NF, O'Connor RL, Fox JM: Arthroscopic treatment of postoperative knee fibroarthrosis. *Clin Orthop* 1982, 166:165–172.

14. Vernace JV, Rothman RH, Booth RE, Balderston RA: Arthroscopic management of the patellar clunk syndrome following posterior stabilized total knee arthroplasty. *J Arthoplasty* 1989, 4:179–182.

15. Wasilewski SA, Frankl U: Arthroscopy of the painful dysfunctional total knee replacement. *Arthroscopy* 1989, 5:294–297.

16. Wasilweski SA, Frankl U: Fracture of polyethylene of patellar component in total knee arthroplasty, diagnosed by arthroscopy. *J Arthroplasty* 1989, 19(suppl):19–22.

17. Williams RJ III, Westrich GH, Siegel J, Windsor RE: Arthroscopic release of the posterior cruciate ligament for stiff total knee arthroplasty. *Clin Orthop* 1996, 331:185–191.

18. Diduch DR, Scuderi GR, Scott WN, *et al.*: The efficacy of arthroscopy following total knee replacement. *Arthroscopy* 1997, 13:166–171.

19. Lonner JH, Parisien JS: Role of arthroscopy in the symptomatic knee arthroplasty. Proceedings of the Annual Meeting of the Arthroscopy Association of North America. San Francisco, CA; May 4–7, 1995.

20. Li PLS, Chakrabarti AJ, Dowell JK: Persistent synovial fistula after arthroscopy: is titanium synovitis a risk factor *J Bone Joint Surg* 1996, 78(suppl B):322–323.

21.•• Lonner JH, Desai P, Dicesare P, *et al.*: The reliability of analysis of intraoperative frozen section for identifying active infection during revision hip or knee arthroplasty. *J Bone Joint Surg* 1996, 78(suppl A):1553–1558.

Prospective study showing that for identifying active infection, it is valuable to obtain tissue for intraoperative frozen sections during revision hip or knee arthroplasty.

22. Lonner JH, Siliski JM, Scott RD: Prodromes of failure in total knee arthroplasty. Proceedings of the Annual Scientific Meeting of the Hospital for Joint Diseases; 1997.

23. Sisto DJ, Cook DL: Infection following knee arthroscopy in joint replacement patients. Proceedings of the Arthroscopy Association of North America. Washington, DC; April 11–14, 1996.

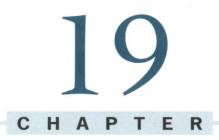

19
CHAPTER

Recent Advances in Ankle Arthroscopic Techniques

JAMES P. TASTO AND PETER D. LAIMINS

F our of the most common conditions in the ankle are ankle instability, syndesmosis injuries, and ankle and subtalar arthritis. The indications for surgery and recent advances in technique provided in this chapter will help the surgeon to improve the ability to care for patients with these ankle conditions.

ANKLE INSTABILITY

Inversion injuries of the ankle are among the most common injuries sustained by athletes and the general population. Although the specific parameters defining this classification are vague and subject to interobserver variation, ankle sprains have been traditionally classified as grade I (mild), grade II (moderate), and grade III (severe). Grade I injuries involve ligaments stretched on a microscopic level with little swelling or tenderness and no mechanical or functional instability. Grade II injuries encompass partial ligament disruption with associated swelling, tenderness, and variable amounts of joint instability. Grade III injuries include a complete rupture of ligaments, more impressive clinical findings, increased joint laxity on physical examination, and possible symptoms of acute or chronic instability.

Most patients who suffer an ankle sprain, especially grades I and II injuries, recover well with nonsurgical management. In cases of more severe ligament disruption, long-term sequelae may develop, leading to a less than ideal outcome. Common complaints from these patients include persistent pain, swelling, stiffness, muscle weakness, and instability. Indeed, many of these symptoms may be causally interrelated. For this reason, it is important to identify the specific offending pathology that is responsible for the persistent symptoms.

Anatomy

The lateral ligamentous complex of the ankle consists of three ligaments: the anterior talofibular ligament (ATFL), the calcaneofibular ligament (CFL), and the posterior talofibular ligament (PTFL) (Fig. 19-1). A study performed by Brostrom [1] found that although isolated tears of the ATFL occurred in 65% of ankle sprains, a combination of ATFL and CFL disruption occurred in 20%. The PTFL was only rarely injured. On physical examination in the acute sprain, areas of tenderness may aid in the diagnosis of specific ligament disruption. In chronic injuries with established subjective and objective instability, tenderness may be less distinct. In these cases, dynamic assessment of instability may be aided by the anterior drawer and talar tilt tests. Findings on physical examination may be compared with stress radiographs. Specific parameters of translation and tilt, which signify ligament disruption, have varied significantly. Many authors have concluded that these maneuvers do not consistently provide reliable diagnostic findings. A prospective study by Johannsen [2] concluded that, based on these two manual tests, it is not possible to differentiate between an isolated lesion of the ATFL and a combined lesion of the ATFL and CFL. In another study, Seligson [3] found that because of the undetermined contribution of subtalar motion to perceived inversion, inversion stress testing (talar tilt) was not helpful in the evaluation of the lateral ligaments.

Arthroscopic Evaluation

In cases of chronic instability, ankle arthroscopy (Fig. 19-2) can provide valuable information and is most useful as a perioperative tool when symptomatic instability requires invasive treatment. Arthroscopic evaluation of the ankle allows inspection of the ATFL and PTFL, the capsular reflection of the CFL, the deep deltoid ligament, the syndesmotic ligament complex, and occasionally, the posterolateral ankle and subtalar capsule. Direct observation of the lateral structures during stress testing (talar tilt, translation, and rotation) is possible during arthroscopy as well. In a recent study, Schafer and Hentermann [4] arthroscopically evaluated 110 symptomatic patients and identified ATFL tears in 64%, CFL disruption in 41%, and deltoid ligament injuries in 6%. Early findings in the authors' series reveal a significant number of partial PTFL, even though the PTFL has previously been described as a ligament rarely involved in lateral ligamentous injury. A number of studies [4–7] have also identified the association of chronic lateral ankle instability with chondral injury. This is an important point to remember because many of these cartilaginous lesions may go undetected without the aid of direct arthroscopic visualization. Cooke [8] reports that stress radiographs and magnetic resonance imaging (MRI) evaluation are normal in more than 50% of cases in which significant intra-articular pathology is subsequently confirmed arthroscopically.

Prior to the arthroscopic procedure, both ankles should be examined under anesthesia. Increased talar translation or tilt of the involved side can be documented with fluoroscopy and compared with that of the uninvolved side. It is important to determine subtalar motion during fluoroscopic inversion stress testing, since increased motion at this joint can be perceived clinically as increased talar tilt. Using standard anteromedial and anterolateral portals, and noninvasive traction of 20 to 25 lbs, all ligamentous structures and chondral surfaces can be evaluated.

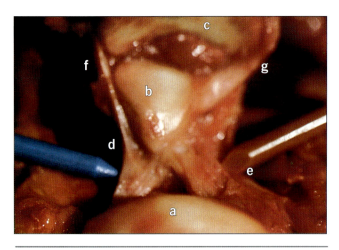

Figure 19-1. Anatomic dissection of ankle showing the talus (*a*), fibula (*b*), tibia (*c*), anterior talofibular ligament (*d*), posterior talofibular ligament (*e*), anterior tibiofibular ligament (*f*), and posterior tibiofibular ligament (*g*).

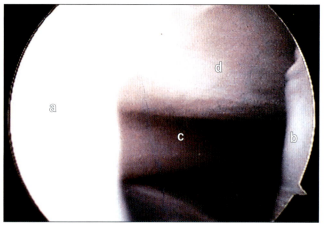

Figure 19-2. Arthroscopic view of the left ankle with posterior capsular disruption and exposure of peroneal tendons, showing the talus (*a*), fibula (*b*), and peroneus longus (*c*) and brevis (*d*).

The advantage of noninvasive traction over the use of a fixed ankle distracter is that it allows for manipulation of the anterolateral portal.

Hawkins [9] has described an arthroscopic lateral ankle stabilization technique that includes removing soft tissue and debris from the ATFL insertion site on the talus, followed by denuding articular cartilage with a burr. An accessory portal is created approximately 1 cm distal to the anterolateral portal so that a staple passed through the accessory portal enters the talus at a right angle. After the foot is brought to a neutral position, the tines of the staple gather capsule and ligament tissue while the staple is secured with a mallet. At this time, the authors do not advocate this procedure. The current recommendation is to use ankle arthroscopy as a perioperative tool in cases of established functional instability. Surgical intervention in the acute ankle sprain, even for a grade III injury, is not advocated. All patients should have formal physical therapy prior to discussion of surgical options. If symptomatic instability persists despite adequate rehabilitative efforts, then an open stabilization procedure should be chosen based on suspected pathology determined through careful history, physical examination, and radiographic studies. Prior to opening the lateral ankle surgically, soft-tissue and chondral injury can be evaluated using anesthesia, fluoroscopy, and ankle arthroscopy. In this manner, precise open stabilization techniques can be used to address all areas of ligamentous insufficiency.

SYNDESMOSIS INJURIES

Isolated ankle syndesmosis sprains and disruptions are uncommon injuries. More frequently, rupture of the syndesmosis is associated with deltoid ligament injury and fractures of the malleoli. These contributing associated injuries naturally increase the suspicion of syndesmosis involvement based on an understanding of the mechanism of injury. However, an ankle sprain with an undetected syndesmosis injury may lead to a prolonged and complicated recovery from an initially benign injury. A high index of suspicion and early recognition leads to improved outcomes in treating this more subtle injury.

The distal tibiofibular syndesmosis consists of three separate ligaments: the anterior inferior tibiofibular (AITF) ligament, the posterior inferior tibiofibular (PITF) ligament, and the interosseous ligament (Figs. 19-3 and 19-4). A distal fascicle of the PITF ligaments has been considered a separate ligament by some authors and has been named the *transverse tibiofibular ligament* [10,11]. Lauge-Hansen describes the mechanism of syndesmosis injury as external rotation of the foot that causes a diastasis of the tibiofibular joint due to pressure exerted by the talus. The ankle is likely to be in a position of full dorsiflexion or plantarflexion at the moment of injury, since these positions place the syndesmosis ligaments under maximal tension [12]. The incidence of ankle diastasis without fracture ranges from 1% to 11% of soft-tissue ankle injuries [13,14].

Clinical Examination

As for all injuries, a careful history and physical examination are essential in diagnosing syndesmotic ligament injuries. Although patients may report a wide variety of mechanisms of injury, trauma that subjects the foot to significant external rotation forces should automatically signal a syndesmosis injury [13]. Patients may complain of

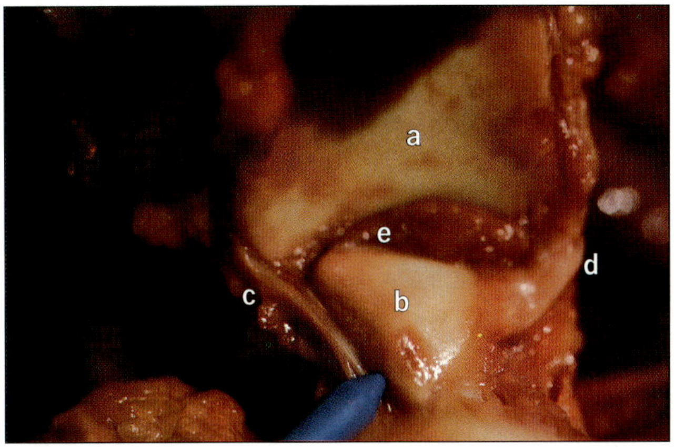

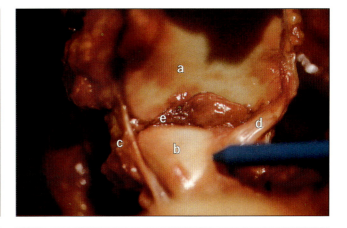

Figure 19-3. Prosected anatomic view of distal tibiofibular joint, internal rotation, showing the tibia (*a*), fibula (*b*), anterior interosseus ligament (*c*), posterior interosseus ligament (*d*), and interosseus ligament (*e*).

Figure 19-4. Prosected anatomic view of distal tibiofibular joint, external rotation, showing the tibia (*a*), fibula (*b*), anterior interosseus ligament (*c*), posterior interosseus ligament (*d*), and interosseus ligament (*e*).

other symptoms, including pain over the anterior syndesmosis, medial deltoid, and tenderness or pain with external rotation of the foot. Two manual tests are helpful in isolating a syndesmosis injury. Hopkinson et al. [13] described the "squeeze test" as compression of the fibula toward the tibia at the distal half of the lower leg that produces pain distally at the syndesmosis. The Cotton test detects increased mediolateral motion of the talus in the mortise. External rotation of the ankle with the knee flexed to 90° also produces pain at the anterior syndesmosis, indicating either an acute or chronic disruption. Edwards and DeLee [15] create two groups based on radiographic evaluation of syndesmotic diastasis. The latent diastasis group exhibits widening of the diastasis only when external rotation or abduction forces are applied. The frank diastasis group presents with syndesmosis widening visible on routine radiographs. Additional information can be obtained from computed tomography (CT) scans, MRI, and ankle arthrography.

In many cases, the clinical findings in syndesmotic ligament injuries can be less clear. In the acute setting, physical examination may reveal diffuse, nonspecific tenderness, and patients may not be able to tolerate stress radiographs. Marymont et al. [16] suggest the use of radionuclide imaging in these cases, citing a 100% sensitivity. They reported two cases of positive scan results and negative stress radiograph results, and Hopkinson et al. [13] identified six of seven patients with similar findings. By maintaining a high index of suspicion in these cases and instituting appropriate treatment, a radiographically occult syndesmosis injury will not be overlooked.

Arthroscopic Technique

Ankle arthroscopy has recently become an important tool in the diagnosis and treatment of syndesmotic ligament injuries. Ogilvie-Harris and Reed [17] arthroscopically evaluated 19 patients with chronic symptoms consistent with syndesmosis disruption. A triad of pathologic findings were identified: disruption of the PITF ligament, disruption of the interosseous ligament, and a posterolateral tibial plafond chondral fracture. Debriding the intra-articular pathology produced good results. In the authors' experience, arthroscopy has been helpful in treating patients who remain symptomatic despite appropriate initial treatment or in cases of a missed diagnosis. Ankle arthroscopy allows static and dynamic inspection of the syndesmotic ligament complex, allowing definitive treatment before the onset of arthritic changes that may result from a chronically incongruent joint. Disruption of the interosseous component of the syndesmotic complex with intact AITF and PITF ligaments has also been observed. The diastasis in the coronal plane is less dramatic than the anterior and posterior and rotational instability patterns noted during direct observation of dynamic stress testing (Figs. 19-5 and 19-6). It is an arthroscopically assisted technique for debridement and stabilization of the disrupted and unstable syndesmosis, which has led to good results in early follow-up and full return to activity. During second-look arthroscopy at the time of hardware removal, complete healing of the syndesmosis has occurred without evidence of persistent instability during dynamic stress testing (Fig. 19-7).

The technique uses noninvasive traction of 20 to 25 lbs with standard anteromedial and anterolateral

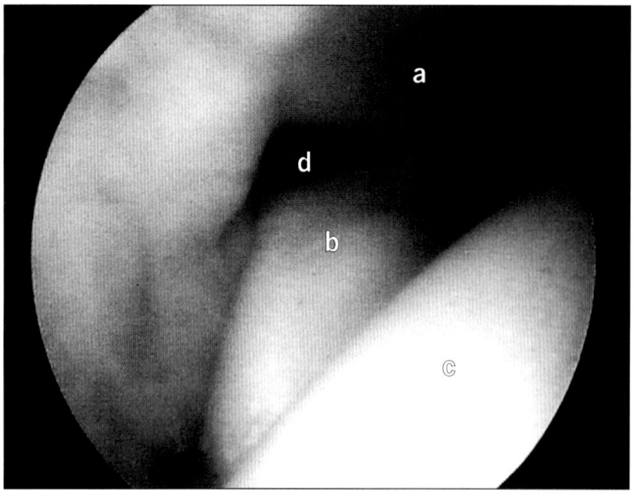

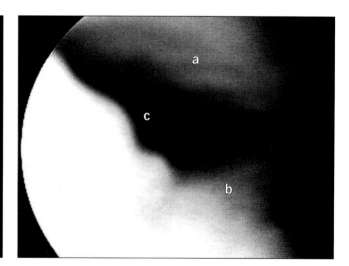

Figure 19-5. Arthroscopic view of the right ankle without stress, showing the tibia (*a*), fibula (*b*), talus (*c*), and interosseus ligament disruption (*d*).

Figure 19-6. Arthroscopic view of the right ankle with external rotation stress and significant anterior and posterior patholaxity, showing the tibia (*a*), talus (*b*), and interosseus ligament disruption (*c*).

portals to examine the ankle joint and syndesmosis. Direct palpation of the syndesmosis is best performed with a probe in the anteromedial portal. Occasionally, the synovium, which overlies the interosseous component of this ligament, may need to be excised to increase the ability to palpate and visualize this area. The AITF and PITF ligaments should be inspected for attenuation, partial tears, and complete disruption. With the camera in the anterolateral portal, the syndesmosis is observed during external rotation of the foot. If the syndesmosis is completely disrupted and a diastasis is present, this position allows visualization proximal to the distal tibiofibular articulation. The complex and interrelated multi-axial motion of the distal fibula, tibia, and talus can be seen at this time.

After arthroscopic confirmation of syndesmotic ligament disruption and instability, the remainder of the ankle joint should be carefully inspected for associated injuries. Chondral injuries and soft-tissue impingement lesions may not be detected by plain radiographs, CT scans, or MRI, but may be picked up arthroscopically. If left untreated, these conditions may cause a poor outcome despite appropriate treatment of the syndesmotic disruption. A systematic inspection of all cartilaginous surfaces should be developed with the ankle in dorsiflexion and plantarflexion to bring the entire weight-bearing portion of the talar dome into view. The most effective way to evaluate the medial gutter and deep fibers of the deltoid ligament is through the anteromedial portal. Although lateral ligamentous injuries are rarely associated with syndesmosis disruption, this area can be inspected and palpated through the anterolateral portal.

In cases of complete or partial disruption of the syndesmosis with observed instability, stabilization of the syndesmosis is indicated. Arthroscopic debridement and curettage of the interosseous component followed by percutaneous screw fixation has led to promising early results, although various open repair and stabilization techniques have been described [12,15,18]. Torn fibers of the interosseous ligament can be removed with a synovial resector. The surgeon should take care to avoid carelessly debriding intact portions of the AITF or PITF ligaments. Next, a curette can debride the distal tibiofibular articulation of remaining interosseous fibers and fibro-osseous debris (Fig. 19-8). The curette is advanced approximately 1 cm proximal to create a bed of cancellous bone throughout the course of the interosseous ligament disruption from anterior to posterior. By placing the camera in the anteromedial portal and looking proximal, the area of debridement between the distal tibia and fibula can be visualized to ensure complete removal of residual ligamentous or cartilaginous debris. Finally, a syndesmotic screw is placed percutaneously while the ankle is held in dorsiflexion and neutral rotation (Figs. 19-9 and 19-10). Fluoroscopy is used to ensure closure of the diastasis, maintenance of an intact mortise, and proper placement of the screw.

Cast immobilization is used in the acute setting of syndesmosis injury without diastasis. Ankle arthroscopy is used for many reasons, including treatment of patients who remain symptomatic after appropriate conservative treatment, for syndesmosis disruption and instability requiring fixation, and for the chronic "high ankle sprain" with clinical evidence of persistent syndesmosis symptoms. Data accumu-

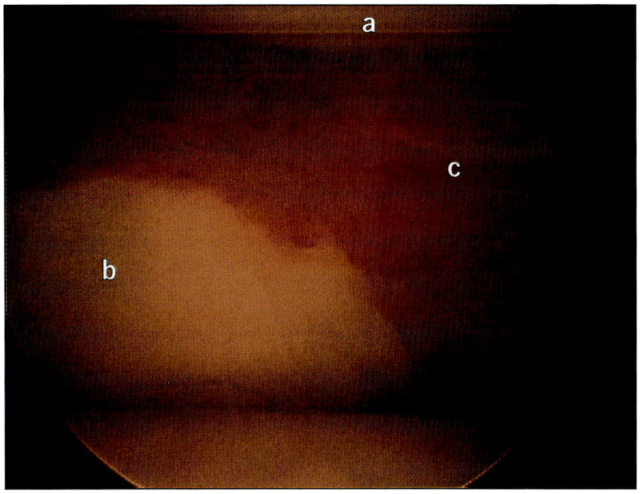

Figure 19-7. Arthroscopic view of healed tibiofibular syndesmosis of the right ankle, showing the tibia (a), fibula (b), and healed interosseus ligament (c).

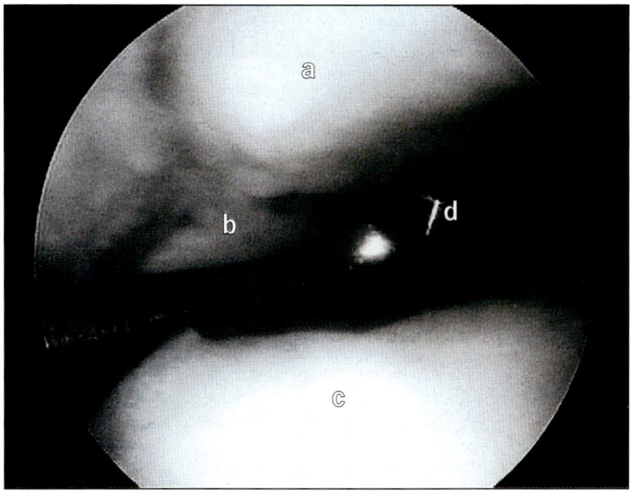

Figure 19-8. Curette debriding the interosseus ligament and space, showing the tibia (a), fibula (b), talus (c), and curette (d).

lated over the past 2.5 years show very promising results, with almost complete return to full activity. There have been no complications to date in this difficult subset of individuals. As experience builds, it is being realized that the distal tibiofibular articulation and syndesmotic ligaments are complex structures with poorly understood biomechanics.

ARTHROSCOPIC ANKLE ARTHRODESIS

Ankle arthrodesis is a time-honored operative procedure designed to deal with the problems of end-stage degenerative joint disease (DJD) of the ankle [19–25]. This procedure does have inherent problems. A review of the open arthroscopic ankle fusion literature [26–32] indicates an overall complication rate exceeding 25%. Recently, a modified mini-open procedure has reduced this complication rate [33,34]. The arthroscopic approach uses soft-tissue distraction, arthroscopic abrasion, creation of vascular channels, and percutaneous screw fixation to achieve arthrodesis. Morbidity is reduced by not using skeletal distraction. This procedure offers the patient advantages such as decreased time necessary to complete union, a higher percentage of successful union, and overall reduction in morbidity.

Arthroscopic ankle arthrodesis has been described by a number of authors [24,35–39] with favorable results and minimal complications. There have been a variety of techniques described in peer review journals that use both skeletal distraction and soft-tissue distraction. The general operative procedure has been quite standard, but fixation techniques have varied [40–43]. For the past 8 years, the authors have prospectively studied and retrospectively analyzed their own series. The following is a description of a technique, results, fusion rate, time until fusion, complications, and suggestions for improvement in the future.

Work-up

The indications for this procedure are end-stage DJD and congenital and paralytic deformities of the ankle not responding to conservative care. Absolute contraindications are infection, pyarthrosis, significant malalignment, and previously failed arthrodesis. Relative contraindications are moderate malalignment and bone loss.

Of the 50 patients who have undergone this procedure, 49 were available for follow-up until either a full fusion, a documented delayed union, or a nonunion was established. A breakdown of the 49 patients shows that 24 had osteoarthritis, 6 had rheumatoid arthritis, and 14 had post-traumatic disorders. Four patients presented with neurologic disorders such as paralytic footdrop and equinus deformity. They requested stabilization to become brace-free. The last patient had unrecognized avascular necrosis of the talus. Three patients underwent a combined arthroscopic ankle and subtalar arthrodesis.

All patients had previously undergone a variety of conservative treatment modalities, including use of nonsteroidal anti-inflammatory drugs (NSAIDs), braces, steroid injections, and shoe modification. They had all reached the stage at which conservative care was no longer effective. Consequently, they consented to arthroscopic ankle arthrodesis with the option of an open procedure if the repair could not be executed arthroscopically. Each case was thought to be a technically successful attempt at arthroscopic ankle

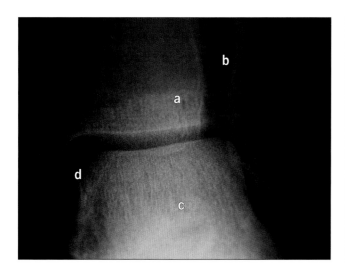

Figure 19-9. Preoperative radiograph of right ankle with diastasis, showing the tibia (*a*), fibula (*b*), talus (*c*), and diastasis (*d*).

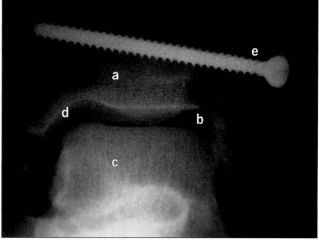

Figure 19-10. Postoperative radiograph of corrected diastasis, showing the tibia (*a*), fibula (*b*), talus (*c*), closure of medial tibial talar defect (*d*), and syndesmosis screw (*e*).

arthrodesis. Only one patient, not included in this series, had an open ankle fusion due to severe arthrofibrosis and a lack of an identifiable joint at the time of surgery.

Arthroscopic Technique

Before surgery, patients receive either spinal or general anesthesia. The anatomic ankle landmarks are clearly delineated with a marking pencil prior to prepping and draping of the extremity. While a traction device is attached to the operating room table, distraction is applied through a soft-tissue distraction strap (Fig. 19-11). There are a variety of commercially available ankle distraction devices that, along with a dorsal containment strap, grasp the superior component of the calcaneus.

Approximately 23 to 25 lbs of traction is applied in a longitudinal axis during the procedure. A knee holder and tourniquet are used for counter traction. Just prior to the surgical procedure, the tourniquet is elevated. After the traction device is applied, the foot of the table is dropped approximately 30° to allow the ankle to remain in a suspended position. Because of the design of the strap, the ability to dorsiflex and plantarflex the ankle is maintained. This facilitates easy access to a number of areas in the ankle.

Approximately 5 to 10 cc of sterile normal saline is instilled into the ankle joint. While a small stab wound is made with a #11 blade over the anteromedial portal, a hemostat is used to bluntly dissect down to the capsule, carefully spreading in a longitudinal axis. The capsule is entered with a dull trocar, and a 2.7-mm wide angle arthroscope is introduced. A 4-mm arthroscope may be used later if the joint expands readily enough to accept it. The arthroscope may be placed into the anterolateral or anteromedial portal, depending upon the surgeon's preference. The authors prefer to use the anteromedial portal initially for viewing because the notch of Hardy provides more room for the arthroscope. This is a two-portal technique, so no accessory portal is established. Generally, a pump is used for fluid and pressure control, but the posterolateral portal may be used for additional drainage. Generous portals allow free-flowing fluid to naturally decompress the joint when the pressure has reached 30 to 35 mm Hg. Fluid extravasation is rare, but the development of a compartment syndrome is possible, so care must be taken when using a pump.

For better visualization, a synovial or full-radius resector blade is used to debride reactive synovium. Resection of the anterior osteophytes of the tibia and talus is achieved with a notchplasty blade or burr. The anterior osteophytes are removed to reduce anterior impingement and to allow full restitution of a neutral position of the tibiotalar joint at the end of the procedure. Failure to do this inhibits access during the procedure and is likely to result in booking of the posterior tibiotalar joint.

Motorized instrumentation or a radiofrequency ablation device is used to denude all the residual articular cartilage, and a motorized burr or notchplasty blade is used to remove 1 to 2 mm of subchondral bone, exposing the soft cancellous bone and vascular bed. Multiple straight and angled curettes are used to debride the medial and lateral gutters, the posterior tibial plafond, and posterior talus (Fig. 19-12). For better visualization, large osseous cartilaginous fragments may be irrigated from the joint with a large suction cannula.

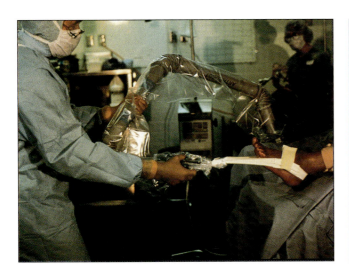

Figure 19-11. Operating room set-up showing the traction device and ankle strap.

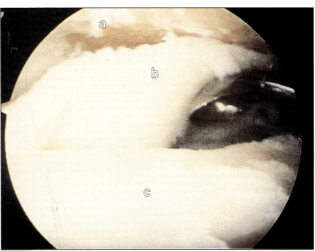

Figure 19-12. Intraoperative debridement of surfaces of ankle joint showing the tibia (*a*), fibula (*b*), and talus (*c*).

When the final phase of alignment has been reached, it is critical to maintain the normal architecture of the tibiotalar joint for better coaptation of the surfaces. It is also extremely important to denude the medial and lateral gutters for better coaptation and seating of the tibial and talar surfaces. The "spot-weld" technique establishes vascularity in the tibial and talar surfaces by creating multiple small holes of 2 to 3 mm in depth with a motorized burr or notchplasty blade. This gives the surgeon a chance to directly visualize the vascularity of both of these areas and to view the blood supply directly when the tourniquet is released.

After the spot-welding technique is completed, the joint is irrigated with copious amounts of normal saline and antibiotic solution. The tourniquet is released, and the joint is observed to ensure that sufficient bleeding of the surfaces has been obtained. Fixation is achieved by holding the ankle in the desired alignment while the first guidewire is placed from the medial border of the tibia directly into the talus approximately 3 to 4 cm above the joint line. The position should be checked with fluoroscopy, and care should be taken to not violate the subtalar joint or to protrude excessively through the soft tissues distally. Appropriate measurements are taken, and two cannulated screws are placed over the guidewires from superomedial to anterolateral. Again, the position of the screws is checked under fluoroscopy to guarantee a neutral position. Initially, a three-screw and crossed-screw system were used early in the development of this technique, but two parallel oblique screws have been used for fixation for the past 6 years without any untoward results (Fig. 19-13).

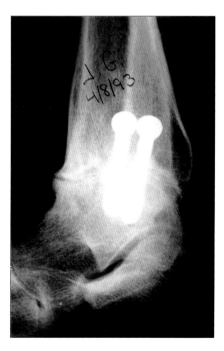

Figure 19-13. Fixation of arthroscopic ankle fusion with two cannulated cancellous screws.

It is common to see a slight tibiotalar gap fluoroscopically and on early radiographs. Early weight bearing should be encouraged, since it fosters coaptation of the two surfaces. This happens fairly rapidly, and surface-to-surface opposition is present in about 3 weeks. As long as the appropriate alignment has been achieved, the surgeon should not be concerned by this gap.

The fusion and portal sites are injected with 20 cc of 0.25% bupivacaine hydrochloride without epinephrine. The wounds are not sutured, but instead are covered with Steri-Strips in order to encourage drainage. A sterile bulky dressing and a bi-valved cast are applied. Postoperative oral medications are used for pain control and 24-hour antibiotic coverage. When stable, the patient is discharged from the outpatient surgery center site. Partial weight bearing with crutches is begun immediately.

Approximately 5 to 7 days postoperatively, the cast is removed, and a custom ankle and foot orthosis (AFO) brace is applied. Full weight bearing is encouraged immediately. The AFO permits bathing and immediate shoe wearing, enhances proprioception, and reduces stress deprivation. It also allows the patient to begin a modified isometric and range-of-motion exercise program. The patient is followed up clinically and radiographically at 2-to 3-week intervals until union has been established. As soon as tolerated, return to work on a modified basis without crutches and full weight bearing on the affected extremity are allowed. The screws are removed only if the patient develops an adverse reaction. Less than 15% of the screws have been removed to date.

Results

The mean follow-up time was 4.2 years (range, 7–96 months). The average time until union was 10.8 weeks. The average hospital stay was 28 hours; however, all patients in the private setting were treated on an outpatient basis. Forty-three of the 49 patients had an uneventful union. There were three patients with delayed union and three patients with nonunion. The three cases of delayed union consisted of two patients with neurologic disorders and one patient with immunosuppression and rheumatoid arthritis. The cases of nonunion represented one patient with avascular necrosis of the talus, one patient with post-traumatic degenerative arthritis, and one patient with a neurologic disorder.

The fusion rate was 96% in the subset of patients with osteoarthritis, rheumatoid arthritis, and post-traumatic arthritis. Delayed union and nonunion were more prevalent in patients with a neurologic defect, immunosuppression, and rheumatoid arthritis with poor osteogenic capabilities. These predisposing factors have been reported in the open ankle arthrodesis literature as well [44–46].

Two patients elected to have a reoperation and successfully underwent open fusion. There were no significant surgical complications in these patients and no significant perioperative morbidity. One patient developed a tarsal tunnel syndrome from excessive swelling around the ankle. This patient eventually had a nonunion. One patient with a neurologic deficit developed a Charcot joint with hypertrophic bone. She was asymptomatic and eventually had some of the excessive bone removed. Seven patients had their screws removed. One patient had persistent pain at his fusion site; the site was explored by another surgeon and found to have a full union. There were no superficial or deep infections in any patients.

Arthroscopic ankle arthrodesis has been described in the literature on a number of occasions, and most series have been able to demonstrate significant advantages with a probable increase in the fusion rate, along with a variety of other advantages. Over an 8-year period, the authors' experience has led to the conclusion that the procedure has a significant reduction in the complication rate compared with procedures discussed in the earlier literature. In addition, the procedure has certainly been well accepted by patients, with a significant reduction in postoperative pain and a much earlier return to function.

The authors have isolated a high-risk group in the series that has been identified as patients who are neurologically compromised, immunosuppressed, have rheumatoid arthritis (and therefore poor osteogenic potential), and are smokers. In the future, these patients may benefit from supplemental bone graft or the use of osteoinductive and osteoconductive materials.

ARTHROSCOPIC SUBTALAR ARTHRODESIS

Operative procedures designed for subtalar fusion have been in existence for nearly 90 years. In 1905, Nieny performed the first subtalar arthrodesis. There have been numerous techniques reported in the literature [47–55] that have used both intra-articular and extra-articular methods. Results have generally been favorable, with a variety of complications reported [56–58]. Data on rate of union, time until union, complications, and long-term follow-up are noticeably missing in the older and the more recent literature. A number of other procedures for subtalar pathology have been described, including arthroscopy, arthroplasty, triple arthrodesis, and sinus tarsi exploration. Surgical open reduction of calcaneal fractures has gained acceptance for attempts at restoring the normal anatomical alignment of the joint surfaces. This is an effort to avoid the sequelae of post-traumatic degenerative arthritis of the subtalar joint. However, both operative and conservative care of calcaneal fractures continue to be plagued with long-term symptomatic degenerative changes in the subtalar joint.

Arthroscopic subtalar arthrodesis (ASTA) as a surgical procedure was developed in 1992 and first reported at the Arthroscopy Association of North America's 1994 Annual Meeting in a preliminary review. The procedure was designed to improve traditional methods by using a microinvasive technique. The decision to proceed with this surgical technique grew out of the success with arthroscopic ankle arthrodesis [59]. ASTA has been described by a number of authors, but no reported cases or attempts at arthroscopic subtalar fusion have been published [60]. Recent work by Solis (Personal communication, 1996) has paralleled some of the authors' earlier work.

The development of an arthroscopic technique was intended to yield less morbidity if it could be performed using the same techniques and principles as those used in arthroscopic ankle fusion. It was hypothesized that perioperative morbidity could be reduced, blood supply preserved, and proprioceptive and neurosensory input enhanced. A prospective study was initiated to document the effectiveness of the procedure and to determine the time until complete fusion, the incidence of delayed and nonunion, and the prevalence of complications.

Indications and Work-up

The indications for ASTA are intractable subtalar pain secondary to rheumatoid arthritis, osteoarthritis, and post-traumatic arthritis. Other indications include neuropathic conditions, gross instability, paralytic conditions, and posterior tibial tendon rupture. Most of the earlier literature in subtalar surgery was centered around the stabilization of paralytic deformities secondary to poliomyelitis. The majority of patients encountered today who require this procedure have post-traumatic and arthritic disorders.

To qualify for arthroscopic subtalar fusion, patients must have failed conservative management. Conservative treatment includes a variety of modalities, including orthotics, use of NSAIDs, activity modification, and occasional cortisone injections into the subtalar joint. They must also be apprised of the possibility of requiring an open procedure if this technique is not technically feasible.

The patient's history is usually one of lateral hindfoot pain, which can be confused quite easily with ankle pathology. Increased symptoms with weight bearing on uneven ground is a classic complaint.

History of a previous calcaneal fracture should immediately alert one to the possibility of subtalar pathology. The clinical findings consist of pain over the sinus tarsi and the posterolateral subtalar joint. They also report a reproduction of the symptoms on inversion and eversion of the subtalar joint with the ankle locked in dorsiflexion

The clinical work-up for this patient profile is quite simple. Often a good history and physical examination, confirmed by plain radiographs, will be sufficient to confirm the diagnosis. On occasion, CT or plain tomography scans may be necessary [61]. There is little need for an MRI scan or arthrography [62]. Differential injections continue to be a valuable diagnostic aid to confirm as well as separate out ankle pain from subtalar pain. Radiographic changes do not have to show profound degenerative changes, since only small alterations in the biomechanics of this joint can produce significant symptoms.

The contraindications to this procedure are previously failed subtalar fusions, gross malalignment requiring correction, infection, and significant bone loss. On occasion, a patient with gross malalignment will be a candidate for *in situ* stabilization. Significant bone loss has not been encountered frequently, and it has not presented a serious problem in a series of arthroscopic ankle arthrodesis [59].

Each procedure was done in an ambulatory surgical center environment, and each patient was discharged on the same day. The only exception to this was the occasional patient who was treated at the Veterans Administration Hospital affiliated with the authors' teaching institution [63]. Because of the use of internal fixation, patients were given preoperative, intraoperative, and postoperative antibiotics for a total of three doses. General anesthesia was used in the majority of the cases.

Arthroscopic Technique

The patient is placed in the lateral decubitus position, lying on the unaffected side. Two pillows are placed between the legs while the affected ankle and subtalar joint are allowed to hang over a blanket roll in a natural position of plantarflexion and inversion. After thoroughly prepping and draping the patient, anatomical landmarks and portal sites are identified and marked with a surgical pen. The tourniquet is then elevated. In general, the operative procedure is completed within one tourniquet time (1 hour and 45 minutes).

Establishing the portal sites is one of the more difficult portions of the procedure. To determine an accurate location for the anterolateral portal, the surgeon places his thumb in the sinus tarsi while attempting to invert and evert the subtalar joint. The portal is in line with the tip of the fibula, approximately 1 cm distal to the anterior border of the fibula (Fig. 19-14). The needle is placed slightly posterior to the sinus tarsi and angled cephalad 20° to 30° and posteromedially approximately 45°. The posterolateral portal is approximately 1 cm superior to the tip and 1 cm posterior to the border of the fibula. This portal may be established at this time, but can also be established under direct visualization after the arthroscope is placed in the anterolateral portal through transillumination. It is critical to predetermine the angles of the subtalar joint because its unique geometry and limited access leave little room for error (Fig. 19-15). If necessary, the surgeon should not hesitate to use fluoroscopy to confirm portal location.

These are the two conventional portals. If necessary, an accessory portal may be established approximately 1 cm posterior to the anterolateral portal. This portal can be used for debridement or for flow or

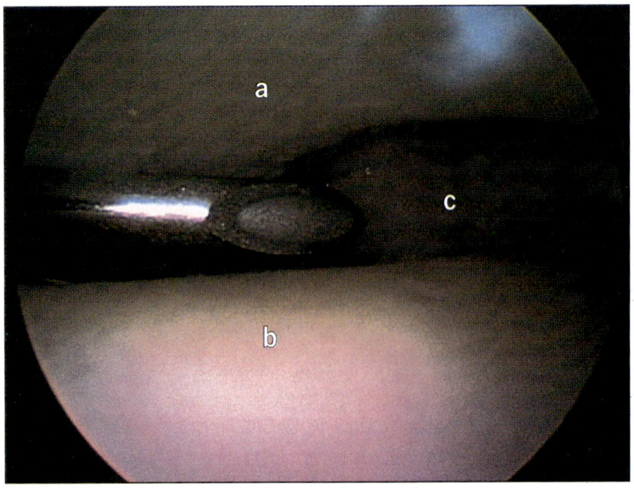

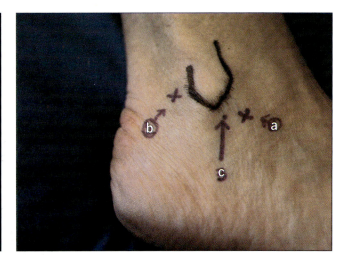

Figure 19-14. Portal sites for subtalar arthrodesis: the anterolateral portal (*a*), posterolateral portal (*b*), and accessory lateral portal (*c*).

Figure 19-15. Arthroscopic view of a right posterior subtalar joint showing the talus (*a*), calcaneus (*b*), and posteromedial corner (*c*).

drainage enhancement. It cannot be used for visualization. During the procedure, both the anterolateral and posterolateral portals are used in an alternating fashion for viewing and for instrumentation. Occasionally, there is significant arthrofibrosis present, making entry and visualization difficult. In these cases, the accessory anterolateral portal is quite useful. The arthroscope used for this procedure should be a 2.7-mm, wide-angled, shortened small-joint arthroscope. It should be equipped with a choice of sheaths to accommodate limited or increased flow. The blunt trocar and sheath is introduced through the anterolateral portal; the posterolateral portal can be established at this time. In the initial cases, a small laminar spreader was used in the anterolateral portal to increase access. This was later abandoned as a routine, but may still be used if distraction is a significant problem. Arthroscopic resection of the interosseous ligament may also be used for additional distraction, but has not been used to date by the authors.

It is important to be absolutely certain that the arthroscope is in the subtalar joint and that the ankle joint or the fibular talar recess have not been inadvertently entered. All debridement and decortication are done posterior to the interosseous ligament because only the posterior facet is fused. The middle and anterior facets are not visualized under normal circumstances unless the interosseous ligament is absent. The majority of the procedure is done with the arthroscope in the anterolateral portal and the instruments in the posterolateral portal. The remaining and final debridement is done by alternating between these two portals.

A primary synovectomy and debridement is necessary for visualization, as is done with other joints. The articular surface is debrided, which makes the joint more capacious, making instrumentation easier. Complete removal of the articular surface down to subchondral bone is the next phase of the procedure (Fig. 19-16). The talocalcaneal geometry is quite unique and requires a variety of instruments. In general, multiangular curettes and a complete set of burrs are sufficient.

After the articular cartilage has been resected, approximately 1 to 2 mm of subchondral bone is removed to expose the highly vascular cancellous bone. Care must be taken not to alter the geometry and not to remove excessive bone; this will lead to poor coaptation of the joint surfaces. After the subchondral plate is removed, small "spot-weld" holes measuring approximately 2 mm in depth are created on the surfaces of the calcaneus and talus to create vascular channels. Careful assessment of the posteromedial corner must be made, since residual bone and cartilage can be left there, which can interfere with coaptation. Often the curette will safely break down

this corner and provide the surgeon with additional tactile feedback. The neurovascular bundle is directly posteromedial and has to be taken into consideration and protected at all times.

After visualization from both portals to ensure complete debridement and decortication, the tourniquet is released, and careful assessment of the vascularity of the calcaneus and talus is made. The joint is then thoroughly irrigated of bone fragments and debris. No autogenous bone graft or bone substitute is needed for this procedure.

The fixation of the fusion is done with a large cannulated 7.0 screw. The guide pin is started at the dorsal anteromedial talus and angled posterior and inferior to the posterolateral calcaneus, but does not violate the calcaneal cortical surface. Under fluoroscopy, the guidewire is placed with the ankle in maximum dorsiflexion to avoid any possible screw head encroachment or impingement on the anterior lip of the tibia. After the guidewire is placed under these conditions, the ankle can be relaxed, the screw inserted under fluoroscopic control, and the fusion site compressed. When using this technique, the screw runs along the natural axis of rotation of the subtalar joint. Starting the screw from the dorsal and medial aspect of the talus avoids painful screw-head prominence over the calcaneus and prevents the need for a second procedure for screw removal. To date, there have been no fractures or complications with this particular fixation technique (Figs. 19-17 and 19-18).

Steri-Strips are used instead of sutures to allow adequate drainage. A bulky dressing and a short leg bi-valve cast are applied. The patient is discharged after appropriate circulatory checks in the recovery

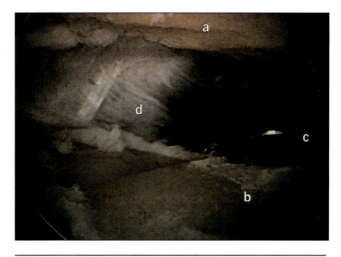

Figure 19-16. Posterior subtalar joint viewed from the posterolateral portal showing the talus (*a*), calcaneus (*b*), sinus tarsi (*c*), and interosseus ligament (*d*).

room. The first clinical evaluation takes place in the office within 48 hours. In approximately 1 week, the cast is removed, and the patient is fitted immediately with an AFO if the swelling is minimal. Full weight bearing is allowed as tolerated at any time following surgery. In general, patients can tolerate full weight bearing without crutch support within 7 to 14 days after surgery. Although patients wear the AFO almost 24 hours a day, they are able to bathe and to take the ankle and foot through a range of motion without the brace. The AFO is removed when full union has been achieved. The standard three views of the ankle plus a Browden view are the radiographs of choice used in follow-up assessment.

Results

Since September of 1992, 18 patients have undergone arthroscopic subtalar fusion with sufficient follow-up time to determine the effectiveness of this procedure. Fusion rate, time until complete union, surgical technique, and complications were analyzed. One standard surgical procedure was used, and the method of internal fixation was not altered during this entire series. The posterior subtalar joint was the only joint fused during this procedure. Three of the 18 patients underwent a combined arthroscopic ankle and subtalar fusion. In this series, there were eight patients with osteoarthritis, eight patients with posttraumatic arthritis, and two with rheumatoid arthritis.

Every patient had a radiographic evaluation at 2-week intervals to determine the rate and quality of fusion. For an arthrodesis to be considered completely fused, it requires both clinical and radiographic support. The parameters required for a successful arthrodesis are evidence of bone consolidation across the subtalar joint, no motion at the screw, the clinical absence of pain with weight bearing, and pain-free forced inversion and eversion. The average mean follow up time is 22

months (range, 6–54 months). In this series, there was clinical and radiographic evidence of union in all 18 patients. The average time until complete fusion was 8.9 weeks (range, 6–16 weeks).

There are considerable advantages to this technique when compared with open procedures. It is a minimally invasive technique that theoretically preserves the blood supply of the calcaneous and talus. This is especially important, considering many of these patients have had previous invasive surgery. Conventional open procedures by definition interrupt the blood supply and compromise vascular ingrowth and eventual fusion. Avoidance of incisions, along with early range of motion and weight bearing, helps to avoid stress deprivation and enhance proprioception, therefore reducing the devastating effects of reflex sympathetic dystrophy.

There were no reoperations, with the exception of one screw removal. One patient had a painful screw at the calcaneus where the screw penetrated the cortex, and the possibility of a stress fracture was considered. Symptoms resolved after screw removal. Two patients had some residual anterolateral pain with some radiographic changes and clinical evidence of minor DJD in the ankle. Both patients responded with complete relief to a diagnostic lidocaine hydrochloride injection into the ankle joint. Valgus tilting of the ankle joint following subtalar arthrodesis has been reported, but it is unclear if this is secondary to the fusion or merely a natural progression of the disease [64]. Two cases not included in this series could not be completed arthroscopically because of significant malformation of the calcaneus and arthrofibrosis of the subtalar joint. These patients underwent a modified mini-open posterior subtalar arthrodesis. Identical screw fixation and postoperative protocol were used in these two patients. Skin problems around the hindfoot can be catastrophic and are obviously avoided using this technique. There were no superficial or deep infections in this series. All

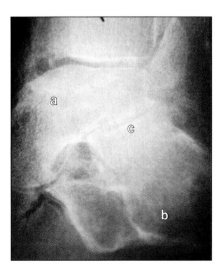

Figure 19-17. Browden view of an arthritic posterior subtalar joint showing the talus (*a*), calcaneus (*b*), and subtalar joint (*c*).

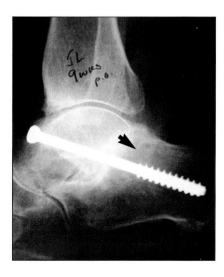

Figure 19-18. Lateral radiograph of a fused subtalar joint with a single cancellous screw across the posterior facet (*arrow*).

arthroscopic procedures have had reported reductions in infection, and one would hope this procedure would also fall into that same category. There have not been sufficient cases, however, to validate this hypothesis.

Most open series show a longer time until union, with some prevalence of nonunions. Although too early to validate, preliminary observations indicate a more rapid time until union, as well as an increased rate of union. There has been a paucity of literature on isolated subtalar arthrodesis with adequate follow-up statistics over the past 25 years.

fore, at this stage, this must be considered an *in situ* fusion. The learning curve is certainly much steeper because of the smaller patient population available for enhancing surgical skills.

Overall, this procedure has stood the test of time and follow-up. The results appear to be excellent in terms of patient satisfaction, fusion rate, time until union, and postoperative morbidity. The recognition and enhancement of this technique and the development of more advanced technology will certainly allow this ASTA technique to improve and be used more often in the future.

Conclusion

Arthroscopic subtalar arthrodesis is a technically demanding procedure that requires some rather advanced arthroscopic skills to perform [65]. Joint access is tight, restricted, and requires small instrumentation. Deformities cannot be corrected; there-

ACKNOWLEDGMENT

The authors would like thank Debbie King, ATC, for her assistance in the production and editing of this manuscript. Thank you also to the Alvarado Hospital Health Foundation, San Diego, for their financial assistance in the form of a grant.

REFERENCES AND RECOMMENDED READING

Recently published papers of particular interest have been highlighted as:
• Of interest
•• Of outstanding interest

1. Brostrom L: Sprained ankles. *Acta Chir Scand* 1964, 128:483–495.

2. Johannsen A: Radiological diagnosis of lateral ligament lesions of the ankle. *Acta Orthop Scand* 1978, 49:295–301.

3. Seligson D, Gassman J, Pope M: Ankle instability: evaluation of the lateral ligaments. *Am J Sports Med* 1980, 8:39–42.

4. Schafer D, Hentermann B: Arthroscopic assessment of the chronic unstable joint. Knee surgery, sports traumatology. *Arthroscopy* 1996, 4:48–52.

5. Kibler WB: Arthroscopic findings in ankle ligament reconstruction. *Clin Sports Med* 1996, 15:799–804.

6. Lundeen RO: Ankle arthroscopy in the adolescent patient. *J Foot Ankle Surg* 1990, 29:510–515.

7. Taga I, Shino K, *et al.*: Articular cartilage lesions in ankles with lateral ligament injury. *Am J Sports Med* 1993, 21:120–126.

8. Cooke: Paper presented at the Combined Meeting on Foot and Ankle Surgery. Dublin, Ireland; 1995.

9. Hawkins RB: Arthroscopic stapling repair for chronic lateral instability. *Clin Podiatr Med Surg* 1987, 4:875–883.

10. Stiehl JB: Complex ankle fracture dislocations with syndesmotic diastasis. *Orthop Rev* 1990, 14:499–507.

11. Taylor DC, Englehardt DL, Bassett FH: Syndesmosis sprains of the ankle. *Am J Sports Med* 1992, 20:146–150.

12. Fritschy D: An unusual ankle injury in top skiers. *Am J Sports Med* 1989, 17:282–285.

13. Hopkinson WJ, St. Pierre P, Ryan JB, Wheeler JH: Syndesmosis sprains of the ankle. *Foot Ankle Int* 1990, 10:325–330.

14. Cedell C: Ankle lesions. *Acta Orthop Scand* 1975, 46:425–445.

15. Edwards GS, DeLee JC: Ankle diastasis without fracture. *Foot Ankle Int* 1984, 4:305–312.

16. Marymont JV, Lynch MA, Henning CE: Acute ligamentous diastasis of the ankle without fracture. *Am J Sports Med* 1986, 14:407–409.

17. Ogilvie-Harris DJ, Reed SC: Disruption of the ankle syndesmosis: diagnosis and treatment by arthroscopic surgery. *Arthroscopy* 1994, 10:561–568.

18. Katznelson A, Lin E, Militiano J: Ruptures of the ligaments about the tibiofibular syndesmosis. *Injury* 1983, 15:170–172.

19. Chen YJ, Huang TJ, Shih HN, *et al.*: Ankle arthrodesis with cross screw fixation. *Acta Orthop Scand* 1996, 67:473–478.

20. Braly WG, Baker JK, Tullos HS: Arthrodesis of the ankle with lateral plating. *Foot Ankle Int* 1994, 15:649–653.

21. Stranks GJ, Cecil T, Jeffery IT: Anterior ankle arthrodesis with cross-screw fixation. *J Bone Joint Surg Br* 1994 76:943–946.

22. Dohm M, Purdy BA, Benjamin J: Primary union of ankle arthrodesis: review of a single institution/multiple surgeon experience. *Foot Ankle Int* 1994, 15:293–296.

23. Mann RA, Van Manen JW, Wapner K, Martin J: Ankle fusion. *Clin Orthop* 1991, 268:49–55.

24. Morgan CD, Henke JA, Bailey RW, Kaufer H: Long-term results of tibiotalar arthrodesis. *J Bone Joint Surg Am* 1985, 67:546–550.

25. Boobbyer GN: The long-term results of ankle arthrodesis. *Acta Orthop Scand*, 1981, 52:107–10.

26. Crosby LA, Yee TC, Formanek TS, Fitzgibbons TC: Complications following arthroscopic ankle arthrodesis. *Foot Ankle Int* 1996, 17:340–342.

27. Frey C, Halikus NM, Vu-Rose T, Ebramzadeh E: A review of ankle arthrodesis: predisposing factors to nonunion. *Foot Ankle Int* 1994, 15:581–584.

28. Cobb TK, Gabrielsen TA, Campbell DC II, *et al.*: Cigarette smoking and nonunion after ankle arthrodesis. *Foot Ankle Int* 1994, 15:64–67.

29. Moran CG, Pinder IM, Smith SR: Ankle arthrodesis in rheumatoid arthritis. *Acta Orthop Scand* 1991, 62:538–543.

30. Helm R: The results of ankle arthrodesis. *J Bone Joint Surg Br* 1990, 71:141–143.

31. Lynch AF, Bourne RB, Rorabeck CH: The long-term results of ankle arthrodesis. *J Bone Joint Surg Br* 1988, 70:113–116.

32. Hagen RJ: Ankle arthrodesis: problems and pitfalls. *Clin Orthop* 1986, 202:152–162.

33. Paremain GD, Miller SD, Myerson MS: Ankle arthrodesis: results after the miniarthrotomy technique. *Foot Ankle Int* 1996, 17:247–252.

34. Miller SD, Paremain GP, Myerson MS: The miniarthrotomy technique of ankle arthrodesis: a cadaver study of operative vascular compromise and early clinical results. *Orthopedics* 1996, 19:425–430.

35. Jerosch J, Steinbeck J, Schroder M, Reer R: Arthroscopically assisted arthrodesis of the ankle joint. *Arch Orthop Trauma Surg* 1996, 115:182–189.

36. Glick JM, Morgan CD, Myerson MS, *et al.*: Ankle arthrodesis using an arthroscopic method. *Arthroscopy* 1996, 12:428–434.

37. Turan I, Wredmark T, Fellander-Tsai L: Arthroscopic ankle arthrodesis in rheumatoid arthritis. *Clin Orthop* 1995, 320:110–114.

38. Corso SJ, Zimmer TJ: Technique and clinical evaluation of arthroscopic ankle arthrodesis. *Arthroscopy* 1995, 11:585–590.

39. Myerson MS, Quill G: Ankle arthrodesis. *Clin Orthop* 1991, 268:84–95.

40. Ogilvie-Harris DJ, Fitsialos D, Hedman TP: Arthrodesis of the ankle. *Clin Orthop* 1994, 304:195–199.

41. Dohm MP, Benjamin JB, Harrison J, Szivek JA: A biomechanical evaluation of three forms of internal fixation used in ankle arthrodesis. *Foot Ankle Int* 1994, 15:297–300.

42. Thordarson DB, Markolf K, Cracchiolo A III: Stability of an ankle arthrodesis fixed by cancellous-bone screws compared with that fixed by an external fixator: a biomechanical study. *J Bone Joint Surg Am* 1992, 74:1050–1055.

43. Holt ES, Hansen ST, Mayo KA, Sangeorzan BJ: Ankle arthrodesis using internal screw fixation. *Clin Orthop* 1991, 268:21–28.

44. Alvarez RG, Barbour TM, Perkins TD: Tibiocalcaneal arthrodesis for nonbraceable neuropathic ankle deformity. *Foot Ankle Int* 1994, 15:354–359.

45. Papa J, Myerson M, Girard P: Salvage, with arthrodesis, in intractable diabetic neuropathic arthropathy of the foot and ankle. *J Bone Joint Surg Am* 1993, 75:1056–1066.

46. Shibata T, Tada K, Hashizume C: The results of arthrodesis of the ankle for leprotic neuroarthropathy. *J Bone Joint Surg Am* 1990, 72:749–756.

47. Thomas FB: Arthrodesis of the subtalar joint. *J Bone Joint Surg* 1967, 1:93–97.

48. Dick IL: Primary fusion of the posterior subtalar joint and the treatment of fractures of the calcaneus. *J Bone Joint Surg* 1953, 35:375.

49. Gallie WE: Subastragalar arthrodesis and fractures of the os calcis. *J Bone Joint Surg* 1943, 25:731.

50. Grice DS: An extra-articular arthrodesis of the subastragalar joint for correction of paralytic flat feet in children. *J Bone Joint Surg* 1952, 34:927.

51. Grice DS: Further experience with extra-articular arthrodesis of the subtalar joint. *J Bone Joint Surg* 1955, 37:246.

52. Hall MC, Pennal GF: Primary subtalar arthrodesis in the treatment of severe fractures of the calcaneus. *J Bone Joint Surg* 1960, 42:336.

53. Geckler EO: Comminuted fractures of the os calcis. *Arch Surg* 1943, 61:469.

54. Harris RI: Fractures of the os calcis. *Ann Surg* 1946, 124:1082.

55. Wilson PD: Treatment of fractures of the os calcis by arthrodesis of the subtalar joint. *JAMA* 1927, 89:1676.

56. Gross RH: A clinical study of bachelor subtalar arthrodesis. *J Bone Joint Surg* 1976, 58:343–349.

57. Mallon WJ, Nunley JA: The Grice procedure, extra-articular subtalar arthrodesis. *Orthop Clin North Am* 1989, 20:649–654.

58. Moreland Jr, Westin GW: Further experience with Grice subtalar arthrodesis. *Clin Orthop* 1986, 207:113–121.

59. Tasto JP: Arthroscopic ankle arthrodesis: a seven year followup. San Diego, CA: American Academy of Orthopaedic Surgery; February, 1997.

60. Ferkel RA: *Arthroscopic Surgery: The Foot & Ankle.* Philadelphia: Lippincott-Raven; 1996.

61. Seltzer SE, Weisman B: CT of the hindfoot with rheumatoid arthritis. *J Arthritis Rheumatol* 1985, 28:12–42.

62. Goosens M: Posterior subtalar joint arthrography: a useful tool in the diagnosis of hindfoot disorders. *Clin Orthop* 1989, 266:248–255.

63. Thomas FB: Arthrodesis of the subtalar joint. *J Bone and Joint Surg* 1967, 1:93–97.

64. Fitzgibbons: Valgus tilting of the ankle joint following subtalar arthrodesis. Paper presented at the International Society of Foot and Ankle Surgery. Dublin, Ireland; August 1995.

65. Tasto JP: Arthroscopic subtalar arthrodesis. In *Foot & Ankle Arthroscopy.* New York: Springer-Verlag; in press.

20
CHAPTER

Arthroscopic Management of Pyarthrosis

HOWARD J. LUKS AND J. SERGE PARISIEN

In 1743, Hunter [1] gave the first description of the pathologic changes that occur when articular cartilage is subject to insult by microbacterial pathogens. The offending agent in the clinical sequelae was not identified until 1924, when Phemister [2] demonstrated the effects of proteolytic enzymes, or "digestive ferments," on articular cartilage. Phemister discovered that the enzymes responsible for destruction of articular cartilage were released by the polymorphonuclear leukocytes present in the environment and not by the bacteria themselves. In 1959, Lack [3] suggested that an increase in plasmin found in the synovial fluid led to destruction of the articular cartilage protein. Van de Loo and van den Berg [4] and Williams *et al.* [5] have demonstrated that in septic arthritis, destruction of articular cartilage is heralded by a profound loss of proteoglycans from both the matrix and the chondrocytes. According to these authors, this loss results from decreased production as well as increased destruction of proteoglycans found in articular cartilage. The metalloproteinase class of enzymes produced within the afflicted joint is responsible for the changes seen in the proteoglycan content of articular cartilage. The production of metalloproteinases (collagenase and neutral protease) by the synovial tissue and the chondrocytes is stimulated by interleukin-1 (IL-1), which is released by the activated mononuclear cells in the infectious environment. After destruction of the cartilaginous matrix, collagen destruction ensues, followed by mechanical and further chemical degradation, resulting in a severely afflicted arthritic joint.

CLINICAL PICTURES

Pyarthrosis may result from direct inoculation of the joint by a puncture wound, laceration, or surgical procedure. It may also be secondary to hematogenous spread from a distant septic focus. The most common offending organisms cultured are gram-positive organisms, such as *Staphylococcus aureus* and *Streptococci*. Gram-negative organisms, such as *Haemophilus influenza*, *Escherichia coli*, and *Pseudomonas aeruginosa* may also cause pyarthrosis, especially among intravenous drug abusers.

Most patients with nongonococcal bacterial arthritis present with only a single joint involved, although 20% to 25% of cases may be polyarticular in nature. The knee joint is most commonly affected. In the polyarticular form, three to four joints are usually affected; such patients frequently have coexisting rheumatologic disease.

There are several predisposing factors that contribute to the risk of developing pyarthrosis. Human immunodeficiency virus (HIV) infection, the presence of a prosthesis in a joint, sickle cell anemia, diabetes mellitus, metastatic carcinoma, intravenous drug abuse, and rheumatoid arthritis all increase the risk of developing an infection within a joint.

Most patients with pyarthrosis present with systemic symptoms, including fevers and chills. Incapacitating pain with joint motion is the most common local sign. The diagnosis of bacterial arthritis is based on a high index of suspicion, which leads to analysis of the synovial fluid from the affected joint. In an immunocompetent host, a leukocyte count greater than 100,000 cells per mL, and a glucose level below the serum level strongly suggest the presence of an infection. Aerobic and anaerobic joint fluid and blood cultures should be obtained at the time of synovial fluid analysis. In complicated cases, a 99-Technetium bone scan in combination with leukocyte-labeled gallium or indium scan can be used to identify an infected joint prosthesis or a distant infectious focus. Early in the course of pyarthrosis, plain radiographs usually show a normal situation but may also reveal subchondral rarefaction, soft-tissue swelling, or localized erosions as the process progresses. Narrowing of the joint space and severe degenerative changes are noted only in advanced cases.

ARTHROSCOPIC MANAGEMENT

Successful management of patients with acute pyarthrosis requires prompt drainage of the purulent material, institution of appropriate antimicrobial therapy, and the beginning of early range-of-motion (ROM) exercises. Nord *et al.* [6••] found that open or arthroscopic drainage was not necessary if the pyarthrosis was addressed with appropriate antibiotics within 72 hours after inoculation. As Nord *et al.* appropriately point out, most clinical presentations occur later than that; therefore, additional study is necessary to delineate the effectiveness of using only antibiotics in infections that have been present longer than 72 hours. Antibiotics alone have been proven to be ineffective in established cases of pyarthrosis in rabbits [7]. Articular aspiration or continuous drainage may not always be appropriate in long-standing cases of pyarthrosis. Loculations within the joint; fibrinous, synovial, or cartilaginous debris; and the presence of fibrous adhesions decrease the effectiveness of repeated needle aspirations. Arthrotomy carries with it significant morbidity in terms of a large dissection, greater postoperative discomfort, and an initially decreased ROM. Arthroscopy offers numerous advantages over arthrotomy and has been used successfully by several authors [8–12] to treat pyarthrosis of the knee, shoulder, ankle, and hip.

Jackson [8] reported on the successful use of the distention and irrigation technique in cases of pyarthrosis of the knee. Ivey [9] and Ivey and Clark [10] showed excellent results using debridement and suction drainage in 11 infected knees with an average follow-up time of 34 months. Smith [11] reported excellent (93.3%) to good (6.7%) results in 30 patients with pyarthrosis of the knee, which were managed arthroscopically. Skyhar and Mubarek [12] reported excellent results in 16 children with septic knee, with an average follow-up period of 36 months. Morbidity from the procedure was low, and recovery was rapid and complete. Only nine patients were place on continuous passive motion (CPM), because it was unavailable earlier in the series. Flood and Kolarik [13] had satisfactory results in two patients with infected total knee arthroplasty. These patients experienced a quick recovery of knee functions and ROM, and on follow-up (an average of 30 months), they were still pain-free and able to continue with their normal activities. Windsor [14], however, thought that arthroscopy had a limited role in the treatment of infected total knee replacement, owing in part to the difficulty of decompressing the posterior compartment. Thiery [15] conducted a multicenter study, through questionnaire, of 46 cases of septic knee treated by arthroscopic means, with an average follow-up period of 7.1 months. After articular lavage and antibiotic therapy (for a mean period of 2 months), results were excellent (78.3%), but with five (10.9%) failures due to persistent infection, and five (10.9%) recurrences. Of the failures, three were infected total joint replacements.

Stanitski *et al.* [16] reported the successful use of arthroscopy in acute septic pediatric knees. Of these 16 knees, 94% resulted from *S. aureus* infection. Foreign bodies were present in the joint in 25% of the patients. No postoperative irrigation or drainage was employed in this group of patients. With an average follow-up of 36.7 months, all patients had full active ROM of their knees without evidence of effusion, synovial thickening, or deformity. Intravenous antibiotics were used for an average of 10 days, followed by oral antibiotics for an additional 2 to 3 weeks in 75% of the patients.

In their series, Parisien and Shaffer [17] reported the treatment of 16 patients with pyarthrosis over a 10-year period, with an average follow-up time of 36 months. All patients were managed with antibiotic therapy, arthroscopic debridement, and the use of CPM, followed by intensive rehabilitation. All patients had excellent to good results.

D'Angelo and Ogilvie-Harris [18] successfully treated nine cases of septic arthritis following arthroscopy using repeat arthroscopy and a suction irrigation system combined with the appropriate antibiotics. Blitzer [19] reported the successful use of arthroscopy in combination with antimicrobial therapy to treat septic arthritis of the hip in four patients. Williams *et al.* [20•] have used arthroscopic techniques successfully in the management of septic arthritis after anterior cruciate reconstruction. Out of seven patients treated with arthroscopic debridement, intravenous antibiotics for 4 to 6 weeks, and protected weight bearing and physical therapy, six had minimal or no pain in their operative knee with satisfactory functional results at a mean follow-up of 29 months. Sanchez and Hennrikus [21•] have used the microjoint arthroscope successfully in the management of acute septic knees in infants (average age, 16 months).

TECHNIQUES

After proper positioning and sterile preparation with the patient under regional or general anesthesia, a large bore inflow sheath is inserted into the joint. The arthroscope is then placed through its sheath, and visualization of the joint is done. Stanitski *et al.* [16] found that 25% of the patients they treated had a foreign body within the knee joint. A thorough, systematic evaluation of the joint must be carried out in cases of a puncture wound or laceration to ensure that no foreign material remains within the joint. Any necrotic material is removed using a motorized shaver, and all loculations and adhesions are removed as they are encountered (Figs. 20-1 to 20-3).

As previously demonstrated by Nelson [22], addition of antibiotics to the irrigation fluid is unnecessary. A synovectomy is not performed routinely because it unnecessarily adds to surgical trauma and may limit attempts at postoperative motion. The joint is irrigated until the effluent is entirely clear, usually requiring 12 liters of fluid. Continuous saline irrigation fluid with two drains has been replaced by the use of a single drain through the anteromedial or anterolateral portal for 48 hours (Figs. 20-4 and 20-5). This postoperative closed-suction drainage is most likely mandatory in joints, such as the hip, that are susceptible to the effects to excess intra-articular pressure.

ANTIBIOTIC ADMINISTRATION

After physical examination of the patient and after the appropriate cultures have been made, intravenous antibiotics are immediately administered. Broad-spectrum cephalosporins may be used pending results of the Gram stain, with adjustment of the specific antibiotic as necessary. The antibiotic regimen can be adjusted

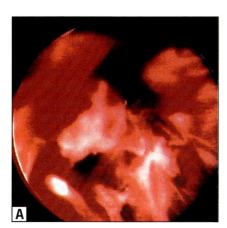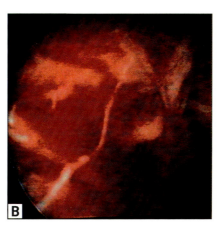

Figure 20-1. Arthroscopic views of necrotic synovium (**A**) and loculated debris (**B**) in pyarthrosis of the knee.

accordingly as the final culture and sensitivity data are evaluated by the surgeon or an infectious disease consultant. Although the practice remains controversial, intravenous antibiotics are generally continued for 10 days; if the patient has responded clinically and the sensitivity data support their use, oral antibiotics are then continued on an outpatient basis for an additional 3 to 4 weeks.

POSTOPERATIVE CARE

In an experimental investigation in the rabbit knee in 1981, Salter *et al.* [23] demonstrated the protective effect of CPM on living articular tissue in acute septic arthritis. For the knee, shoulder, and hip, CPM is begun immediately after surgery. Under the guidance of a physical therapist, active motion is encouraged, beginning on the first postoperative day and continuing until full ROM is achieved. Partial weight bearing, progressing to full weight bearing, is allowed.

CONCLUSION

When treated improperly or too late in its course, acute septic arthritis can cause irreversible damage to the articular cartilage or any synovial joint. Arthroscopic debridement of the acutely septic knee, shoulder, hip, and ankle may be safely carried out and is useful as an adjunct to antibiotic joint sterilization. Copious high-flow irrigation, foreign body removal, synovial biopsy, and synovial debridement with a minimum of the morbidity associated with a formal arthrotomy can be achieved. This, in turn, allows for rapid joint and patient mobilization, which are key features in the overall treatment of the patient with an acute pyarthrosis.

Prompt recognition and treatment of an infected joint are critical to achieving a successful outcome. Arthroscopy merely represents one interventional treatment modality that is useful as an adjunct to the overall management of these patients.

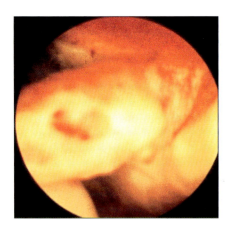

Figure 20-2. Necrotic synovium in pyarthrosis of the knee.

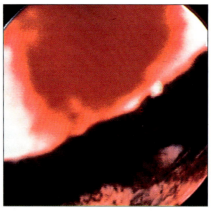

Figure 20-3. Arthroscopic view after debridement of necrotic synovium.

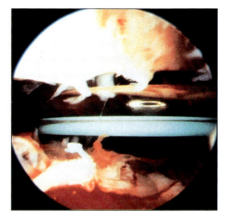

Figure 20-4. Intra-articular drain placed through inferior arthroscopic portal.

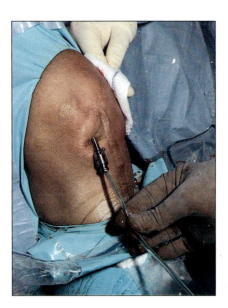

Figure 20-5. Insertion of suction drain at the completion of the arthroscopic procedure.

REFERENCES AND RECOMMENDED READING

Recently published papers of particular interest have been highlighted as:
- • Of interest
- •• Of outstanding interest

1. Hunter W: The structure and disease of articulating cartilage. *Philos Trans R Soc Lond (Biol)* 1743, 42:514.

2. Phemister DB: The effect of pressure on articular surfaces in pyogenic and tuberculous arthritides and its bearing on treatment. *Ann Surg* 1924, 80:481–500.

3. Lack CH: Chondrolysis in arthritis. *J Bone Joint Surg* 1959, 41(suppl B):384–387.

4. van de Loo AA, van den Berg WB: Effects of murine recombinant interleukin-1 on the synovial joints in mice: measurement of patella cartilage metabolism and joint inflammation. *Ann Rheum Dis* 1990, 49:238–245.

5. Williams RJ III, Smith RF, Shurman DJ: Septic arthritis: Staphylococcal induction of chondrocyte proteolytic activity. *Arthritis Rheum* 1990, 33:533–541.

6.•• Nord KD, Dore DD, Deeney VF, *et al.*: Evaluation of treatment modalities for septic arthritis with histological grading and analysis of levels of uronic acid, neutral protease and interleukin-1. *J Bone Joint Surg* 1995, 77(suppl A):258–265.
Excellent study of the various treatment modalities of acute septic arthritis in goat models.

7. Riegels-Nielsen P, Frimodt-Moller N, Sorenson M, Jensen JS: Antibiotic treatment insufficient for established septic arthritis. *Acta Orthop Scand* 1989, 60:113–115.

8. Jackson RW: Arthroscopic treatment of the septic knee. *Arthroscopy* 1985, 1:194–197.

9. Ivey M: The infected knee. In *Arthroscopic Surgery*. Edited by Parisien JS. New York: McGraw-Hill; 1988:155–161.

10. Ivey M, Clark R: Arthroscopic debridement of the knee for septic arthritis. *Clin Orthop* 1985, 199:201–206.

11. Smith MJ: Arthroscopic treatment of the septic knee. *Arthroscopy* 1986, 2:30–34.

12. Skyhar MJ, Mubarek SJ: Arthroscopic treatment of septic knee in children. *J Pediatr Orthop* 1987, 7:647–651.

13. Flood JN, Kolarik DB: Arthroscopic irrigation and debridement of infected total knee arthroplasty: report on two cases. *Arthroscopy* 1988, 4:182–186.

14. Windsor R: Arthroscopic diagnosis and treatment of the infected knee. In *Arthroscopy of the Knee*. Edited by Scott WN. Philadelphia: WB Saunders; 1990:207–213.

15. Thiery JA: Arthroscopic drainage in septic arthritides of the knee: a multicenter study. *Arthroscopy* 1989, 5:65–69.

16. Stanitski CL, Harvell JC, Fu FH: Arthroscopy in acute septic knees: management in pediatric patients. *Clin Orthop* 1989, 241:209–212.

17. Parisien JS, Shaffer B: Arthroscopic management of pyarthrosis. *Clin Orthop* 1992, 275:243–247.

18. D'Angelo GL, Ogilvie-Harris DJ: Septic arthritis following arthroscopy with cost/benefit analysis of antibiotic prophylaxis. *Arthroscopy* 1988, 4:10–14.

19. Blitzer CM: Arthroscopic management of septic arthritis of the hip. *Arthroscopy* 1993, 9:414–416.

20.• Williams RJ, Laurencin CT, Warren RF, *et al.*: Septic arthritis after arthroscopic anterior cruciate ligament reconstruction. *Am J Sports Med* 1997, 25:261–267.
Excellent report on the use of arthroscopic techniques in the management of infection following anterior cruciate ligament reconstruction.

21.• Sanchez AA, Hennrikus WL: Arthroscopically assisted treatment of acute septic knees in infants using the microjoint arthroscope. *Arthroscopy* 1997, 13:350–354.
Report on acute septic knees in infants (average age, 16 months) being managed successfully with the microjoint arthroscope.

22. Nelson JD: Antibiotic concentrations in septic joint effusions. *N Engl J Med* 1971, 284:349–352.

23. Salter RB, Bell RS, Kelley FW: The protective effect of continuous passive motion in living articular cartilage in acute septic arthritis: an experimental investigation in the rabbit. *Clin Orthop* 1989, 159:223–247.

Index

Page numbers followed by *f* and *t* indicate figures and tables, respectively.

indications for, 8
rehabilitation after, 9
technique for, 8–9, 8f–12f
partial meniscectomy for, 7
regeneration of after total knee arthroplasty, arthroscopic diagnosis
and treatment of, 176, 176f
Metal suture anchors, 74, 77
Miner's elbow, arthroscopic diagnosis and treatment of, 132–133, 132f–133f
Mini-open incision, for rotator cuff repair
diagnostic arthroscopy in, 104
open repair vs, 103–104
patient position for, 104, 104f
repair technique in, 106–107, 106f–107f
results of, 108
subacromial bursectomy and decompression in, 104–106, 104f–106f
Mitek suture anchors, for arthroscopic rotator cuff repair, 79, 84f

N

Nerve block, in shoulder arthroscopy, complications due to, 111, 113
Neurapraxia, due to hip arthroscopy, 157
Neurologic complications, due to shoulder arthroscopy, 110–111
Niky knot, 62f–65f, 66–67
Nitinol guidewire, 21
in hip arthroscopy, 150f, 152, 152f
Notchplasty
in anterior cruciate ligament reconstruction, 19
in anterior cruciate ligament revision, 30, 30f

O

Office-based ambulatory surgical center, anterior cruciate ligament
reconstruction performed in, 15–26
Olecranon bursitis, arthroscopic diagnosis and treatment of, 132–133, 132f–133f
Operating room, layout of, for hip arthroscopy, 150–151
Osteoarthritis
of elbow, arthroscopic treatment of, 130–131
of hip, arthroscopic debridement for, 155f, 155–156
of posterior subtalar joint, arthroscopic treatment for, 166
Osteochondral fracture, of carpal bones, 141t
Osteochondral lesion, of talocalcaneal joint, arthroscopic excision of, 166, 167f
Osteochondritis dissecans, of hip joint, arthroscopic assessment and
debridement in, 156
Osteochondromatosis, synovial, arthroscopic removal of loose bodies
in, 155f, 156
Osteochondrosis, of femoral head, arthroscopic removal of loose bodies
in, 157
Osteophytosis, of hip, arthroscopy contraindicated in, 157
Os trigonum tarsi, arthroscopic excision of, 166
Outerbridge-Kashiwagi procedure, arthroscopic variation of, 134f

P

Pain, after anterior cruciate ligament reconstruction, control of, 18
Palsy
due to hip arthroscopy, 157
due to interscalene block, 111
Patellar clunk syndrome, after total knee arthroplasty, arthroscopic
diagnosis and treatment of, 177
Patellar dysfunction, after total knee arthroplasty, arthroscopic diagnosis and treatment of, 177

Patellar tendon allograft, for knee ligament reconstruction, 48f
Patholaxity, determination of, in reconstruction of anterior cruciate lig-
ament in children, 40, 40t
PCL see Posterior cruciate ligament (PCL)
PDS sutures, 82, 83f–84f
Perilunate injury pattern, 141t
Perineal tears, due to hip arthroscopy, 157
Peroneus brevis, 182f
Peroneus longus, 182
Perthes disease, arthroscopic removal of loose bodies in, 157
PGA (polyglyconate) suture anchors, 74–75
Phrenic nerve palsy, due to interscalene block, 111
Physis
drill holes through, 40, 40t
surgery near, principles regarding, 40, 40t
PITF (posterior inferior tibiofibular ligament), 183
disrupted, 184
Plantar aponeurosis, structure of, 2
Plantar fasciitis
conservative treatment of, 1, 3–4
defined, 1
endoscopic release for, 4–5, 4f–5f
nerves at risk in, 2, 2f
partial vs total, 5–6
Plastic suture anchors, 74, 77
PLA (polylactate) suture anchors, 74–75
PLC (posterolateral complex), reconstruction of, allograft tissue for, 47
Pneumothorax, due to interscalene block, 113
POL (posterior oblique ligament), reconstruction of, in anterior cruciate
ligament revision, 33
Polyethylene fragments, in knee joint, after total knee arthroplasty,
arthroscopic diagnosis and removal of, 177
Polyethylene wear, after total knee arthroplasty, diagnosis and treat-
ment of, 176, 177f
Polyglyconate (PGA) suture anchors, 74–75
Polylactate (PLA) suture anchors, 74–75
Popliteus tendon, snapping of, after total knee arthroplasty, arthroscop-
ic treatment for, 178
Portal placement
for hip joint arthroscopy, 150f, 152f, 152–153
for posterior subtalar joint arthroscopy, 162–163, 163f
for shoulder arthroscopy, 111–113, 112f
Postanesthesia recovery, scoring of, 22t
Posterior antebrachial cutaneous nerve, 127f
Posterior capitellar joint, arthroscopic visualization of, 125
Posterior cruciate ligament (PCL)
reconstruction of, allograft tissue for, 47, 53
tight, after total knee arthroplasty, arthroscopic release of, 178
Posterior inferior tibiofibular ligament (PITF), 183
disrupted, 184
Posterior interosseous ligament, 183f
Posterior oblique ligament (POL), reconstruction of, in anterior cruciate
ligament revision, 33
Posterior subtalar joint, osteoarthritis of, arthroscopic treatment for,
166
Posterior talofibular ligament (PTFL), 181, 182f
Posterior tibiofibular ligament, 182f
Posterolateral complex (PLC), reconstruction of, allograft tissue for, 47
Posterolateral instability, of elbow, test for, 128
Postsurgical infection, foreign material removal required in, 73
Pound-in suture anchors, 72f, 72–73
Power shaver, in hip arthroscopy, 150f
Protrusio acetabuli, hip arthroscopy contraindicated in, 157
Proximal radioulnar joint, arthroscopic visualization of, 125, 126f
PTFL (posterior talofibular ligament), 181, 182f